MR Imaging of the Pancreas

Editors

KUMAR SANDRASEGARAN
DUSHYANT V. SAHANI

MAGNETIC RESONANCE IMAGING CLINICS OF NORTH AMERICA

www.mri.theclinics.com

Consulting Editors
SURESH K. MUKHERJI
LYNNE S. STEINBACH

August 2018 • Volume 26 • Number 3

ELSEVIER

1600 John F. Kennedy Boulevard • Suite 1800 • Philadelphia, Pennsylvania, 19103-2899

http://www.mri.theclinics.com

MRI CLINICS OF NORTH AMERICA Volume 26, Number 3
August 2018 ISSN 1064-9689, ISBN 13: 978-0-323-61398-9

Editor: John Vassallo (j.vassallo@elsevier.com)
Developmental Editor: Meredith Madeira

Magnetic Resonance Imaging Clinics of North America (ISSN 1064-9689) is published quarterly by Elsevier Inc., 360 Park Avenue South, New York, NY 10010-1710. Months of issue are February, May, August, and November. Business and Editorial Offices: 1600 John F. Kennedy Blvd., Ste. 1800, Philadelphia, PA 19103-2899. Customer Service Office: 3251 Riverport Lane, Maryland Heights, MO 63043. Periodicals postage paid at New York, NY and additional mailing offices. Subscription prices are $395.00 per year (domestic individuals), $701.00 per year (domestic institutions), $100.00 per year (domestic students/residents), $437.00 per year (Canadian individuals), $913.00 per year (Canadian institutions), $545.00 per year (international individuals), $913.00 per year (international institutions), and $275.00 per year (international and Canadian students/residents). International air speed delivery is included in all *Clinics* subscription prices. All prices are subject to change without notice. **POSTMASTER:** Send address changes to *Magnetic Resonance Imaging Clinics*, Elsevier Health Sciences Division, Subscription Customer Service, 3251 Riverport Lane, Maryland Heights, MO 63043. Customer Service (orders, claims, online, change of address): Elsevier Health Sciences Division, Subscription **Customer Service, 3251 Riverport Lane, Maryland Heights, MO 63043. Tel:1-800-654-2452 (U.S. and Canada); 314-447-8871 (outside U.S. and Canada). Fax: 314-447-8029. E-mail: journalscustomer service-usa@elsevier.com (for print support); journalsonlinesupport-usa@elsevier.com (for online support).**

Reprints. For copies of 100 or more of articles in this publication, please contact the Commercial Reprints Department, Elsevier Inc., 360 Park Avenue South, New York, NY 10010-1710. Tel.: 212-633-3874; Fax: 212-633-3820; E-mail: reprints@elsevier.com.

Magnetic Resonance Imaging Clinics of North America is covered in the *RSNA Index of Imaging Literature, MEDLINE/PubMed (Index Medicus),* and *EMBASE/Excerpta Medica.*

Contributors

CONSULTING EDITORS

SURESH K. MUKHERJI, MD, MBA, FACR
Professor and Chairman, Walter F. Patenge
Endowed Chair, Department of Radiology,
Michigan State University, Chief Medical
Officer and Director of Health Care Delivery,
Michigan State University Health Team, East
Lansing, Michigan, USA

LYNNE S. STEINBACH, MD, FACR
Professor of Radiology and Orthopaedic
Surgery, Department of Radiology and
Biomedical Imaging, University of California,
San Francisco, San Francisco, California, USA

EDITORS

KUMAR SANDRASEGARAN, MD
Section Chief, Abdominal Imaging,
Department of Radiology and Imaging
Sciences, Indiana University, Indianapolis,
Indiana, USA

DUSHYANT V. SAHANI, MD
Director of Computed Tomography, Associate
Professor, Department of Radiology, Division
of Abdominal Imaging, Massachusetts General
Hospital, Boston, Massachusetts, USA

AUTHORS

KRISTINE S. BURK, MD
Department of Radiology, Massachusetts
General Hospital, Boston, Massachusetts,
USA

DANIEL E. CASON, MD
Department of Radiology, The University of
Alabama at Birmingham, Birmingham,
Alabama, USA

ARGHA CHATTERJEE, MD
Research Fellow, Department of
Radiology, Northwestern Memorial
Hospital, Northwestern University Feinberg
School of Medicine, Chicago, Illinois,
USA

ERIC COLLISSON, MD
Associate Professor, Department of Medicine,
University of California, San Francisco,
San Francisco, California, USA

ANIL K. DASYAM, MD
Associate Professor, Department of Radiology,
University of Pittsburgh Medical Center,
Pittsburgh, Pennsylvania, USA

CHRISTOPHER FUNG, MD
Department of Radiology and Diagnostic
Imaging, University of Alberta, Edmonton,
Alberta, Canada

ALEXANDER R. GUIMARAES, MD, PhD
Assistant Professor of Radiology, Department
of Diagnostic Radiology, Oregon Health &
Science University, Portland, Oregon, USA

NIMA HAFEZI-NEJAD, MD
Russell H. Morgan Department of Radiology,
Johns Hopkins School of Medicine, Baltimore,
Maryland, USA

THOMAS A. HOPE, MD
Assistant Professor in Residence, Department
of Radiology and Biomedical Imaging,
University of California, San Francisco, San
Francisco, California, USA

PRIYANKA JHA, MD
Assistant Professor, Department of Radiology
and Biomedical Imaging, University of
California, San Francisco, San Francisco,
California, USA

AVINASH KAMBADAKONE, MD, FRCR
Assistant Professor, Department of Radiology, Massachusetts General Hospital, Boston, Massachusetts, USA

VENKATA S. KATABATHINA, MD
Section Chief, Abdominal Radiology, Department of Radiology, University of Texas Health Science Center at San Antonio, San Antonio, Texas, USA

DAVID KNIPP, MD
Department of Radiology, Massachusetts General Hospital, Boston, Massachusetts, USA

GRACE C. LO, MD
Assistant Professor, Department of Radiology, Weill Cornell Medical College, New York, New York, USA

NADINE MALLAK, MD
Assistant Professor of Radiology, Department of Diagnostic Radiology, Oregon Health & Science University, Portland, Oregon, USA

ROHAN MANICKAM, BS
Department of Radiology, The University of Texas MD Anderson Cancer Center, Houston, Texas, USA

CHRISTINE O. MENIAS, MD
Professor, Department of Radiology, Mayo Clinic's Campus in Arizona, Scottsdale, Arizona, USA

FRANK H. MILLER, MD
Lee F. Rogers MD Professor of Medical Education, Chief, Body Imaging Section and Fellowship Program, Medical Director, MRI, Department of Radiology, Northwestern Memorial Hospital, Northwestern University Feinberg School of Medicine, Chicago, Illinois, USA

DESIREE E. MORGAN, MD
Department of Radiology, The University of Alabama at Birmingham, Birmingham, Alabama, USA

BHAVIK N. PATEL, MD, MBA
Assistant Professor in Diagnostic Radiology, Body Imaging Division, Stanford University Medical Center, Stanford, California, USA

KRISTIN K. PORTER, MD, PhD
Department of Radiology, The University of Alabama at Birmingham, Birmingham, Alabama, USA

SRINIVASA R. PRASAD, MD
Professor, Department of Radiology, The University of Texas MD Anderson Cancer Center, Houston, Texas, USA

OMID Y. RIKHTEHGAR, MD
Department of Radiology, University of Texas Health Science Center at San Antonio, San Antonio, Texas, USA

DUSHYANT V. SAHANI, MD
Director of Computed Tomography, Associate Professor, Department of Radiology, Division of Abdominal Imaging, Massachusetts General Hospital, Boston, Massachusetts, USA

ANUP S. SHETTY, MD
Assistant Professor of Radiology, Mallinckrodt Institute of Radiology, Washington University School of Medicine, St Louis, Missouri, USA

NASIR SIDDIQUI, MD
Department of Radiology, DuPage Medical Group, Lisle, Illinois, USA

VIKESH K. SINGH, MD, MSc
Department of Internal Medicine, Pancreatitis Center, Johns Hopkins Medical Institutions, Division of Gastroenterology, Johns Hopkins School of Medicine, Baltimore, Maryland, USA

NAOKI TAKAHASHI, MD
Department of Radiology, Mayo Clinic, Rochester, Minnesota, USA

TEMEL TIRKES, MD
Department of Radiology and Imaging Sciences, Indiana University School of Medicine, IU Health University Hospital, Indianapolis, Indiana, USA

CAMILA LOPES VENDRAMI, MD
Research Fellow, Department of Radiology, Northwestern Memorial Hospital, Northwestern University Feinberg School of Medicine, Chicago, Illinois, USA

ZHEN J. WANG, MD
Associate Professor, Department of Radiology
and Biomedical Imaging, University of
California, San Francisco, San Francisco,
California, USA

BENJAMIN M. YEH, MD
Professor, Department of Radiology
and Biomedical Imaging, University of
California, San Francisco, San Francisco,
California, USA

RONALD ZAGORIA, MD
Professor, Department of Radiology and
Biomedical Imaging, University of California,
San Francisco, San Francisco, California, USA

ATIF ZAHEER, MD, FSAR
Russell H. Morgan Department of Radiology,
Johns Hopkins School of Medicine,
Department of Internal Medicine, Pancreatitis
Center, Johns Hopkins Medical Institutions,
Baltimore, Maryland, USA

Contributors

ZHEN J. WANG, MD
Associate Professor, Department of Radiology
and Biomedical Imaging, University of
California, San Francisco, San Francisco,
California, USA

BENJAMIN M. YEH, MD
Professor, Department of Radiology
and Biomedical Imaging, University of
California, San Francisco, San Francisco,
California, USA

RONALD ZAGORIA, MD
Professor, Department of Radiology and
Biomedical Imaging, University of California,
San Francisco, San Francisco, California, USA

ATIF ZAHEER, MD, FSAR
Russell H. Morgan Department of Radiology,
Johns Hopkins School of Medicine,
Department of Internal Medicine, Pancreatitis
Center, Johns Hopkins Medical Institutions,
Baltimore, Maryland, USA

Contents

non–contour-deforming tumors and for characterizing indeterminate pancreatic findings at computed tomography. MR imaging can also improve the detection of distant metastases, especially in the liver, thereby facilitating the appropriate selection of surgical candidates.

Venkata S. Katabathina, Omid Y. Rikhtehgar, Anil K. Dasyam, Rohan Manickam, and Srinivasa R. Prasad

There is a wide spectrum of pancreatic neoplasms with characteristic genetic abnormalities, tumor pathways, and histopathology that primarily determine tumor biology, treatment response, and prognosis. Although most pancreatic tumors are sporadic, 10% of neoplasms occur in the setting of distinct hereditary syndromes. Detailed studies of these rare syndromes have allowed researchers to identify a myriad of specific genetic signatures of pancreatic tumors. A better understanding of tumor genomics may have significant clinical implications in the diagnosis and management of patients with pancreatic tumors. Evolving knowledge has paved the way to screening paradigms and protocols in individuals at higher risk of developing pancreatic tumors.

Grace C. Lo and Avinash Kambadakone

Imaging plays a crucial role in the identification, diagnosis, treatment, and surveillance of pancreatic neuroendocrine tumors (PNETs). Although computed tomography has been traditionally used for the evaluation of PNETs, evolving techniques with MR imaging have broadened and strengthened its role as an important tool in the diagnosis, staging, and assessment of response to therapy.

Kristine S. Burk, David Knipp, and Dushyant V. Sahani

Cystic pancreatic lesions are common and often incidentally detected on cross-sectional examinations of the abdomen. Most lesions are asymptomatic and benign. However, some carry a significant risk of malignant degeneration, so correct identification, complete characterization, and adequate follow-up/management of these lesions are paramount. MR imaging/magnetic resonance cholangiopancreatography is an ideal single imaging modality for complete characterization and follow-up of cystic pancreatic lesions. This article discusses the epidemiology, pathology, and imaging characteristics of the most common cystic pancreatic neoplasms and concludes with a discussion of the most up-to-date follow-up imaging guideline recommendations.

Anup S. Shetty and Christine O. Menias

Although pancreatic ductal adenocarcinoma is the most common type of pancreatic cancer, a variety of rarer benign and malignant tumors of the pancreas have been identified. Computed tomography (CT) and MR imaging are the primary modalities for further noninvasive characterization of these lesions. This article presents an approach to imaging of rare pancreatic tumors, including the CT and MR imaging technique, key imaging features and examples, and differential diagnosis.

MR imaging is useful for diagnosing acute pancreatitis when the clinical situation is unclear, for elucidating the underlying cause of acute pancreatitis, for evaluating complications and disease severity, and for guiding intervention. MR imaging allows for noninvasive evaluation of the pancreatic parenchyma, biliary and pancreatic ducts, exocrine function, peripancreatic soft tissues, and vascular structures in a single examination. MR imaging is emerging as the imaging examination of choice in acute pancreatitis. In this article, the role of imaging in acute pancreatitis is reviewed with an emphasis on the advantages of MR imaging.

Diagnosis of chronic pancreatitis requires a complete medical history and clinical investigations, including imaging technologies and function tests. MR imaging/magnetic resonance cholangiopancreatography is the preferred diagnostic tool for the detection of ductal and parenchymal changes in patients with chronic pancreatitis. Ductal changes may not be present in the initial phase of chronic pancreatitis. Therefore, early diagnosis remains challenging.

Autoimmune pancreatitis (AIP) is characterized by autoimmune inflammatory destruction of the pancreatic tissue. Imaging plays an essential role in the diagnosis. AIP type 1 is the pancreatic manifestation of immunoglobulin G4 (IgG4)–related disease and is associated with IgG4-positive plasma cell infiltration and fibrosis of multiple organ systems. Type 2 is a related disease with pancreatic inflammation with or without concurrent inflammatory bowel disease. The authors demonstrate the imaging findings that are associated with the pancreatic and extrapancreatic manifestations of AIP. They emphasize the common MR imaging and magnetic resonance cholangiopancreatography findings to help make the diagnosis of AIP.

MAGNETIC RESONANCE IMAGING CLINICS OF NORTH AMERICA

VISIT THE CLINICS ONLINE!
Access your subscription at:
www.theclinics.com

PROGRAM OBJECTIVE

The goal of *Magnetic Resonance Imaging Clinics of North America* is to keep practicing physicians up to date with current clinical practice by providing timely articles reviewing the state of the art in patient care.

TARGET AUDIENCE

All practicing physicians and healthcare professionals who provide patient care utilizing findings from Magnetic Resonance Imaging.

LEARNING OBJECTIVES

Upon completion of this activity, participants will be able to:
1. Review MRI techniques for pancreas imaging
2. Discuss MRI in pancreatic cancer and autoimmune pancreatitis
3. Recognize cystic pancreatic tumours and rare pancreatic tumours

ACCREDITATION

The Elsevier Office of Continuing Medical Education (EOCME) is accredited by the Accreditation Council for Continuing Medical Education (ACCME) to provide continuing medical education for physicians.

The EOCME designates this enduring material for a maximum of 15 *AMA PRA Category 1 Credit*(s)™. Physicians should claim only the credit commensurate with the extent of their participation in the activity.

All other healthcare professionals requesting continuing education credit for this enduring material will be issued a certificate of participation.

DISCLOSURE OF CONFLICTS OF INTEREST

The EOCME assesses conflict of interest with its instructors, faculty, planners, and other individuals who are in a position to control the content of CME activities. All relevant conflicts of interest that are identified are thoroughly vetted by EOCME for fair balance, scientific objectivity, and patient care recommendations. EOCME is committed to providing its learners with CME activities that promote improvements or quality in healthcare and not a specific proprietary business or a commercial interest.

The planning committee, staff, authors and editors listed below have identified no financial relationships or relationships to products or devices they or their spouse/life partner have with commercial interest related to the content of this CME activity:

Kristine S. Burk, MD; Daniel E. Cason, MD; Argha Chatterjee, MD; Eric Collisson, MD; Anil K. Dasyam, MD; Christopher Fung, MD; Alexander R. Guimaraes, MD, PhD; Nima Hafezi-Nejad, MD; Priyanka Jha, MD; Avinash Kambadakone, MD, FRCR; Venkata S. Katabathina, MD; Alison Kemp; David Knipp, MD; Pradeep Kuttysankaran; Grace C. Lo, MD; Nadine Mallak, MD; Rohan Manickam, BS; Christine O. Menias, MD; Frank H. Miller, MD; Suresh K. Mukherji, MD, MBA, FACR; Desiree E. Morgan, MD; Bhavik N. Patel, MD, MBA; Kristin K. Porter, MD, PhD; Srinivasa R. Prasad, MD; Omid Y. Rikhtehgar, MD; Dushyant V. Sahani, MD; Kumar Sandrasegaran, MD; Anup S. Shetty, MD; Nasir Siddiqui, MD; Vikesh K. Singh, MD, MSc; Lynne S. Steinbach, MD, FACR; Naoki Takahashi, MD; Temel Tirkes, MD; Camila Lopes Vendrami, MD; John Vassallo; Zhen J. Wang, MD; Benjamin M. Yeh, MD; Ronald Zagoria, MD; Atif Zaheer, MD, FSAR.

The planning committee, staff, authors and editors listed below have identified financial relationships or relationships to products or devices they or their spouse/life partner have with commercial interest related to the content of this CME activity:

Thomas A. Hope, MD: has received research support from General Electric Company.

UNAPPROVED/OFF-LABEL USE DISCLOSURE

The EOCME requires CME faculty to disclose to the participants:
1. When products or procedures being discussed are off-label, unlabelled, experimental, and/or investigational (not US Food and Drug Administration [FDA] approved); and
2. Any limitations on the information presented, such as data that are preliminary or that represent ongoing research, interim analyses, and/or unsupported opinions. Faculty may discuss information about pharmaceutical agents that is outside of FDA-approved labelling. This information is intended solely for CME and is not intended to promote off-label use of these medications. If you have any questions, contact the medical affairs department of the manufacturer for the most recent prescribing information.

TO ENROLL

To enroll in the *Magnetic Resonance Imaging Clinics of North America* Continuing Medical Education program, call customer service at 1-800-654-2452 or sign up online at http://www.theclinics.com/home/cme. The CME program is available to subscribers for an additional annual fee of USD 260.

METHOD OF PARTICIPATION

In order to claim credit, participants must complete the following:

1. Complete enrolment as indicated above.
2. Read the activity.
3. Complete the CME Test and Evaluation. Participants must achieve a score of 70% on the test. All CME Tests and Evaluations must be completed online.

CME INQUIRIES/SPECIAL NEEDS

For all CME inquiries or special needs, please contact elsevierCME@elsevier.com.

Foreword
MR Imaging of the Pancreas

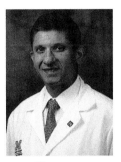

Suresh K. Mukherji, MD, MBA, FACR
Consulting Editor

I would like to thank my two friends and colleagues, Drs Sandrasegaran and Sahani, for editing this wonderful issue of *Magnetic Resonance Imaging Clinics of North America* entitled, "MR Imaging of the Pancreas." This is a very important issue that provides the audience with a state-of-the-art update on new imaging techniques and their applications to the various complex pathologies of the pancreas. This issue is a collection of eleven review articles covering the entire gamut of pancreatic diseases with a focus on MR imaging technique and diagnosis.

These articles are authored by international leaders in the field of MR imaging and pancreas imaging. I want to thank the authors for their efforts in creating such outstanding contributions. The information is timely and relevant, which will add value to our daily clinical practice.

On a personal note, this topic is especially poignant for me as my father died of pancreatic cancer. I hope the information provided in this important issue by these world experts will help provide earlier diagnosis and improved outcomes for patients with such a devastating disease. Thank you, again, to all who participated for your meaningful contributions.

Suresh K. Mukherji, MD, MBA, FACR
Department of Radiology
Michigan State University
Michigan State University Health Team
846 Service Road
East Lansing, MI 48824, USA

E-mail address:
mukherji@rad.msu.edu

Magn Reson Imaging Clin N Am 26 (2018) xiii
https://doi.org/10.1016/j.mric.2018.05.002
1064-9689/18/© 2018 Published by Elsevier Inc.

Preface
MR Imaging of the Pancreas

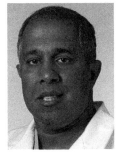 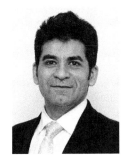

Kumar Sandrasegaran, MD   Dushyant V. Sahani, MD
Editors

It has been our pleasure to serve as guest editors for the current issue of *Magnetic Resonance Imaging Clinics of North America* entitled, "MR Imaging of the Pancreas." Pancreatic pathologies have some major ramifications on patient management. MR imaging is accepted as a key component of diagnosis of pancreatic diseases, particularly for evaluating focal masses, cystic lesions, and inflammatory conditions such as chronic pancreatitis. The ability of MR imaging to detect pancreatic ductal disease is superior to computed tomography or conventional sonography. There has been evolution in MR imaging technology with the introduction of newer sequences and techniques, which have been adopted as part of MR imaging protocols. However, the pace of innovation in MR imaging continues with hybrid techniques that are likely to play a greater role in the future of pancreas imaging. There has also been rising demand in streamlining the MR imaging exams by applying more time-efficient and clinically relevant abbreviated protocols in certain situations like following pancreatic cystic lesions. The present issue is a collection of eleven review articles covering the entire gamut of pancreatic diseases with a focus on MR imaging technique and diagnosis. These articles are authored by international leaders in the field of MR imaging and pancreas imaging. It is our hope that readers will find the wealth of information to be a substantial enhancement to their daily clinical practice. Following is a brief outline of the articles in this issue:

1. "Routine MR Imaging for Pancreas" by Bhavik Patel discusses standard MR imaging and magnetic resonance cholangiopancreatography (MRCP) of pancreas, including the use of gadolinium, as well as aspects of 3-T MR imaging of pancreas.

2. "Advanced MR Imaging Techniques for Pancreas Imaging" by Frank Miller and colleagues looks at the value of diffusion-weighted imaging, secretin-enhanced MRCP, MR perfusion, T1 mapping, and MR elastography in a variety of pancreatic diseases.

3. "PET/MR Imaging of the Pancreas" by Alexander Guimaraes and colleagues analyzes the latest research on PET MR imaging, including the use of newer radiopharmaceuticals, such as fluorothymidine, hypoxia agents, and somatostatin receptor imaging.

4. "The Role of MR Imaging in Pancreatic Cancer" by Zhen Wang and colleagues elaborates the uses and limitations of MR imaging for diagnosis, staging, and monitoring treatment response of this deadly cancer.

5. "Genetics of Pancreatic Neoplasms and Role of Screening" by Srinivasa Prasad and colleagues reviews the genetics of pancreas cancer, particularly hereditary and familial syndromes of this disease as well as genetics of cystic pancreatic lesions and neuroendocrine tumor. They explore the role of screening for pancreas cancer.

6. "MR Imaging of Pancreatic Neuroendocrine Tumors" by Avinash Kambadakone and Grace Lo reviews the optimal MR imaging technique, diagnosis, differential diagnosis, staging, and treatment response of pancreatic neuroendocrine tumors.

Magn Reson Imaging Clin N Am 26 (2018) xv–xvi
https://doi.org/10.1016/j.mric.2018.05.001
1064-9689/18/© 2018 Published by Elsevier Inc.

mri.theclinics.com

7. "Cystic Pancreatic Tumors" by coeditor Dushyant Sahani and colleagues illustrates the pathology, imaging appearances, and management of pancreatic cystic lesions, including intraductal mucinous cystic neoplasm, mucinous cystic tumors, serous cystadenoma, and solid pseudopapillary tumor.

8. "Rare Pancreatic Tumors" by Christine Menias and Anup Shetty focuses on the imaging features and approach to uncommon tumors such as lymphoma, mesenchymal tumors, acinar cell cancer, and pancreaticoblastoma.

9. "Acute Pancreatitis: How Can MR Imaging Help" by Desiree Morgan and colleagues dissertates the course of interstitial and necrotic pancreatitis and how imaging, particularly MR imaging, helps with the diagnosis and choice of management.

10. "Chronic Pancreatitis: What the Clinician Wants to Know from MR Imaging" by Temel Tirkes examines the information the clinician would like to see from MR imaging of this disease and elaborates on MR imaging–based classification of the severity of chronic pancreatitis.

11. "MR Imaging of Autoimmune Pancreatitis" by Atif Zaheer and colleagues examines new concepts of this entity, including types I and II diseases and the use of MR imaging in the diagnosis and assessment of treatment response of autoimmune pancreatitis.

We believe this issue will be valuable to practicing radiologists at all levels. We appreciate the editorial assistance from Elsevier in preparing this issue, especially Meredith Madeira, Kristen Helm, and Dr Mukherji. We hope you enjoy reading this issue of *Magnetic Resonance Imaging Clinics of North America* as much as we have.

Kumar Sandrasegaran, MD
Abdominal Imaging
Department of Radiology and Imaging Sciences
Indiana University School of Medicine
550 North University Boulevard
Indianapolis, IN 46202, USA

Dushyant V. Sahani, MD
Radiology Department–
Division of Abdominal Imaging
Massachusetts General Hospital
55 Fruit Street, White Building, Room 270
Boston, MA 02114, USA

E-mail addresses:
ksandras@iupui.edu (K. Sandrasegaran)
DSAHANI@mgh.harvard.edu (D.V. Sahani)

Routine MR Imaging for Pancreas

Bhavik N. Patel, MD, MBA

KEYWORDS

• MR imaging • Pancreas • T1 weighted • T2 weighted • MRCP

KEY POINTS

- MR imaging with magnetic resonance cholangiopancreatography (MRCP) serves as both a primary diagnostic and problem-solving tool for comprehensive evaluation of the pancreas.
- T1- and T2-weighted images comprise the routine protocol, which are performed at 1.5 T or 3.0 T.
- Higher image quality for evaluation of the pancreas can be achieved with 3.0 T compared with 1.5 T.
- A normal pancreas has a high T1 signal, and pre–contrast- and post–contrast-enhanced T1-weighted images are useful for identifying neoplastic and inflammatory pathologies.
- MRCP allows excellent visualization of the pancreatic duct.

INTRODUCTION

Given the fastidious nature of the gland and the often diagnostically challenging and complex disease processes that can involve the pancreas, a combination of multiple imaging modalities (eg, dual-energy computed tomography, ultrasound, endoscopic retrograde cholangiopancreatography) are often required for diagnostic evaluation.

MR imaging serves as a unique and valuable diagnostic tool allowing high-resolution imaging of the pancreas and simultaneous evaluation of the pancreatic parenchyma, peripancreatic soft tissues, pancreatic duct, biliary duct, and the surrounding rich neurovascular bundles. Recent technical advances have further boosted the clinical utility of MR imaging for the evaluation of the pancreas, now with shorter scan times and larger bores allowing scanning of large and claustrophobic patients.[1] In fact, scanners with a field strength of 7 T, 60-cm bore size, more than 200 coil elements, and up to 128 radiofrequency (RF) channels are now available for clinical use. New sequences, such as diffusion-weighted, 3-dimensional (3D), T1-weighted, and magnetic resonance (MR) cholangiopancreatography (MRCP) images allows accurate detection and characterization of neoplastic as well as inflammatory processes. MR imaging is commonly used for evaluation and further characterization of cystic pancreatic lesions and chronic pancreatitis. It serves as a problem-solving tool in patients with elevated liver enzymes, acute right upper quadrant pain, acute pancreatitis, and pancreatic cancer. This review highlights the routine MR imaging protocol for evaluating the pancreas.

MR IMAGING TECHNIQUE

The author's routine MR imaging protocol of the pancreas includes 2-dimensional (2D) and 3D spin echo (SE) coronal MRCP, T2-weighted 2D axial and coronal fat-suppressed fast SE, non–fat-suppressed T2-weighted axial fast SE, 2D axial diffusion-weighted, T1-weighted 2D axial in-phase and opposed-phase gradient echo (GE), and pregadolinium and postgadolinium 3D axial T1-weighted GE sequences. **Tables 1** and **2** outline the technical parameters of these sequences using 1.5 and 3.0 T MR imaging.

1.5 VERSUS 3.0 T MR IMAGING

Signal-to-noise ratio (SNR) varies linearly with field strength. Thus, the largest advantage of scanning

Disclosure Statement: The author has nothing to disclose.
Body Imaging Division, Stanford University Medical Center, 300 Pasteur Drive, H1307, Stanford, CA 94305, USA
E-mail address: bhavikp@stanford.edu

Magn Reson Imaging Clin N Am 26 (2018) 315–322
https://doi.org/10.1016/j.mric.2018.03.009

Table 1
Scanner parameters for routine pancreatic imaging on 3.0-T MR imaging

Parameter	T2 2D SSFSE	T2 2D SSFSE	T2 2D SSFSE (Fat Sat)	2D SE MRCP	3D FSE MRCP	2D SE DWI	2D SPGR I/O	T1 3D SPGR[a]
Plane	Axial	Coronal	Axial	Coronal	Coronal	Axial	Axial	Axial
No. of echoes	1	1	1	1	1	1	2	2
TE/TR (ms)	100/min	120/min	min/min	200/min	min/—	min/3748	—/150	min/—
Flip angle	—	—	—	—	—	—	—	15
RBW	83.33	83.33	100.00	83.33	62.5	—	—	166.67
FOV	34.0	42.0	38.0	38.0	36.0	42.0	38.0	32.0
ST/SP	4.0/2.0	4.0/0.0	7.0/1.0	5.0/0/0	2.0/—	7.0/0.0	5.0/0.5	3.0/—
Frequency direction	R/L	S/I	R/L	S/I	S/I	R/L	R/L	R/L
Matrix	352 × 256	416 × 256	384 × 224	320 × 224	320 × 256	80 × 128	256 × 256	320 × 224
NEX	0.75	1	1	1	1	1	1	1
Respiration	BH	BH	BH	BH	Nav	BH	BH	BH

Abbreviations: DWI, diffusion-weighted images; FOV, field of view; I/O, in- and opposed phase; NEX, number of excitations; RBW, receiver bandwidth; Sat, saturation; SPGR, spoiled gradient echo; SSFSE, single shot fast spin echo; ST/SP, slice thickness/slice spacing; TE/TR, echo and repetition time.
[a] Represents pregadolinium and postgadolinium.

at 3.0 T compared with 1.5 T is the increased SNR.[2] Theoretically, the increase in SNR should be 2-fold. However, because of technical factors, such as RF field inhomogeneities, increased susceptibility effects, and limitations of the amount of energy deposited, the actual SNR is closer to 1.7 times higher than at 1.5 T.[3–5] This increased SNR can be used to improve spatial resolution, increase temporal resolution, or decrease acquisition time, or both.[3,5] Clinically, this could allow improved lesion visibility or reduced motion artifact. At 3.0 T, T1 relaxation of tissues increases; if imaged at similar repetition times (TRs) to 1.5 T, this would result in lower soft tissue contrast

Table 2
Scanner parameters for routine pancreatic imaging on 1.5-T MR imaging

Parameter	T2 2D SSFSE	T2 2D SSFSE (Fat Sat)	2D SE MRCP	3D FSE MRCP	2D SE DWI	2D SPGR I/O	T1 3D SPGR[a]
Plane	Axial	Axial	Coronal	Coronal	Axial	Axial	Axial
No. of echoes	1	1	1	1	1	2	1
TE/TR (ms)	90/min	90/—	90/min	min/—	min/6000	—/150	min/—
Flip angle	—	—	—	—	—	—	15
RBW	35.71	50.00	31.25	62.50	—	—	125.00
FOV	36.0	38.0	36.0	35.0	38.0	38.0	38.0
ST/SP	4.0/0.0	6.0/1/0	4.0/0.0	2.2/—	7.0/0.0	5.0/0.5	5.0/—
Frequency direction	R/L	R/L	S/I	S/I	R/L	R/L	R/L
Matrix	320 × 256	384 × 256	320 × 256	352 × 224	80 × 128	256 × 256	288 × 224
NEX	1	2	1	1	1	1	1
Respiration	BH	BH	BH	Nav	BH	BH	BH

Abbreviations: DWI, diffusion weighted images; FOV, field of view; I/O, in- and opposed phase; NEX, number of excitations; RBW, receiver bandwidth; Sat, saturation; SPGR, spoiled gradient echo; SSFSE, single shot fast spin echo; ST/SP, slice thickness/slice spacing; TE/TR, echo and repetition time.
[a] Represents before gadolinium and after gadolinium.

at 3.0 T.[3,6,7] In order to generate comparable T1 soft tissue contrast, TRs could be increased at 3.0 T.[5] However, in doing so, the acquisition time would increase.[2] A solution to this is to use parallel imaging techniques, which decrease acquisition time by sampling the signal from phased-array coils in a parallel fashion with increased distance between phase-encoding lines in k-space.[3,8,9] Two major drawbacks of this technique are aliasing or wraparound artifact and decreased SNR. However, higher inherent SNR at 3.0 T and spatial dependence of the phased-array coil elements overcome these limitations.[1,8,9]

T1 shortening of gadolinium-based contrast agents are not affected by the increase in magnetic field strength.[5] However, because of the relatively less intrinsic T1 contrast at higher field strengths, the effect of gadolinium enhancement is more pronounced leading to a higher contrast-to-noise ratio at 3.0 T compared with 1.5 T.[10] For pancreatic imaging, this can translate to improved lesion conspicuity, particularly of hypervascular tumors. Overall, T2 relaxation times and signal intensity do not change significantly at higher field strengths.[7] Although some earlier studies suggested no significant advantage of imaging at 3.0 T compared with 1.5 T,[1,3,11] more recent studies, particularly as they apply to pancreatic imaging, have shown superior image quality at 3.0 T.[12–14]

PATIENT PREPARATION

Before MR imaging scanning, patients are asked to have nothing by mouth for 4 hours. This requirement allows adequate gallbladder distension. It also allows for an adequate assessment of the response to secretin should secretin MRCP be performed, though this is not part of the routine protocol. Negative oral contrast allows distension of the upper gastrointestinal tract and can aid in better visualization of the pancreas as a result. Pineapple and blueberry juice have been reported to be used as oral contrast agents.[15–17] However, it has been reported that manganese contained within these agents can affect signal intensities on T1- and T2-weighted sequences.[1] Several oral contrast agents, both positive and negative, have been reported to have adequate results for MR imaging of the upper abdomen, including diluted gadolinium, barium, and oral magnetic particles, to name a few.[1,18–20]

T1-WEIGHTED IMAGING

T1-weighted images are generated using breath-hold spoiled gradient recall echo, which allows a short echo time (TE) and faster acquisition.[21] Flip angle of these sequences should be 70° or greater, and fat suppression techniques should be applied.[22] This combination results in adequate T1 signal of the pancreas as well as improved delineation of the pancreatic parenchyma from the surrounding low-intensity fat.[23] Two-point Dixon images can be used for fat suppression, in which two 2D GE sequences with different TEs are used to exploit the differences in chemical shift between water and fat protons.[1,24] This ability results in in- and opposed-phase images by which fat shows signal drop-off on opposed-phase images. The 3D two-point Dixon techniques have the added advantage of yielding thinner, contiguous slices from a single breath hold. A main disadvantage of 2-point Dixon techniques is their susceptibility to magnetic field inhomogeneities, which can result in incomplete fat suppression. Three-point Dixon techniques are now available that correct for T2* decay and magnetic field inhomogeneities by acquiring a third image.[1,24,25] The 3-point Dixon technique achieves water and fat separation using iterative decomposition with echo asymmetric and least-squares estimation (IDEAL).[24,25] Dixon fat-water separation techniques have traditionally been limited to single-coil aquisitions.[26] However, IDEAL techniques have been shown to work well with multi-coil acquisitions and parallel imaging, though at a cost of a longer minimum scan time.[24,26]

The normal pancreas has a high intrinsic T1 signal due to its protein and endoplasmic reticulum content (**Fig. 1**).[27] Using the aforementioned sequences to maximize T1 signal, a homogenously bright normal pancreas will be sharply delineated from the adjacent low-intensity fat. Additionally, inflammatory processes, such as

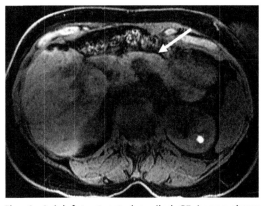

Fig. 1. Axial fat-saturated spoiled GE image shows intrinsic high T1 signal intensity of the pancreas (*arrow*). Note its similar high T1 signal to the liver parenchyma.

pancreatitis, as well as exocrine tumors (ie, pancreatic adenocarcinoma) will appear hypointense (**Fig. 2**).[23] The normal diffusely increased T1 signal of the pancreatic parenchyma may decrease with increasing fibrosis seen with aging or in patients with long-standing obstruction, either from pancreatitis or an obstructing pancreatic stone or mass.[28]

CONTRAST-ENHANCED T1 IMAGES

The author's pancreas MR imaging protocol routinely uses dynamic, breath-hold extracellular, gadolinium-enhanced sequences, though it is common at some centers to obtain MR imaging without contrast if the clinical indication is solely to evaluate for choledocholithiasis. The 3D spoiled GE (SPGR) with fat suppression is usually used. Depending on the vendor, postcontrast T1-weighted sequences may be named differently, such as volume interpolated breath-hold F-GRE (VIBE), liver acquisition with volume acceleration (LAVA), and T1-weighted high-resolution isotropic volume examination (THRIVE).[1] Intravenous gadolinium is injected through a 20-gauge catheter at a volume of 0.1 mL/kg body weight using an MR imaging–compatible injector with a flow rate of 2.0 mL/s. This injection is followed by a 20-mL saline flush. After obtaining an unenhanced sequence, dynamic enhanced sequences after administration of gadolinium are typically acquired in the arterial (20–25 seconds after contrast injection), portal venous (55–60 seconds after injection of contrast), and delayed venous (90–180 seconds after injection) sequences.[1,29]

Gadolinium-enhanced sequences maximize the T1 signal intensity of normal pancreatic parenchyma. This effect increases the lesion conspicuity of pancreatic adenocarcinomas (see **Fig. 2**), which are typically hypointense or might otherwise not be readily apparent on CT. Additionally, it may also aid

in detecting suspicious features of cystic lesions (ie, enhancing mural nodularity).[30] Contrast-enhanced sequences may also aid in improved detection of pancreatic necrosis in cases of acute pancreatitis. Finally, hypervascular tumors, such as small, functioning neuroendocrine and renal cell carcinoma metastases, are more conspicuous with the administration of gadolinium (**Fig. 3**).[31]

T2-WEIGHTED IMAGING

T2-weighted images have a longer TR and TE (ie, TR >1800 milliseconds and TE >60 milliseconds) than T1-weighted images. Traditionally, SE pulse sequences were used, but these were more prone to motion artifact from longer acquisition times. Fast and turbo SE (FSE and TSE) have replaced conventional SE, as they require less acquisition time.

Single-shot FSE (SSFSE) or half-Fourier acquisition single-shot turbo SE sequences are the preferred methods of obtaining breath-held T2-weighted images, which acquire half of the k-space in one long echo train after a single excitation.[32] SSFSEs have superior image quality than TSE sequences and can be used to obtain T2-weighted images with a TE of 100 milliseconds.[1,33] Compared with conventional sequences, fat has a higher signal intensity necessitating fat-suppression techniques. Additionally, because of less signal acquisition and T2 decay during the long echo train, these sequences have relatively lower SNR and contrast-to-noise ratio (CNR) of tissue with shorter T2.[1,34] In fact, it has been shown that the CNR of solid liver lesions, such as colorectal metastases, are lower with SSFSE sequences.[35]

Fat suppression can be achieved with either chemical shift or inversion recovery (IR). Chemical shift suppression takes advantage of the small difference in resonance frequency between water

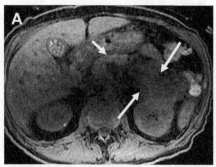 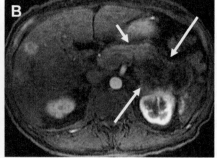

Fig. 2. A 67-year-old man with pancreatic tail adenocarcinoma. Note on the axial T1 spoiled GE (*A*) normal high T1 signal within the pancreatic head and neck (*short arrow*). Postcontrast image (*B*) shows a hypointense mass, path proven to be a pancreatic adenocarcinoma (*long arrows*).

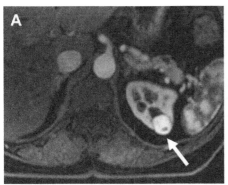
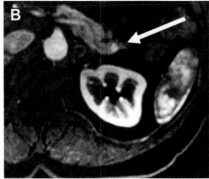

Fig. 3. A 57-year-old man with left renal cell carcinoma. Axial fat-saturated T1 3D SPGR during the arterial phase shows an enhancing left renal mass (*A, arrow*). Axial image in the same patient (*B*) shows a hypervascular lesion within the pancreas (*arrow*), consistent with renal cell metastasis.

and fat protons. In this technique, before applying the slice-selection pulse, a frequency selective saturation pulse with the same resonance frequency is applied to each slide selection RF pulse. Spoiled gradient pulses are immediately applied thereafter to diphase signal from lipids. This technique, however, is susceptible to magnetic field inhomogeneities, which could lead to incomplete fat suppression.[36]

With the IR fat-suppression technique, suppression of fat is based on the fact that fat has shorter T1 than water. Thus, after a 180° inversion, magnetization of fat will recover quicker than water. Thus, a 90° pulse applied at the null point of fat will allow water to recover and produce a signal, whereas fat will not. The null point of T1 from fat depends on the magnetic field strength. Typically, inversion times of greater than 150 milliseconds are used at 1.5 T.[1,36]

On T2-weighted images, the normal pancreas shows low to intermediate signal, usually lower than the liver and spleen (**Fig. 4**). Cystic lesions and fluid collection within and around the pancreas can be well demonstrated on T2-weighted images. Additionally, the pancreatic duct is usually well outlined in cross section with a high signal from the pancreatic fluid. This high signal can be used to guide acquisition of the MRCP series.[23]

MAGNETIC RESONANCE CHOLANGIOPANCREATOGRAPHY

MRCP allows excellent visualization of the pancreatic duct, and techniques used to obtain it vary but are all heavily T2 weighted and usually performed with either FSE or SSFSE sequences. Typically, a single 90° pulse is followed by multiple 180° refocusing pulses applied to generate single-section thick slab and multi-section thin slabs. FSE MRCP is performed with respiratory gating using long echo train and TRs. The long echo train reduces imaging time compared with traditional T2-weighted SE but results in blurring of the image from averaging the signal from multiple respiratory cycles. SSFSE MRCP is advantageous over FSE because of acquisition using a single breath hold, resulting in superior image quality SNR from decreased motion artifacts, such as respiration and peristalsis. However, this advantage comes at a cost of slightly decreased spatial resolution.[37] SSFSE MRCP uses a half Fourier technique by filling half of the k-space data and filling the rest by extrapolation.

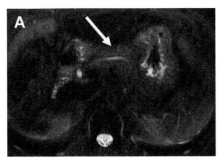
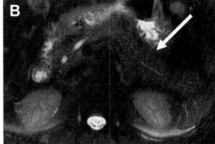

Fig. 4. Two axial 2D SSFSE T2-weighted images (*A, B*) showing normal intermediate signal of the pancreas (*arrow*).

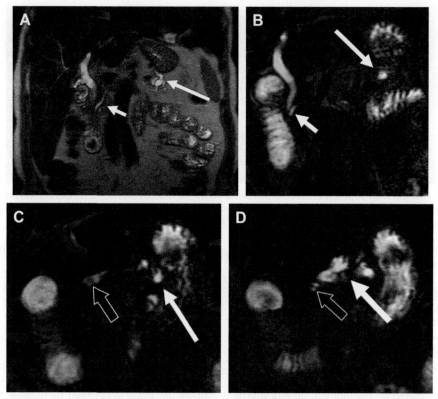

Fig. 5. A 4-year-old boy with choledocholithiasis. Coronal 2D SE MRCP (*A*) shows normal caliber duct in the head (*short arrow*) and dilated main duct and side branches in the tail (*long arrow*). Coronal 3D FSE MRCP in the same patient (*B–D*) shows normal pancreatic duct in the head (*short arrow*) and dilatation in the tail (*longer arrow*). A filling defect is seen in the midbody duct (*open arrow*), consistent with a stone.

Three-dimensional FSE has several advantages over 2D MRCP, including thin contiguous slices resulting in improved image quality of the oblique reconstructions performed from the acquisition plane. Specifically, it has been shown that 3D MRCP allows better assessment of pancreatic side branches, ductal stones, as well as biliary anatomy.[38,39] The author uses a navigator-based triggering. This triggering requires relatively uniform and regular breathing for adequate image quality. Newer 3D FRFSE sequences are available that result in contiguous, registered images allowing multi-planar reformation performed in a single breath hold.[38]

The normal caliber of the pancreatic duct is 3.5 mm in the head, 2.5 mm in the body, and 1.5 mm in the tail of the pancreas.[40,41] Typically, the entire duct is not seen on a single source image because of its anatomic course. However, thin sequential images can allow excellent visualization of the duct and evaluate it for strictures, stones, anomalies, and cystic lesions (**Figs. 5** and **6**).

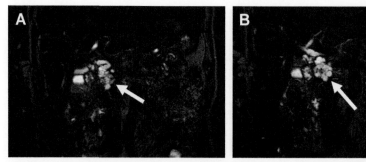

Fig. 6. A 1-year-old girl with serous cystadenoma in the pancreatic head. Two coronal 3D FSE MRCP images (*A, B*) show a multi-lobulated lesion (*arrow*) in the pancreatic head with central low signal intensity from calcification.

Occasionally, it is normal for the duct to not be visible, as patients are routinely imaged in the physiologic, nondistended state. Secretin may be administered as part of MRCP, though this is not the author's routine protocol. A dose of 1 mL of secretin per 10 kg of body weight can be administered intravenously, and preadministration and postadministration MRCP images are compared to determine if after 2 to 3 minutes there is a response in the pancreatic duct. Normally after secretin administration, the duct will enlarge followed by a return to baseline with increased T2 signal within the duodenum from emptying of the pancreatic juices. A lack of response or persistent dilation without a return to baseline (>3 mm at 10 minutes) is considered abnormal.[23,37]

SUMMARY

MR imaging of the pancreas is a valuable diagnostic tool, allowing problem-solving of complex cases as well as serving as a first-line modality of choice for certain indications. The noninvasive nature allows a comprehensive evaluation of the pancreatic parenchyma, the pancreatic duct, biliary anatomy, as well as the adjacent soft tissues. Recent advances in MR imaging techniques over the last decade have resulted in superior image quality with faster acquisition times. A routine MR imaging protocol at its core should include T1- and T2-weighted sequences with MRCP and gadolinium-enhanced sequences.

REFERENCES

1. Sandrasegaran K, Lin C, Akisik FM, et al. State-of-the-art pancreatic MRI. AJR Am J Roentgenol 2010;195(1):42–53.
2. Barth MM, Smith MP, Pedrosa I, et al. Body MR imaging at 3.0 T: understanding the opportunities and challenges. Radiographics 2007;27(5):1445–62 [discussion: 1462–4].
3. Erturk SM, Alberich-Bayarri A, Herrmann KA, et al. Use of 3.0-T MR imaging for evaluation of the abdomen. Radiographics 2009;29(6):1547–63.
4. Merkle EM, Dale BM. Abdominal MRI at 3.0 T: the basics revisited. AJR Am J Roentgenol 2006; 186(6):1524–32.
5. Chang KJ, Kamel IR, Macura KJ, et al. 3.0-T MR imaging of the abdomen: comparison with 1.5 T. Radiographics 2008;28(7):1983–98.
6. Soher BJ, Dale BM, Merkle EM. A review of MR physics: 3T versus 1.5T. Magn Reson Imaging Clin N Am 2007;15(3):277–90, v.
7. de Bazelaire CM, Duhamel GD, Rofsky NM, et al. MR imaging relaxation times of abdominal and pelvic tissues measured in vivo at 3.0 T: preliminary results. Radiology 2004;230(3):652–9.
8. Glockner JF, Hu HH, Stanley DW, et al. Parallel MR imaging: a user's guide. Radiographics 2005;25(5): 1279–97.
9. Deshmane A, Gulani V, Griswold MA, et al. Parallel MR imaging. J Magn Reson Imaging 2012;36(1): 55–72.
10. Elster AD. How much contrast is enough? Dependence of enhancement on field strength and MR pulse sequence. Eur Radiol 1997;7(Suppl 5): 276–80.
11. Kim SY, Byun JH, Lee SS, et al. Biliary tract depiction in living potential liver donors: intraindividual comparison of MR cholangiography at 3.0 and 1.5 T. Radiology 2010;254(2):469–78.
12. Isoda H, Kataoka M, Maetani Y, et al. MRCP imaging at 3.0 T vs. 1.5 T: preliminary experience in healthy volunteers. J Magn Reson Imaging 2007;25(5): 1000–6.
13. Onishi H, Kim T, Hori M, et al. MR cholangiopancreatography at 3.0 T: intraindividual comparative study with MR cholangiopancreatography at 1.5 T for clinical patients. Invest Radiol 2009;44(9):559–65.
14. Edelman RR, Salanitri G, Brand R, et al. Magnetic resonance imaging of the pancreas at 3.0 tesla: qualitative and quantitative comparison with 1.5 tesla. Invest Radiol 2006;41(2):175–80.
15. Coppens E, Metens T, Winant C, et al. Pineapple juice labeled with gadolinium: a convenient oral contrast for magnetic resonance cholangiopancreatography. Eur Radiol 2005;15(10):2122–9.
16. Papanikolaou N, Karantanas A, Maris T, et al. MR cholangiopancreatography before and after oral blueberry juice administration. J Comput Assist Tomogr 2000;24(2):229–34.
17. Riordan RD, Khonsari M, Jeffries J, et al. Pineapple juice as a negative oral contrast agent in magnetic resonance cholangiopancreatography: a preliminary evaluation. Br J Radiol 2004;77(924):991–9.
18. Vlahos L, Gouliamos A, Athanasopoulou A, et al. A comparative study between Gd-DTPA and oral magnetic particles (OMP) as gastrointestinal (GI) contrast agents for MRI of the abdomen. Magn Reson Imaging 1994;12(5):719–26.
19. Ros PR, Steinman RM, Torres GM, et al. The value of barium as a gastrointestinal contrast agent in MR imaging: a comparison study in normal volunteers. AJR Am J Roentgenol 1991;157(4):761–7.
20. Oksendal AN, Jacobsen TF, Gundersen HG, et al. Superparamagnetic particles as an oral contrast agent in abdominal magnetic resonance imaging. Invest Radiol 1991;26(Suppl 1):S67–70 [discussion: S71].
21. Martin J, Sentis M, Puig J, et al. Comparison of in-phase and opposed-phase GRE and conventional SE MR pulse sequences in T1-weighted imaging of

liver lesions. J Comput Assist Tomogr 1996;20(6): 890–7.

22. Kim YK, Kim CS, Lee JM, et al. Value of adding T1-weighted image to MR cholangiopancreatography for detecting intrahepatic biliary stones. AJR Am J Roentgenol 2006;187(3):W267–74.

23. Matos C, Cappeliez O, Winant C, et al. MR imaging of the pancreas: a pictorial tour. Radiographics 2002;22(1):e2.

24. Reeder SB, McKenzie CA, Pineda AR, et al. Water-fat separation with IDEAL gradient-echo imaging. J Magn Reson Imaging 2007;25(3):644–52.

25. Reeder SB, Pineda AR, Wen Z, et al. Iterative decomposition of water and fat with echo asymmetry and least-squares estimation (IDEAL): application with fast spin-echo imaging. Magn Reson Med 2005;54(3):636–44.

26. Reeder SB, Wen Z, Yu H, et al. Multicoil Dixon chemical species separation with an iterative least-squares estimation method. Magn Reson Med 2004;51(1):35–45.

27. Pamuklar E, Semelka RC. MR imaging of the pancreas. Magn Reson Imaging Clin N Am 2005; 13(2):313–30.

28. Winston CB, Mitchell DG, Outwater EK, et al. Pancreatic signal intensity on T1-weighted fat saturation MR images: clinical correlation. J Magn Reson Imaging 1995;5(3):267–71.

29. Kuhn JP, Hegenscheid K, Siegmund W, et al. Normal dynamic MRI enhancement patterns of the upper abdominal organs: gadoxetic acid compared with gadobutrol. AJR Am J Roentgenol 2009;193(5): 1318–23.

30. Patel BN, Gupta RT, Zani S, et al. How the radiologist can add value in the evaluation of the pre- and post-surgical pancreas. Abdom Imaging 2015;40(8): 2932–44.

31. Raman SP, Hruban RH, Cameron JL, et al. Pancreatic imaging mimics: part 2, pancreatic neuroendocrine tumors and their mimics. AJR Am J Roentgenol 2012;199(2):309–18.

32. Kim BS, Kim JH, Choi GM, et al. Comparison of three free-breathing T2-weighted MRI sequences in the evaluation of focal liver lesions. AJR Am J Roentgenol 2008;190(1):W19–27.

33. Bosmans H, Van Hoe L, Gryspeerdt S, et al. Single-shot T2-weighted MR imaging of the upper abdomen: preliminary experience with double-echo HASTE technique. AJR Am J Roentgenol 1997;169(5):1291–3.

34. Semelka RC, Kelekis NL, Thomasson D, et al. HASTE MR imaging: description of technique and preliminary results in the abdomen. J Magn Reson Imaging 1996;6(4):698–9.

35. Lee SS, Byun JH, Hong HS, et al. Image quality and focal lesion detection on T2-weighted MR imaging of the liver: comparison of two high-resolution free-breathing imaging techniques with two breath-hold imaging techniques. J Magn Reson Imaging 2007; 26(2):323–30.

36. Delfaut EM, Beltran J, Johnson G, et al. Fat suppression in MR imaging: techniques and pitfalls. Radiographics 1999;19(2):373–82.

37. Vitellas KM, Keogan MT, Spritzer CE, et al. MR cholangiopancreatography of bile and pancreatic duct abnormalities with emphasis on the single-shot fast spin-echo technique. Radiographics 2000;20(4): 939–57 [quiz: 1107–8, 1112].

38. Sodickson A, Mortele KJ, Barish MA, et al. Three-dimensional fast-recovery fast spin-echo MRCP: comparison with two-dimensional single-shot fast spin-echo techniques. Radiology 2006;238(2): 549–59.

39. Yoon LS, Catalano OA, Fritz S, et al. Another dimension in magnetic resonance cholangiopancreatography: comparison of 2- and 3-dimensional magnetic resonance cholangiopancreatography for the evaluation of intraductal papillary mucinous neoplasm of the pancreas. J Comput Assist Tomogr 2009;33(3): 363–8.

40. Soto JA, Barish MA, Yucel EK, et al. MR cholangiopancreatography: findings on 3D fast spin-echo imaging. AJR Am J Roentgenol 1995;165(6): 1397–401.

41. Mortele KJ, Rocha TC, Streeter JL, et al. Multimodality imaging of pancreatic and biliary congenital anomalies. Radiographics 2006;26(3):715–31.

Advanced MR Imaging Techniques for Pancreas Imaging

Nasir Siddiqui, MD[a], Camila Lopes Vendrami, MD[b],
Argha Chatterjee, MD[b], Frank H. Miller, MD[b],*

KEYWORDS

- MR imaging pancreas • Diffusion-weighted imaging • Secretin enhanced MRCP • MR perfusion
- MR elastography • Pancreatitis • Pancreatic neoplasms

KEY POINTS

- Advances in pancreatic MR imaging, specifically using diffusion-weighted imaging and secretin-enhanced MR cholangiography, have improved the diagnostic performance of MR in the evaluation of pancreatic diseases.
- Diffusion-weighted imaging has the potential to identify and characterize both focal and diffuse pancreatic processes.
- Diffusion-weighted imaging has better sensitivity than conventional computed tomography in detecting causal pancreatic tumors in acute pancreatitis, and is more accurate in identifying infected peripancreatic fluid collections.
- Diffusion-weighted imaging can help to distinguish chronic pancreatitis from normal pancreas, and may aid in identifying and monitoring treatment response in the setting of autoimmune pancreatitis.

INTRODUCTION

Advances in imaging techniques have led to an increased use of MR imaging in the evaluation of the pancreas[1] (Table 1). Optimization of diffusion-weighted imaging (DWI) has allowed for an increasing role in body applications, especially in the detection and characterization of pancreatic disorders.[2–4] Several studies have demonstrated promising results in using DWI for the detection and staging of acute pancreatitis (AP), grading chronic pancreatitis (CP), and detecting as well as monitoring treatment response for autoimmune pancreatitis (AIP).[5–8] Also, there is an increasing role of DWI in detecting and characterizing pancreatic lesions, identifying early hepatic and nodal metastases, and assessing for malignant degeneration in cystic pancreatic neoplasms.[9–11] MR cholangiography (MRCP) is an established, noninvasive alternative to endoscopic retrograde cholangiography (ERCP) for the evaluation of anatomic variation and diseases of the biliary and pancreatic ducts. More recently, secretin-enhanced MRCP (S-MRCP) has emerged as a useful adjunct in assessing pancreatic disorders with improved detection of morphologic abnormalities of the pancreatic duct and evaluating acute and CP.[12–15] Additionally, emerging MR techniques show promise in evaluating pancreatic diseases. MR perfusion techniques including

Disclosures: The authors have nothing to disclose.
[a] Department of Radiology, DuPage Medical Group, 430 Warrenville Road, Lisle, IL 60532, USA; [b] Department of Radiology, Northwestern Memorial Hospital, Northwestern University Feinberg School of Medicine, 676 North St. Clair Street Suite 800, Chicago, IL 60611, USA
* Corresponding author.
E-mail address: frank.miller@nm.org

Magn Reson Imaging Clin N Am 26 (2018) 323–344
https://doi.org/10.1016/j.mric.2018.03.002

Table 1
Advanced MR techniques for pancreatic imaging

Advanced MR Techniques	Description
Diffusion-weighted imaging	• Depicts the random microscopic motion of water molecules, which depend on tissue cellularity and cell membrane integrity. • Tissue types that exhibit restricted diffusion include tumor, inflammation, infections, and fibrosis. • Use of multiple b-values and generation of ADC maps allow for qualitative and quantitative assessment of pancreatic disease processes.
MRCP	• Exploits heavily T2-weighted imaging to evaluate the pancreatic duct and biliary tract. • Strong correlation between MRCP and ERCP in regards to pancreatic duct assessment.
S-MRCP	• Secretin distends the pancreatic duct allowing for better delineation of ductal anatomy on MRCP. • S-MRCP can identify subtle side branch dilatation in mild chronic pancreatitis, complex ductal anomalies and stenosis of the pancreatic duct. • S-MRCP can be used to evaluate the exocrine response of the pancreas.
MR perfusion	• MR perfusion assesses regional tissue perfusion based on the dynamics of uptake and washout of contrast agents. • MR perfusion may be useful in evaluating for pancreatic cancer and assessing treatment response to antiangiogenic therapies.
T1 mapping/relaxometry	• T1 relaxation time of pancreatic parenchyma increases with fibrosis, atrophy and edema. • Detection of subtle changes in T1 relaxation may be helpful in the early detection of pancreatic parenchymal diseases.
MRE	• MRE detects changes in tissue stiffness, which may result from fibrosis, inflammation or edema. • Detection of increased stiffness could indicate and potentially quantify pancreatic parenchymal diseases such as chronic pancreatitis.

Abbreviations: ADC, apparent diffusion coefficient; MRCP, MR cholangiography; MRE, MR elastography; S-MRCP, secretin-enhanced MRCP.

dynamic-contrast enhancement (DCE) are mostly in the early phases of investigation, but show potential in assessing tumor perfusion, especially in evaluating treatment response to antiangiogenic therapies.[16] T1 mapping/relaxometry of the pancreas has demonstrated promising results in distinguishing between mild CP and disease-free pancreas.[17] MR elastography (MRE) has been shown to be the most accurate noninvasive test to assess hepatic fibrosis in chronic liver disease, and the application to deeper organs such as the pancreas are being developed.[18] In this article, we discuss the advances in pancreatic imaging using the aforementioned techniques.

DIFFUSION-WEIGHTED IMAGING
Principles

Diffusion-weighted MR imaging exploits the random thermally induced mobility of water molecules, known as Brownian motion, in the biological environment. The restriction of water molecules

results in high signal intensity on DW images and low signal on apparent diffusion coefficient (ADC) maps, whereas the unimpeded movement of water results in high signal intensity on DW images, which has decreased signal at higher b-values and high signal on ADC maps.[19]

Technical Considerations

Improvements in MR technology with the optimization of "ultrafast" echoplanar and parallel imaging, and refinements in high-density surface coils and respiratory navigation have allowed for an increased role of DWI in body applications.[20,21] The fast spin-echo T2-weighted sequence allows for the measurement of diffusion by using a pair of gradients that are applied before and after the 180° refocusing radiofrequency pulse. In restricted diffusion, the phase shift caused by the first gradient is canceled by the second gradient, resulting in no significant loss of signal.[2–4] Conversely, in free diffusion, the interval movement of water between the applied gradients will not fully rephase, resulting in reduced signal on DWI. The major technical limitations of DWI is the inherent low signal to noise ratio and susceptibility artifact associated with echoplanar imaging. **Table 2** reviews scanning parameters that may be optimized to mitigate these limitations,[19,22,23] and **Table 3** outlines a sample of acquisition parameters used for DWI.

The b-value is a technical parameter indicating the degree of diffusion weighting and, therefore, indicates the sensitivity of the sequence to restricted diffusion.[23] DWI is obtained using at least 2 distinct b-values, one low (<200 s/mm^2) and another high (800 or 1000 s/mm^2, for example). However, images of 3 or more b-values are often generated. High b-value images have higher contrast resolution but lower spatial resolution, whereas low b-value images have generally higher spatial resolution and better image quality,

Table 3
Diffusion-weighted MR imaging acquisition parameters

Parameters	Description
Sequence	SS-EPI
Disposition	Free breathing
TR (ms)	6000
TE (ms)	59
Slice thickness (mm)	5
Gap (mm)	1
FOV (cm)	360
Parallel imaging factor	2
Matrix size	128 × 128
b-Values	50, 500, and 1000

Abbreviations: FOV, field of view; SS-EPI, single-shot spin-echo echo-planar.

Table 2
DWI technical limitations and potential solutions

Technical Challenge	Potential Solutions
Inherent low SNR	To optimize SNR consider: • Imaging at a higher magnetic field strength (3.0 T vs 1.5 T) but 3.0 T may have more artifacts • Minimizing TE (<100 ms) • Increasing number of excitations • Decreasing matrix size • Increase slice thickness and/or field of view • Use free breathing or respiratory triggered techniques with potentially longer acquisition times
Susceptibility to artifact	To minimize DWI artifacts consider: • Long repetition time to minimize T1 saturation effects, usually 3 times the T1 of a typical liver metastasis (>2500 ms) • Use fat suppression techniques to reduce ghosting artifact from chemical shift and respiratory motion • Consider breath-hold imaging to reduce artifact from motion

Abbreviations: DWI, diffusion-weighted imaging; SNR, signal to noise ratio.

being comparable with T2-weighted fat-suppressed images.[19] At low b-values, lesions with high free water have higher signal intensity because of the effect of T2 weighting on the image contrast. This phenomenon is known as T2 shine-through and can be seen in benign cystic lesions and hemangiomas.[19–22] As the b-value is increased, tissues with high diffusivity (such as cysts) demonstrate signal loss, whereas tissues with restricted diffusion (such as tumor tissue) maintain a high signal intensity.[23] Therefore, qualitative and quantitative assessment of diffusion restriction requires examination of images at different b-values.[3]

The interpretation of DWI requires the generation of ADC maps. The term apparent is used in ADC because the true coefficient cannot be measured using MR imaging. ADC maps are automatically generated by commercial MR workstations. Quantitative analysis of ADC values may be estimated by drawing regions of interest (ROIs) on both normal and abnormal tissue.

Clinical Applications

The potential clinical uses of pancreatic DWI are summarized in **Table 4**. These are discussed in greater detail herein.

Normal pancreatic parenchyma

There is significant variability in the reported ADC values of normal pancreatic parenchyma.[24] Nonetheless, the majority of studies demonstrate relative intrastudy similarity between the different pancreatic segments (ie, head, neck, body, and tail).[24] Therefore, the pancreas can be considered to be homogenous in ADC distribution,

Table 4
Potential uses of DWI in pancreatic imaging

Condition	Applications for DWI
AP	• Improved detection of AP, particularly when T1 and T2 findings are subtle or contrast cannot be given • Aid in differentiating between infected and noninfected PFCs
CP	• Distinguish CP and normal pancreas, but cannot distinguish between mild and severe CP • May be useful in quantifying the extent of pancreatic exocrine dysfunction when used with secretin
AIP	• Useful in diagnosing AIP and identifying focal pancreatic involvement • Effective in monitoring response to treatment
Pancreatic adenocarcinoma	• High diagnostic performance for detection of pancreatic adenocarcinoma • Improved staging accuracy by identifying small liver and lymph node metastasis • May identify small lesions before conventional MR sequences
PNETs	• Can help identify small PNET • More sensitive in detecting liver metastasis compared with T2-weighted imaging and DCE-MR • May be useful in distinguishing tumor grades
Cystic pancreatic lesions	• Often not useful for differentiating between cystic lesions but may help in detecting malignant degeneration or identifying mural nodularity

Abbreviations: AIP, autoimmune pancreatitis; AP, acute pancreatitis; CP, chronic pancreatitis; DCE-MR, dynamic contrast-enhanced MR imaging; PNETS, pancreatic neuroendocrine tumors.

and normal pancreatic parenchyma can be used as an internal standard when evaluating a focal abnormality.[3] However, caution should be used when evaluating diffuse pancreatic diseases or a focal abnormality in the setting of diffuse pancreatic disease.

Inflammatory conditions

Acute pancreatitis AP can occur once or repetitively and can be associated with mild to severe inflammatory edema. AP usually is a self-limiting process; however, it may progress to necrotizing pancreatitis resulting in necrosis of the pancreas and/or peripancreatic tissue.[25] Typically, the pancreatic parenchyma seems to be enlarged with increased signal on T2-weighted images (T2WI) and abnormally low signal on T1-weighted images (T1WI). Diagnostic features include stranding of the peripancreatic fat tissue with low signal intensity on T1WI, and edema and fluid around the pancreas on fat-suppressed T2WI.[25] Necrotizing pancreatitis is characterized by nonenhancing or severely hypoenhancing pancreatic tissue.[26] Patients with AP may develop complications, such as bleeding, infected fluid collections, and vascular complications (thrombosis or pseudoaneurysm).[25,26]

On DWI, AP results in parenchymal restricted diffusion with corresponding lower ADC values than that of normal parenchyma (**Fig. 1**).[27] In some patients, DWI may best show findings of AP, because the findings on conventional T1WI and T2WI may be subtle. In comparable studies performed at 1.5 T, lower ADC values were found in individuals with AP when compared with normal individuals. In their studies, a threshold ADC value of 1.60×10^{-3} mm^2/s and 1.62×10^{-3} mm^2/s demonstrated sensitivities of 93% and 84.1%, and specificities of 87% and 90.5% for the detection of pancreatitis, respectively.[5,27] Unenhanced MR imaging with DWI was found to be equivalent to contrast-enhanced computed tomography (CT) and outperformed unenhanced CT in the detection of AP.[5] In addition, DWI has the potential of detecting pancreatic tumors that result in AP at a higher sensitivity than conventional CT.[5]

In the setting of AP complicated by a peripancreatic fluid collection (PFC), DWI can aid in the differentiation of infected and noninfected PFCs.[28] The early and noninvasive determination of superimposed infection is of paramount clinical importance because treatment and prognosis differ from noninfected PFCs. Infection is suspected on DWI when the PFC demonstrates restricted diffusion seen as hyperintense signal on high b-values and corresponding low signal on ADC maps (**Fig. 2**). The ADC values were significantly lower for infected PFCs compared with noninfected PFCs with a reported accuracy of 95.2% in 1 study.[29] Additionally, the accuracy

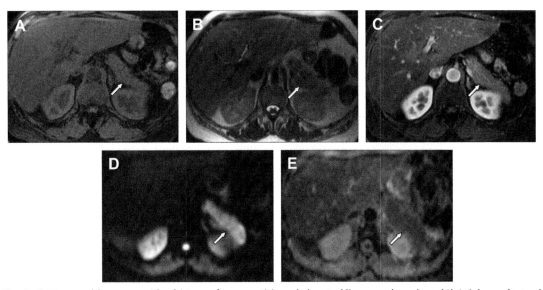

Fig. 1. A 54-year-old woman with a history of pancreatitis and elevated lipase and amylase. (A) Axial unenhanced T1-weighted fat saturated MR image shows subtle decreased signal intensity of pancreatic tail (arrow) with fairly normal signal intensity on (B) T2-weighted MR imaging (arrow). (C) Axial contrast-enhanced MR image shows decreased enhancement of the pancreatic tail (arrow). (D, E) Diffusion-weighted MR image (D) shows markedly abnormal pancreatic tail (arrow) with high signal intensity on b = 500 s/mm^2 image, which is dark (arrow) on the (E) apparent diffusion coefficient (ADC) map image with ADC measuring 0.1 × 10^{-3} mm^2/s.

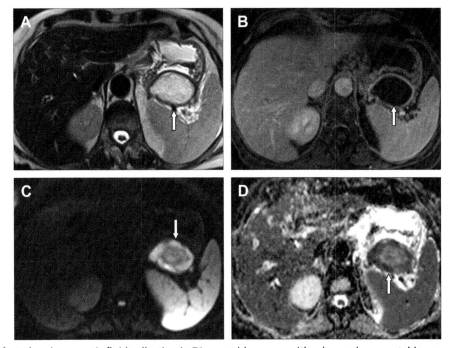

Fig. 2. Infected peripancreatic fluid collection in 71-year-old woman with advanced unresectable pancreatic can-cer with known malignant duodenal stricture and biliary stent placement, with a history of intermittent diarrhea, periodic bilious emesis, and weight loss of 30 pounds. (A) Axial T2-weighted MR image shows high signal inten-sity fluid collection and low signal intensity rim (arrow). (B) Axial contrast-enhanced T1-weighted fat-saturated image shows fluid collection with mildly enhancing wall (arrow). Based on conventional imaging, the lesion is not clearly infected. (C) Axial diffusion-weighted MR image (b = 800 s/mm^2) shows the abnormality (arrow) as high signal intensity, which is dark on the (D) apparent diffusion coefficient map (arrow) with the ADC measuring 1.3 × 10^{-3} mm^2/s from restricted diffusion. Aspiration showed infected fluid.

and sensitivity of DWI-MR surpassed CT in identifying the presence of infection in PFCs.[29]

Chronic pancreatitis CP encompasses a broad range of progressive fibroinflammatory diseases of the exocrine pancreas that ultimately result in damage to the pancreatic structure and function. On MR imaging, there is loss of the normal high T1WI signal of the pancreatic parenchyma secondary to fibrosis, and diminished enhancement on the arterial phase with progressive delayed enhancement.[30] Additionally, changes to the pancreatic duct such as dilatation, strictures, and dilated side branches can be seen.[30]

DWI has shown promise as a parametric imaging marker in evaluating the severity of the disease, as pancreatic tissue sampling for analysis and diagnosis is invasive and often impractical. ADC values have been found to be lower in patients with CP when compared with normal patients; however, no significant difference in ADC values was noted between mild and severe forms of pancreatitis.[6,7] The decreased ADC values in CP may relate to the replacement of pancreatic parenchyma with fibrotic tissue and/or decreased pancreatic exocrine function, resulting in decreased diffusion of water in the gland. An ADC threshold value of 2.20×10^{-3} mm^2/s was found to have 100% sensitivity and 73% specificity for discriminating normal pancreas from CP at 3.0 T.[7]

The use of secretin to stimulate pancreatic secretions, in conjunction with DWI, can provide useful information regarding physiologic alterations caused by CP.[6,7,29,31] The dynamic changes to ADC values after the administration of secretin are felt to correlate with pancreatic exocrine function.[6,7,31] In the setting of CP, there is a delayed peak in ADC values relative to the normal peak ADC values in healthy pancreatic parenchyma.[29] The delayed peak in ADC measurements may be beneficial in quantifying the extent of pancreatic exocrine dysfunction; however, more research must be performed in determining its clinical usefulness. Currently, DWI can help to distinguish between CP and normal pancreas, but cannot distinguish between mild and severe CP.[6,7]

Autoimmune pancreatitis AIP is a type of CP owing to a postulated autoimmune mechanism that is characterized by extensive fibrosis with mixed inflammatory cell infiltration along the pancreatic ducts, and responsiveness to steroid treatment. Serum immunoglobulin G4 levels are usually elevated in AIP serving as biomarker for the disease, and can be monitored to assess treatment response and disease activity.[8,32,33] DWI may be the first study to suggest this diagnosis, and is beneficial in identifying focal pancreatic involvement and assessing treatment response.[8] AIP may present as focal pancreatic enlargement with mass effect and restricted diffusion, which can make it difficult to differentiate it from pancreatic cancer[34] (**Fig. 3**). Studies have shown that AIP demonstrates restricted diffusion with ADC values lower than pancreatic carcinoma. In particular, 1 study demonstrated a sensitivity of 100% and specificity of 98% with a markedly low ADC threshold value of 0.88×10^{-3} mm^2/s.[35] However, the small sample sizes and limited number of studies makes it difficult to draw definitive conclusions and other specific imaging features such as capsule-like rim enhancement, skipped strictures of the common bile duct, and/or main pancreatic duct and renal/retroperitoneal involvement should be used in conjunction with DWI to suggest AIP.[8,34,35] Furthermore, the combination of MR DWI and CT imaging has been found to be more accurate in distinguishing between AIP and pancreatic cancer than by using either modality alone.[35]

DWI has been effective in monitoring treatment response in AIP.[8,36] AIP demonstrates gradual improvement in restricted diffusion, presumably related to amelioration of inflammation, after the administration of steroid therapy. Symptomatic AIP patients have been found to present with significantly lower ADC values than asymptomatic patients.[36] Also, ADC values and immunoglobulin G4 index values have shown an inverse correlation suggesting that ADC values can be reflective of disease activity.[8]

Solid pancreatic lesions

Pancreatic adenocarcinoma Pancreatic adenocarcinoma is the most common malignant neoplasm of the pancreas. The majority of early and curable tumors are associated with nonspecific and mild symptoms and, therefore, survival depends on early detection and accurate staging.[37] DWI may increase early detection by identifying a mass with restricted diffusion before other imaging features are manifested (**Fig. 4**). Additionally, DWI may be helpful in the detection of metastasis to the liver and lymph nodes, thus, improving staging accuracy, as well as allowing small metastasis, not well-seen in other sequences, to be identified and characterized (**Fig. 5**).[38]

Pancreatic adenocarcinoma is typically hypointense to normal pancreas on T1 fat-suppressed sequences, and demonstrates decreased enhancement on the arterial phase with subsequent progressive enhancement on delayed phases.[38] Small pancreatic masses can be difficult

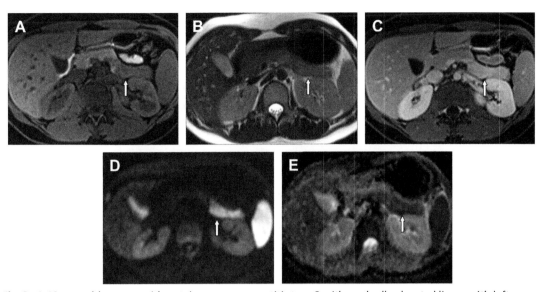

Fig. 3. A 19-year-old woman with autoimmune pancreatitis type 2 with markedly elevated lipase with left upper quadrant pain and normal serum immunoglobulin G4. (*A*) Axial T1-weighted fat-saturated MR image shows hypointense pancreatic tail (*arrow*) with slightly increased signal intensity on (*B*) T2-weighted MR image (*arrow*). (*C*) Axial contrast-enhanced MR image shows enhancement of the lesion on the pancreatic tail (*arrow*). (*D*) Diffusion-weighted MR image (b = 800 s/mm^2) best shows the abnormality as markedly increased signal intensity (*arrow*) with decreased signal intensity (*arrow*) on the (*E*) apparent diffusion coefficient (ADC) map with the ADC measuring 1.0×10^{-3} mm^2/s.

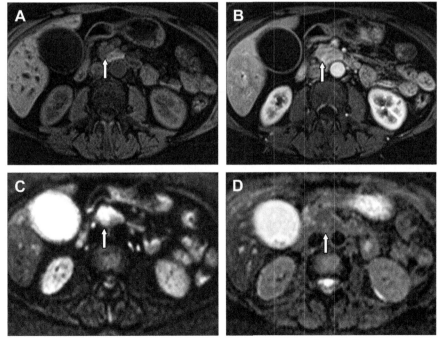

Fig. 4. A 57-year-old woman with jaundice from a high-grade infiltrating ductal adenocarcinoma (grade 3). (*A*) Axial T1-weighted fat-saturated MR image shows subtle small hypointense lesion (*arrow*) that enhances on (*B*) contrast-enhanced MR imaging, but was more difficult to see (*arrow*). (*C*) Axial diffusion-weighted MR image (b = 500 s/mm^2) shows a high signal intensity mass (*arrow*) measuring 1.7 cm, which is dark (*arrow*) on the (*D*) apparent diffusion coefficient (ADC) map (ADC of 1.2×10^{-3} mm^2/s).

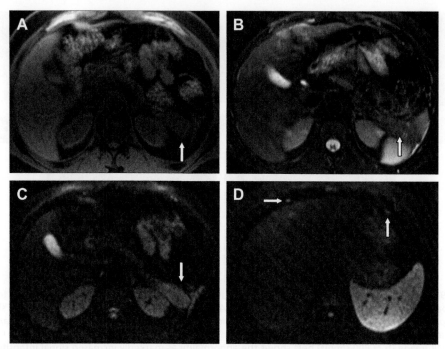

Fig. 5. A 56 year-old man in evaluation of a left kidney mass demonstrated on computed tomography scanning. (*A*) Axial T1-weighted MR image shows enlargement (*arrow*) of the pancreatic tail, which is also seen on (*B*) T2-weighted fat-suppressed image (*arrow*). (*C*) Axial diffusion-weighted MR image (b = 500 s/mm²) image shows a focal area of increased signal in the tail (*arrow*). (*D*) Axial diffusion-weighted MR image (b = 500 s/mm²) shows small tumoral implants (*arrows*). The presence of omental tumor implants best seen on diffusion-weighted imaging suggests that the pancreatic tail lesion is from pancreatic cancer instead of autoimmune pancreatitis, which can also have a bulbous appearance to the pancreatic tail.

to detect because of minimal mass effect and pancreatic contour deformity. Commonly, secondary signs such as focal pancreatic atrophy or pancreatic duct dilatation are used to identify a small underlying mass.[38] DWI can facilitate the detection of small lesions by exploiting the hypercellular and fibrotic nature of the tumor. With high b-values, there is increased conspicuity of the small fibrotic mass, which demonstrates hyperintense signal relative to the normal pancreas and correspondingly low ADC.

The use of MR DWI has demonstrated a high diagnostic performance for the detection of pancreatic adenocarcinoma with a reported accuracy of 96%.[39] DWI using a b-value of 500 s/mm² was found to be equivalent to gadolinium-enhanced MR imaging; however, the best reported values for the detection of pancreatic adenocarcinoma were using a b-value of 1000 s/mm² demonstrating a sensitivity and specificity of 96% and 99%, respectively.[39,40] Large pancreatic adenocarcinomas or treated disease may have necrotic components that demonstrate increased ADC values owing to the free motion of water. Additionally, the colloid form of adenocarcinoma and pseudocysts secondary to ductal

obstruction can result in heterogeneous signal alteration on DWI.[3] Therefore, the disparity in reported ADC values for pancreatic adenocarcinoma in the literature likely relates to variability in the extent of fibrosis, necrosis, and cellular density within the tumors.[41] The clinical use of ADC values to predict the prognosis of newly diagnosed pancreatic adenocarcinoma has yet to be established. In 1 study, no association between tumor grade and ADC values was identified.[42] In contrast, Wang and colleagues[43] demonstrated a significant difference in ADC values between poorly and well- or moderately differentiated pancreatic ductal adenocarcinoma.

Distinguishing mass-forming pancreatitis from pancreatic carcinoma remains a diagnostic dilemma owing to overlapping imaging features on cross-sectional imaging.[38] The role of DWI in distinguishing these entities is unclear, with conflicting and inconsistent results in ADC values.[9,44,45] The variation between studies and overlap of ADC values between pancreatic adenocarcinoma and mass-forming pancreatitis likely relates to the variable proportion of fibrosis and inflammation associated with the diseases processes. Consequently, the use of MR DWI by itself to prospectively distinguish pancreatic adenocarcinoma and mass-forming pancreatitis in clinical practice is not recommended.

Pancreatic neuroendocrine tumors Pancreatic neuroendocrine tumors (PNETs) account for 1% to 2% of all pancreatic neoplasms.[46] Symptoms of functioning endocrine tumors relate to the secreted hormones rather than mass effect, and thus small functioning endocrine tumors may be undetectable on conventional MR imaging. Typically, PNETs demonstrate hypointense signal relative to normal pancreas on unenhanced fat-suppressed T1WI, and hypervascular enhancement during the arterial phase after the administration of gadolinium contrast.[38] However, small neoplasms can have variable presentations and may not have the typical hypervascular imaging appearance of PNETs on contrast-enhanced examinations nor high signal on T2WI.[47] In this setting, DWI has been found to significantly improve the detection of PNETs; particularly, neoplasms that are isointense on T2WI[38] (**Fig. 6**). Additionally, DWI is more sensitive in detecting liver metastasis from PNETs than T2WI and DCE MR imaging,[10] thus, allowing for more accurate staging.

The ADC values of PNETs can be variable owing to the underlying histopathologic characteristics of the lesion, such as the degree of necrosis and hemorrhage. However, in the absence of significant necrosis or hemorrhage, DWI may be useful in further characterizing the malignant potential of the endocrine neoplasm.[48] On DWI, small benign endocrine neoplasms may have a relatively high ADC value with hyperintense signal on low b-values (0–50 s/mm^2), whereas malignant endocrine neoplasms may demonstrate low ADC values with hyperintense signal on high b-values (>500 s/mm^2). Although a consensus regarding the usefulness of DWI in predicting tumor grade has not been reached, it may be helpful in differentiating benign and malignant PNETs without hemorrhage or cystic degeneration by ADC values.[48–50]

Uncommon solid pancreatic lesions Solid pseudopapillary neoplasm (SPN) is a rare tumor with a low malignant potential predominantly affecting young women.[51] SPN typically present as a heterogeneous encapsulated mass that may contain solid, cystic, and/or hemorrhagic components.[38] The presence of a fibrous capsule and intratumoral hemorrhage are important morphologic features in differentiating SPN from other pancreatic lesions. SPN have been shown to have lower ADC values compared with normal parenchyma; however, the composition of the neoplasm (solid vs cystic or hemorrhagic fluid) determines the degree of restricted diffusion and ADC values.[38]

Intrapancreatic accessory spleen, although not a neoplastic process, is a differential consideration for a solid pancreatic tail mass. Intrapancreatic

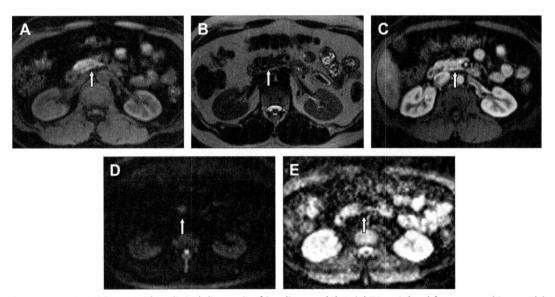

Fig. 6. A 48-year-old man with a clinical diagnosis of insulinoma. (*A*) Axial T1-weighted fat-saturated image, (*B*) axial T2-weighted MR image, and (*C*) contrast-enhanced T1-weighted do not show any obvious lesion in the uncinate process of pancreas (*arrow, A-C*). (*D*) Axial diffusion-weighted MR image (b = 1000 s/mm^2) image shows a hyperintense lesion (*arrow*) in the uncinate process which shows (*E*) low signal intensity (*arrow*) on the apparent diffusion coefficient (ADC) map with the ADC measuring 1.0×10^{-3} mm^2/s, showing the usefulness of the diffusion-weighted MR image. The lesion was pathologically proven to be an insulinoma.

accessory spleen typically follows the signal intensity of the spleen on all imaging sequences. DWI and ADC maps showing values similar to spleen have demonstrated a high diagnostic performance in differentiating intrapancreatic accessory spleen from other solid pancreatic neoplasms.[52] Therefore, in addition to convention MR imaging, DWI is an additional tool that can be used in differentiating intrapancreatic accessory spleen from other solid pancreatic lesions.

CYSTIC PANCREATIC LESIONS

DWI may be beneficial in identifying cystic pancreatic lesions owing to the free movement of water resulting in hyperintense signal on low b-values and relatively high ADC values; however, because of considerable overlap in ADC values, its role in differentiating between cystic lesions is limited.[11,53–55] Currently, the use of DWI in characterizing cystic lesions is not established owing to significant variability and conflicting results in the reported literature.[3] As discussed, DWI is a useful tool in differentiating infected and noninfected PFCs and pseudocysts. In addition, DWI may be beneficial in detecting malignant degeneration of mucinous cystadenomas or identifying mural nodularity in high-grade versus low-grade intraductal papillary mucinous neoplasms (IPMNs).[11] In such cases, the solid neoplastic component may demonstrate restricted diffusion raising concern for malignant transformation (**Fig. 7**).

Secretin-Enhanced MR Cholangiography

Principles
MRCP is a noninvasive technique for assessing the pancreatic ducts with established correlation with ERCP in evaluating anatomic variation and disease processes.[12] Secretin is a peptide hormone produced in the intestinal mucosa, which stimulates the secretion of bicarbonate-rich fluid into the pancreatic ducts and transiently increases the tone of the sphincter of Oddi. The increased fluid distention of the pancreatic duct allows for improved detection of pancreatic ductal anomalies, and perhaps in the diagnosis of pancreatic cystic lesions.[13] Additionally, S-MRCP can assess pancreatic glandular function, monitor pancreatic flow dynamics and can be beneficial in evaluating the remnant pancreas after pancreatoduodenectomy.[13]

Technical considerations
S-MRCP is typically performed on a 1.5 T or 3.0 T magnet using phased-array multichannel coils. Imaging protocols commonly consist of T1-weighted gradient echo, T2-weighted axial and coronal sequences, 2-dimensional and 3-dimensional MRCP, and T1-weighted gradient echo before

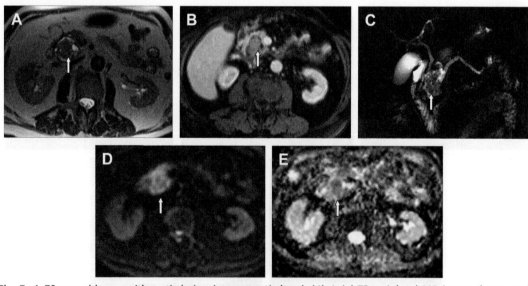

Fig. 7. A 79-year-old man with cystic lesion in pancreatic head. (*A*) Axial T2-weighted MR image shows cystic pancreatic head lesion with a large low signal intensity component (*arrow*). (*B*) Axial contrast-enhanced MR image shows enhancing lesion (*arrow*). (*C*) MR cholangiography shows large filling defect (*arrow*) in the pancreatic duct. (*D*) Axial diffusion-weighted MR image (b = 500 s/mm²) shows high signal intensity in the lesion (*arrow*) with a corresponding low signal intensity on the (*E*) apparent diffusion coefficient (ADC) map (*arrow*) with the ADC measuring 1.2×10^{-3} mm²/s. The lesion was a side branch intraductal papillary mucinous neoplasm with malignant solid component that had restricted diffusion.

and after gadolinium contrast. A typical protocol used for S-MRCP is outlined in **Table 5**. Additionally, at our institution, after administration of secretin, dynamic imaging is performed with coronal single shot turbo spin echo sequences obtained at 30-second intervals for 10 minutes covering the pancreas and adjacent small bowel, and subsequently a respiratory-triggered 3-dimensional turbo spin echo sequence is obtained. The peak effect of secretin is usually seen 3 to 5 minutes after injection, at which time the main pancreatic duct can increase by 1 mm or more from baseline and side branch radicals may become visible. Additionally, secretin can be used to assess pancreatic exocrine response, either quantitatively or semiquantitatively, by evaluating duodenal filling after secretin administration.

To enhance the exocrine response to secretin, patients should fast for at least 4 hours before MR imaging.[13] Administration of a negative contrast agent to suppress the high-intensity fluid in the stomach and duodenum on MRCP images is recommended. This result can be achieved with diluted gadolinium in water or pineapple juice at 100% concentration (320 mL).[13,56,57] Antiperistaltic agents such as glucagon can be used to avoid motion artifact from bowel peristalsis.

The recommended manufacturer's dose of secretin is 0.2 µg/kg, which is administered through slow intravenous injection over a period of 1 minute to mitigate the potential side effect of abdominal pain seen with bolus administration. Secretin has a safe drug profile with mild adverse effects of nausea, flushing, and vomiting seen in 0.5% of patients. Secretin is relative contraindicated in the setting of severe AP; however, it has

routinely been used safely in the setting of mild pancreatitis.[13,15]

Clinical applications
The potential clinical uses of S-MRCP are summarized in **Table 6**. These are discussed in more detail herein.

Acute pancreatitis The initial evaluation of AP is typically performed with CT to assess the severity of disease and identify the presence of complications. However, MRCP is preferred to CT owing to better sensitivity when evaluating for underlying biliary disease or anatomic variation.[58] In particular, in the setting of recurrent AP (patients with >1 episode of AP), S-MRCP has been found to be more sensitive in detecting an underlying cause for recurrent AP when clinical and laboratory findings are inconclusive.[15]

The use of S-MRCP improves the visualization of the pancreatic ductal system, allowing for better delineation of morphologic variations when compared with MRCP. The improved visualization of the pancreatic duct increases diagnostic confidence in confirming or excluding clinically significant entities such as pancreatic divisum, santorinicele or an anomalous pancreaticobiliary junction.[15,56,59]

Pancreatic divisum Pancreatic divisum (PD) is the most common congenital anatomic variant caused by the lack of fusion between the dorsal and ventral pancreatic anlages resulting into 2 distinct pancreatic ducts. This can predispose the patient to obstructive pancreatopathy resulting in pancreatitis or pancreatic-type pain. PD is seen in about 15% to 20% of patients with unexplained pancreatitis, and 5% to 10% of the general population.[57,60] An incomplete PD, also known as a dominant dorsal duct, characterized by a diminutive communication between the dorsal and ventral pancreatic ducts has been reported in 10% to 15% of patients on ERCP studies, and may have similar clinical implications to patients with a "complete" PD (**Fig. 8**).[57] S-MRCP demonstrates superior sensitivity compared with MRCP with a recent study demonstrating a sensitivity of 86% for PD on S-MRCP compared with 57% for PD on MRCP, and only a minimal loss of specificity (92% vs 96%).[15] Other studies have demonstrated similar diagnostic accuracy with reported sensitivities of 73% and 100% and specificity of 97% to 100%.[61,62] The lower sensitivity for detecting PD in one study was attributed to the presence of CP. Thus, the use of S-MRCP improves the detection of PD in 5% - 29% of patients when compared with conventional MRCP.[12,15,61,62]

Table 5 Secretin-enhanced rare MRCP parameters	
Parameters	**Description**
Disposition	Breath-holding
TR (ms)	4500
TE (ms)	735
Slice thickness (mm)	30–70
FOV (cm)	300
Fat suppression	Spectral selected
Parallel imaging factor	2
Matrix size	269 × 384
Number of signal averages acquired	1

Abbreviations: FOV, field of view; MRCP, MR cholangiography.

Table 6
Potential uses of S-MRCP in pancreatic imaging

Condition	Applications for S-MRCP
AP	• Improved detection for anatomic variations including pancreas divisum, Santorinicele and APBJ • More sensitive in detecting an underlying cause for recurrent AP
CP	• Aid in early detection of CP by better delineation of abnormal side branch dilatation • Assess and potentially quantify pancreatic exocrine dysfunction in CP, and may be used to evaluate progression of disease and treatment response • Identifying pancreatic exocrine dysfunction may be beneficial in detecting CP in the absence of morphologic abnormalities
IPMN	• May help in differentiating side branch IPMNs from other cystic pancreatic lesions by improving visibility of communication between main pancreatic duct and cystic lesion
Inflammatory pancreatic mass	• May aid in distinguishing benign from malignant strictures by better assessment for the duct-penetrating sign
Postoperative pancreas	• Superior visualization of the pancreatic duct and anastomosis may aid in the detection of an anastomotic stricture • May help in identifying a pancreatic duct leak

Abbreviations: AP, acute pancreatitis; APBJ, anomalous pancreaticobiliary junction; CP, chronic pancreatitis; IPMN, intraductal papillary mucinous neoplasm; S-MRCP, secretin-enhanced MRCP.

Santorinicele Santorinicele is a focal dilatation of the distal dorsal (Santorini) duct, just proximal to the duodenal wall, presumably related to relative stenosis of the minor papilla. In the setting of PD or a dominant dorsal duct, the increased pressure in the dorsal duct secondary to impaired flow thorough the accessory papilla results in recurrent episodes of AP, which is typically treated with

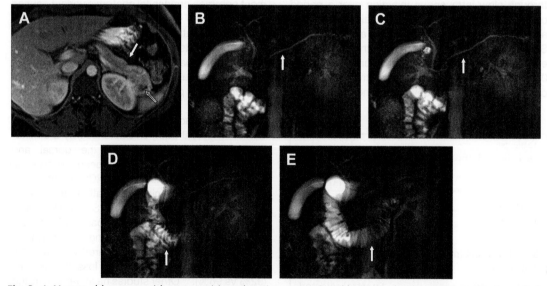

Fig. 8. A 41-year-old woman with pancreatitis and cystic pancreatic tail lesion underwent MR imaging to exclude chronic pancreatitis. (*A*) Axial contrast-enhanced T1-weighted fat-saturated image shows normal size, shape, signal intensity, and enhancement of the pancreas (*arrow*) with a cystic lesion in the pancreatic tail (*open arrow*). (*B-E*) Coronal thick-slab heavily T2-weighted MR images (2D-RARE) taken serially after secretin injection. Initial images demonstrate improved visualization of the downstream portion of the main pancreatic duct (*arrow, B-C*) from (*B*) 0 minute to (*C*) 1 minute post-injection. Later images show progressive luminal opacification of the duodenum (*arrow, D-E*) up to the fourth portion at (*D*) 5 minutes and (*E*) 10 minutes; this is compatible with grade 4 duodenal filling, suggestive of normal pancreatic function.

endoscopic sphincterotomy of the minor papilla.[13] S-MRCP is beneficial in identifying the presence of Santorinicele in the setting of recurrent AP. In one study, S-MRCP was found to be more sensitive than MRCP identifying a Santorinicele in seven out of 107 (6%) patients compared with 3 out of 107 (3%) patients on MRCP.[61]

Anomalous pancreaticobiliary junction An anomalous pancreaticobiliary junction is a rare congenital variant of clinical importance because it predisposes the patient to a higher incidence of pancreatic diseases (38%), typically pancreatitis, and also an increased risk of cholangiocarcinoma (15.6%) and choledochal cysts.[63,64] In anomalous pancreaticobiliary junction, the main pancreatic duct and common bile duct join outside of the duodenal wall, resulting in a common channel predisposing the patient to bidirectional flow owing to lack of sphincter muscle function. The reflux of pancreatic juices into the biliary tree has been proposed as the cause for the increase risk in cholangiocarcinomas. S-MRCP can improve the detection of anomalous pancreaticobiliary junction, and may demonstrate reflux of pancreatic juices into the biliary tree and gallbladder.[65]

Chronic pancreatitis In the early phase of CP, the fibroinflammatory process can be identified by abnormal side branch dilatation assuming a club-like configuration, which is a hallmark feature of CP on ERCP. Because of the small size, the detection of abnormal side branch dilatation can be difficult on MRCP, and may lead to a high false-negative rate.[14] S-MRCP with improved distention of the ductal system allows for better delineation of abnormal side branch dilatation, and hence improved detection of early CP.[14] Sandrasegaran and colleagues[15] demonstrated a significant increase in sensitivity of S-MRCP compared with MRCP (71.4% vs 21.4%) for the detection of side branch dilatation in a blinded comparison using ERCP as a reference standard. An additional study demonstrated improved visualization of side branch dilatation from 4% to 63% when comparing MRCP with S-MRCP.[14] Therefore, S-MRCP with the improved detection of side branch dilatation aids in identifying early CP, limiting the need for invasive procedures and their potential complications.

In the setting of severe CP, the fibroinflammatory process results in main pancreatic ductal dilatation and irregularity with the development of main duct strictures. S-MRCP causes distention of the main pancreatic duct by stimulating the exocrine secretion of fluid. Therefore, the loss of distensibility can be used as a surrogate marker for CP.[66] However, a potential pitfall can be seen in the setting of a stricture or obstruction in the distal duct or ampulla, which may result in upstream ductal distention after S-MRCP. Because strictures are often seen in the setting of CP, ductal distention after S-MRCP may be falsely reassuring.[13]

Typically, in severe CP the pancreatic ductal system is already dilated and the pancreatic exocrine function is reduced. Therefore, S-MRCP may not significantly aid in making the diagnosis of severe CP compared with MRCP based on ductal abnormalities.[56] However, S-MRCP may be beneficial in identifying flow-limiting strictures of the main pancreatic duct and noninvasively estimating the pancreatic exocrine function.[67] The evaluation of the pancreatic exocrine reserve can be used to assess progression of disease and evaluate treatment response. Additionally, identifying pancreatic exocrine dysfunction may be beneficial in detecting CP in the absence of morphologic abnormalities.[58] The pancreatic exocrine function can be estimated by measuring the duodenal filling after secretin stimulation and may be evaluated in a semiquantitative or quantitative manner (**Fig. 9**). For the semiquantitative evaluation of the pancreatic exocrine function, the amount of duodenal and small bowel filling with pancreatic fluid after secretin administration is analyzed.[68] Filling of the duodenum is graded according to duodenal anatomic imaging findings and defined as grade 1, pancreatic fluid excretion is confined to the duodenal bulb; grade 2, fluid reached the second portion of the duodenum; grade 3, duodenal filling is seen as far the third portion of the duodenum; and grade 4 with observed filling of duodenum and jejunum (**Fig. 10**). Although normal filling of the duodenum may be seen, impairment of the pancreatic exocrine function cannot be excluded.[13,69] Other methods of quantification using volume of fluid excreted in the duodenum or peak flow rate have been proposed.[67,70]

Pancreatic lesions
Intraductal papillary mucinous neoplasm IPMN is the most common cystic neoplasm of the pancreas, representing 36% of incidental pancreatic cystic lesions seen on imaging.[71] The reported risk of in situ or invasive malignancy associated with a main duct IPMN (57%–92%) is significantly higher than a side branch IPMN (<20%).[72] S-MRCP may aid in distinguishing a side branch IPMN from other cystic pancreatic lesions including main duct IPMN and mucinous cystic neoplasms, which have a relatively greater

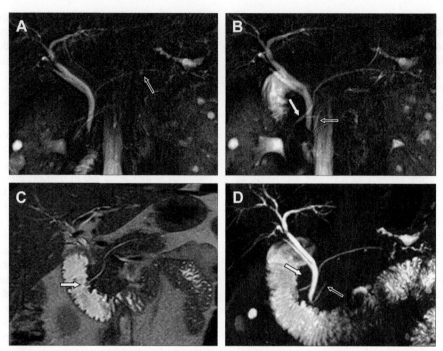

Fig. 9. Pancreatic divisum in a 39-year-old man with recurrent acute pancreatitis. (*A*) Coronal thick-slab heavily T2-weighted MR image (2D-RARE) before the injection of secretin shows the common bile duct (CBD) and proximal portion of the main pancreatic duct (MPD) (*open arrow*), but the distal portion of the MPD is not seen well. (*B*) Coronal 2D-RARE image 1 minute after the injection of secretin clearly show the dorsal duct of Santorini (*solid arrow*), crossing over the distal portion of CBD, and the small ventral duct of Wirsung (*open arrow*). (*C*) Coronal T2-weighted MR image shows the dorsal duct (*solid arrow*) draining into the minor papilla. (*D*) Postsecretin coronal maximum intensity projection of 3-dimensional-RARE image shows both dorsal (*solid arrow*) and ventral (*open arrow*) pancreatic ducts clearly.

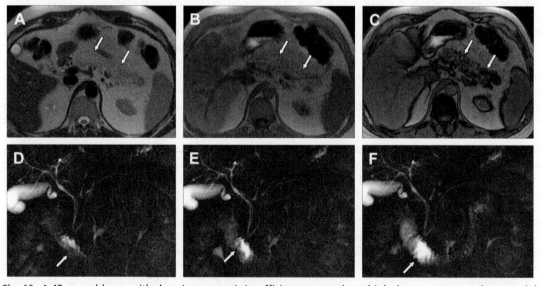

Fig. 10. A 43-year-old man with chronic pancreatic insufficiency currently on high-dose enzyme supplements. (*A*) Axial T2-weighted MR image and (*B*) T1-weighted in-phase and (*C*) opposed-phase MR images show high T2 signal intensity of pancreatic parenchyma with diffuse decrease in signal intensity in opposed phase image suggesting fatty replacement of pancreas (*arrows*). (*D–F*) Coronal thick-slab heavily T2-weighted MR images (2D-RARE) taken serially after secretin injection show no significant increase in the caliber of main pancreatic duct and luminal filling only up to the second portion even after 10 minutes postinjection with no or minimal filling of third and fourth portions (*arrow*) (grade 2 duodenal filling), suggestive of mild pancreatic insufficiency.

malignant potential.[57] The presence of a direct communication with the main pancreatic duct is a distinguishing feature of a side branch IPMN, and S-MRCP may improve the visibility of a communication between the main pancreatic duct and the cystic lesion (**Fig. 11**). Additionally, improved visualization may allow for improved detection of ductal irregularity and may aid in distinguishing a side branch IPMN from a mixed type IPMN. However, the role of S-MRCP in evaluating pancreatic cystic lesions is debatable because there are no controlled studies comparing S-MRCP with MRCP.[12,57]

Inflammatory pancreatic mass Pancreatic ductal strictures are a secondary sign of pancreatic adenocarcinoma and PNETs[73,74]; however, a benign ductal stricture can be seen in the setting of CP or AIP. Studies have shown that a benign stricture tends to have a nonobstructed main pancreatic duct that may penetrate the inflammatory mass on ultrasound imaging, ERCP, or MRCP, termed the duct-penetrating sign. Ichikawa and colleagues[75] demonstrated that the duct-penetrating sign was present in 85% of benign strictures and was absent in 96% of malignant strictures, with a diagnostic accuracy

of 94% for an inflammatory pancreatic mass. S-MRCP results in increased fluid distension of the pancreatic ductal system allowing for a better assessment for the presence or absence of the duct-penetrating sign, thus, assisting in differentiating benign from malignant strictures.[56]

Postoperative pancreas

S-MRCP is the preferred noninvasive method for evaluating the postoperative pancreas, because ERCP can be technically difficult to perform on a patient after a pancreatic surgical procedure.[13] Monill and colleagues[76] demonstrated a significant improvement in pancreatic duct and anastomotic site visualization with S-MRCP, which may aid in the detection of an anastomotic stricture. Progressive distention of the pancreatic duct upstream from the anastomosis and a decreased excretory response are features that can be seen with an anastomotic stricture. Additionally, S-MRCP may be beneficial in identifying a pancreatic duct leak by demonstrating accumulation of fluid along the pancreas during dynamic imaging after secretin administration.[13]

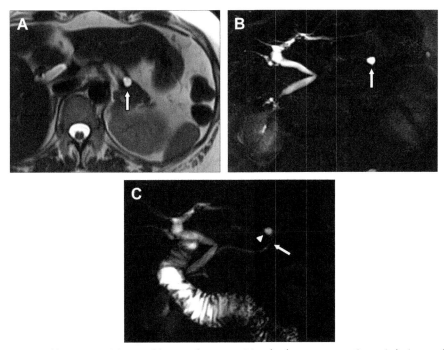

Fig. 11. A 56-year-old woman without a history of pancreatitis who has a pancreatic cystic lesion under evaluation for possible ductal communication. (*A*) Axial T2-weighted MR image shows a hyperintense lesion in the distal pancreatic body/tail (*arrow*). (*B, C*) Coronal thick-slab heavily T2-weighted MR images (RARE) (*B*) before secretin injection does not show communication between the main pancreatic duct and the lesion (*arrow*) but image at (*C*) 10 minutes post-injection demonstrates communication between the main pancreatic duct (*arrow*) and the lesion (*arrowhead*) confirming it is a branch duct intraductal papillary mucinous neoplasm.

MR Perfusion

Principles

Perfusion MR imaging assesses regional tissue perfusion based on the dynamics of uptake and washout of contrast agents. MR perfusion has the advantage of being free of radiation exposure and, in some cases, does not require the injection of a contrast agent. MR perfusion is a potentially useful tool in the assessment of pancreatic perfusion, evaluation of pancreatic cancer, and assessment of response to antiangiogenic therapies.

Technical Considerations

MR perfusion can be performed by 3 techniques (Table 7). DCE, dynamic susceptibility contrast, and arterial spin labeling. DCE is most commonly used for abdominal applications. Limited literature is found on arterial spin labeling in pancreas imaging[77,78] as well as on pancreatic dynamic susceptibility contrast,[79] both techniques being commonly used in neuroradiology but requiring further validation for abdominal applications.

DCE uses a T1-weighted gradient echo based sequence, which is repeated at short intervals on a predetermined section of the body after the injection of gadolinium. Repeat imaging of the same section monitors the appearance of contrast, gradual enhancement, peak enhancement, and subsequent washout from the organ of interest. This information can be evaluated qualitatively by simple observation at different phases or can be presented semiquantitatively as a time versus signal intensity curve. Semiquantitative parameters that can be calculated from the curve include onset time (time of first arrival of gadolinium after injection), maximal initial slope, peak signal intensity, and washout gradient. However, these parameters are limited by observer variations, imaging protocol and hardware. Quantitative parameters (Table 8) are less dependent on these factors. The most commonly used parameter is K^{trans} or the volume transfer constant, which indicates the rate of transfer of solute between plasma and extravascular extracellular space.[16] K^{trans} is a function of the capillary permeability when the tissue permeability is very low; however, when tissue permeability is very high it is reflective of tissue blood flow.[80] Other parameters include the fractional volume of extravascular extracellular space and fractional volume of plasma.

Table 7
MR perfusion techniques

MR Perfusion Techniques	Description
Dynamic contrast enhancement	• Repeated T1 gradient echo imaging is performed every few seconds over a period of 3–5 min to capture the change in tissue signal intensity over time after contrast administration • Changes in signal intensity can be evaluated qualitatively by evaluating enhancement patterns, semiquantitatively by tracking signal intensity over time, or quantitatively by using mathematical models to derive tissue perfusion and permeability parameters • Can help to differentiate lesions with different perfusion characteristics, which have other overlapping imaging features • May provide information regarding tumor perfusion and microvascular to aid in treatment planning, and may be used to evaluate treatment response after antiangiogenic therapies
Dynamic susceptibility contrast	• Contrast agent creates local magnetic susceptibility (T2*) by passing through the intravascular space resulting in a transient signal drop during the first pass of the contrast agent • Allows evaluation of overall tumor vascularity and an indirect assessment of tumor angiogenesis, which may be helpful in identifying aggressive neoplasms
Arterial spin labeling	• Noncontrast technique that can quantify blood flow by saturating protons in the arterial blood by radiofrequency inversion, thus allowing quantitative assessment of tissue perfusion • Could be used to evaluate perfusion disorders in inflammatory pancreatic pathologies or endocrine and exocrine pancreatic diseases as well as in pancreatic transplants • May aid in evaluating treatment response after antiangiogenic therapies

Table 8
Quantitative parameters of dynamic contrast-enhanced MR

Parameter	Description
Transfer constant (K^{Trans})	• Volume transfer coefficient between blood plasma and extravascular extracellular space • Characterizes the diffusive property of contrast across the capillary endothelium for a tissue or lesion
Volume of extravascular extracellular space (v_e)	• Volume of extravascular extracellular space per unit volume of tissue
Volume of blood plasma (v_p)	• Volume of blood plasma per unit volume of tissue
Rate constant (k_{ep})	• Rate constant between extravascular extracellular space and blood plasma • $k_{ep} = K^{Trans}/v_e$

Clinical Applications

Pancreatic perfusion may be an indicator of overall pancreatic secretory function with studies demonstrating increased perfusion on DCE-MR in normal patients after secretin stimulation.[81] In patients with coronary artery disease and type 2 diabetes mellitus, the pancreas shows increased endothelial permeability (K^{Trans}) and decreased plasma volume. This increase in endothelial permeability may relate to endothelial dysfunction, which could be used to monitor the progression or response to treatment in patients with type 2 diabetes mellitus.[82]

The evaluation of pancreatic tumor perfusion is useful in assessing treatment response and predicting efficacy of antiangiogenic therapies.[83,84] Akisik and colleagues[84] showed a decrease in K^{Trans} after therapy for pancreatic carcinoma, and found pretreatment K^{Trans} to be significantly higher in patients who showed a marked response to therapy. Also, K^{Trans} was found to be significantly lower in pancreatic carcinoma when compared with normal pancreas, and K^{Trans} had a negative correlation with tumor fibrosis content.[83,85] This latter finding may be beneficial in determining which patients respond to antifibrotic therapy. Although promising, further research is still needed before using DCE in clinical practice to differentiate between solid pancreatic lesions.[85]

Perfusion studies have shown value in the evaluation of the transplanted pancreas with DCE-MR demonstrating a high sensitivity for the early detection of acute allograft rejection.[86] In addition, DCE-MR in combination with S-MRCP was found to further aid in differentiating well-functioning from dysfunctional transplants.[87]

T1 Mapping/Relaxometry

Pancreatic parenchyma has a short T1 relaxation time compared with other abdominal organs and is relatively hyperintense in T1WI owing to the presence of a high amount of acinar protein and rough endoplasmic reticulum in the pancreatic cells.[88] The T1 relaxation time of pancreatic parenchyma increases with disease processes such as atrophy, fibrosis, and edema. Consequently, diffuse pancreatic parenchymal diseases, especially CP, and focal pancreatic lesions show hypointensity relative to the normal pancreas on fat-suppressed T1WI. Detection of subtle changes in T1 relaxation by semiquantitative and quantitative techniques may be helpful in the early diagnosis of pancreatic parenchymal disease.

Semiquantitative estimation of T1 signal intensity evaluating the signal intensity ratio between the pancreas and muscle in patients who underwent pancreatectomy correlated with parenchymal fibrosis on histopathology showing a decrease in signal intensity ratio with progression and degree of fibrosis.[88] However, the T1 signal intensity ratio between pancreas and spleen found no statistically significant difference between groups with normal and abnormal pancreatic function.[89] Nevertheless, these semiquantitative estimations do not measure the absolute T1 relaxation time and are limited by image contrast and scanner variation.[17]

Quantitative measurement of T1 relaxation time was limited in abdominal applications because of the long scanning time of spin echo images and resultant respiratory and motion artifacts. Newer scanning protocols using 3-dimensional gradient echo and parallel imaging techniques are capable of generating parametric maps of T1 relaxation time in a single breathhold. Tirkes and colleagues[17] used a double flip angle gradient echo sequence to compare the T1 relaxation time of pancreatic parenchyma in normal controls and in patients with mild CP (**Fig. 12**). They found a statistically significant increase of T1 relaxation time in the group with mild CP. A T1 relaxation time cutoff of 900 milliseconds was 80% sensitive and 69% specific in the diagnosis of mild CP (**Fig. 13**).

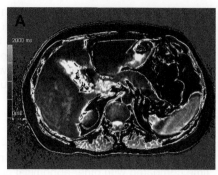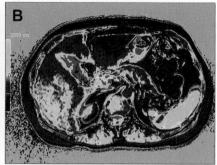

Fig. 12. A 55-year-old woman with right upper quadrant pain. (*A*) Grayscale and (*B*) color T1 maps (both scaled from 0 to 2000 ms). Average T1 relaxation time was 681 milliseconds, which is normal and unlikely to indicate chronic pancreatitis. (*Courtesy of* Temel Tirkes, MD, Department of Radiology, Indiana University School of Medicine.)

MR Elastography

MRE detects changes in tissue stiffness. Disease processes such as fibrosis, inflammation, and edema increases tissue stiffness and the detection of increased stiffness could act as a surrogate marker of the presence and quantification of these disease processes. In abdominal MRE, a pneumatic driver is placed on the abdominal wall that produces primary waves of a predetermined frequency. These waves travel through the organs of interest and generated secondary sheer waves. The wavelength and velocity of the waves are a function of the stiffness of the tissue through which the wave travels. MRE uses a modified phase contrast technique that determines the wavelength and velocity of the waves and, in turn, the stiffness of the tissue. Stiffness of the tissue is measured in kilopascals. MRE generates a parametric color map for the qualitative evaluation of the stiffness of the examined section of the abdomen. Tissue stiffness can be quantitatively measured by placing an region of interest over the organ.

The retroperitoneal location of pancreas poses a challenge to the delivery of waves to the organ. For pancreatic applications, a special pneumatic driver that conforms to the anterior abdominal wall is placed in the subxiphoid region. Mean stiffness of the normal pancreas ranges from 1.11 to 1.15 kilopascals at a driver frequency of 40 Hz and 2.09 to 2.47 kilopascals at a driver frequency of 60 Hz.[18,90,91] Pancreatic stiffness is lower than that of the liver at 40 Hz, but similar to that of the liver at 60 Hz. However, more consistent measurement can be acquired at 40 Hz.[90] Stiffness measurements are higher in the pancreas with cancer and CP.[91] Imaging of the pancreas is currently significantly limited by bowel gas and its deep location so currently the technique is not widely used as compared with hepatic imaging.

SUMMARY

Recent advances in pancreatic MR imaging, specifically using DWI and S-MRCP, have improved the diagnostic performance of MR imaging in the evaluation of pancreatic diseases. DWI has the potential to identify and characterize both focal and diffuse pancreatic processes. DWI has better sensitivity to conventional CT scanning in detecting causal pancreatic tumors in the setting of AP, and is more accurate in identifying infected PFCs. DWI can help to distinguish CP from the normal pancreas, and may aid in identifying and monitoring treatment response in the setting of AIP. Additionally, DWI can aid in identifying, characterizing, and staging a variety of pancreatic tumors, and may be beneficial in detecting malignant degeneration of cystic pancreatic neoplasms. However, DWI remains limited in

Fig. 13. A 41-year-old woman with a history of chronic pancreatitis. Color map T1 map (scaled from 0 to 2000 milliseconds). Average T1 relaxation time was 1482 milliseconds, which is prolonged and, therefore, consistent with the patient's history. (*Courtesy of* Temel Tirkes, MD, Department of Radiology, Indiana University School of Medicine.)

accurately distinguishing pancreatic ductal adenocarcinoma from mass-forming pancreatitis, and in distinguishing between cystic pancreatic lesions. Secretin enhances the diagnostic performance of MRCP in the evaluation of recurrent AP, anatomic ductal variants, CP, and main pancreatic ductal stenosis. In addition, S-MRCP can provide functional information of the exocrine pancreas.

Emerging MR imaging techniques show promise in evaluating the pancreas. MR perfusion is a potentially useful technique in diagnosing pancreatic cancer and as a biomarker to assess treatment response to antiangiogenic and antifibrotic therapies. The use of T1 mapping/relaxometry and MRE are in the early phases of investigation but show promising results in differentiating between CP and disease-free pancreas.

REFERENCES

1. Tirkes T, Menias CO, Sandrasegaran K. MR imaging techniques for pancreas. Radiol Clin North Am 2012; 50(3):379–93.
2. Koh DM, Collins DJ. Diffusion-weighted MRI in the body: applications and challenges in oncology. AJR Am J Roentgenol 2007;188(6):1622–35.
3. Barral M, Taouli B, Guiu B, et al. Diffusion-weighted MR imaging of the pancreas: current status and recommendations. Radiology 2015;274(1):45–63.
4. Bammer R. Basic principles of diffusion-weighted imaging. Eur J Radiol 2003;45(3):169–84.
5. Shinya S, Sasaki T, Nakagawa Y, et al. The efficacy of diffusion-weighted imaging for the detection and evaluation of acute pancreatitis. Hepatogastroenterology 2009;56(94–95):1407–10.
6. Akisik MF, Aisen AM, Sandrasegaran K, et al. Assessment of chronic pancreatitis: utility of diffusion-weighted MR imaging with secretin enhancement. Radiology 2009;250(1):103–9.
7. Akisik MF, Sandrasegaran K, Jennings SG, et al. Diagnosis of chronic pancreatitis by using apparent diffusion coefficient measurements at 3.0-T MR following secretin stimulation. Radiology 2009; 252(2):418–25.
8. Taniguchi T, Kobayashi H, Nishikawa K, et al. Diffusion-weighted magnetic resonance imaging in autoimmune pancreatitis. Jpn J Radiol 2009;27(3): 138–42.
9. Lee SS, Byun JH, Park BJ, et al. Quantitative analysis of diffusion-weighted magnetic resonance imaging of the pancreas: usefulness in characterizing solid pancreatic masses. J Magn Reson Imaging 2008;28(4):928–36.
10. d'Assignies G, Fina P, Bruno O, et al. High sensitivity of diffusion-weighted MR imaging for the detection of liver metastases from neuroendocrine tumors:

comparison with T2-weighted and dynamic gadolinium-enhanced MR imaging. Radiology 2013;268(2):390–9.
11. Sandrasegaran K, Akisik FM, Patel AA, et al. Diffusion-weighted imaging in characterization of cystic pancreatic lesions. Clin Radiol 2011;66(9):808–14.
12. Akisik MF, Sandrasegaran K, Aisen AA, et al. Dynamic secretin-enhanced MR cholangiopancreatography. Radiographics 2006;26(3):665–77.
13. Tirkes T, Sandrasegaran K, Sanyal R, et al. Secretin-enhanced MR cholangiopancreatography: spectrum of findings. Radiographics 2013;33(7): 1889–906.
14. Manfredi R, Costamagna G, Brizi MG, et al. Severe chronic pancreatitis versus suspected pancreatic disease: dynamic MR cholangiopancreatography after secretin stimulation. Radiology 2000;214(3): 849–55.
15. Sandrasegaran K, Tahir B, Barad U, et al. The value of secretin-enhanced MRCP in patients with recurrent acute pancreatitis. AJR Am J Roentgenol 2017;208(2):315–21.
16. Sandrasegaran K. Functional MR imaging of the abdomen. Radiol Clin North Am 2014;52(4): 883–903.
17. Tirkes T, Lin C, Fogel EL, et al. T1 mapping for diagnosis of mild chronic pancreatitis. J Magn Reson Imaging 2017;45(4):1171–6.
18. Itoh Y, Takehara Y, Kawase T, et al. Feasibility of magnetic resonance elastography for the pancreas at 3T. J Magn Reson Imaging 2016;43(2):384–90.
19. Qayyum A. Diffusion-weighted imaging in the abdomen and pelvis: concepts and applications. Radiographics 2009;29(6):1797–810.
20. Ichikawa T, Haradome H, Hachiya J, et al. Diffusion-weighted MR imaging with single-shot echo-planar imaging in the upper abdomen: preliminary clinical experience in 61 patients. Abdom Imaging 1999; 24(5):456–61.
21. Kanematsu M, Goshima S, Watanabe H, et al. Diffusion/perfusion MR imaging of the liver: practice, challenges, and future. Magn Reson Med Sci 2012;11(3):151–61.
22. Koh DM, Takahara T, Imai Y, et al. Practical aspects of assessing tumors using clinical diffusion-weighted imaging in the body. Magn Reson Med Sci 2007;6(4):211–24.
23. Patterson DM, Padhani AR, Collins DJ. Technology insight: water diffusion MRI–a potential new biomarker of response to cancer therapy. Nat Clin Pract Oncol 2008;5(4):220–33.
24. Schoennagel BP, Habermann CR, Roesch M, et al. Diffusion-weighted imaging of the healthy pancreas: apparent diffusion coefficient values of the normal head, body, and tail calculated from different sets of b-values. J Magn Reson Imaging 2011;34(4): 861–5.

25. Banks PA, Bollen TL, Dervenis C, et al. Classification of acute pancreatitis–2012: revision of the Atlanta classification and definitions by international consensus. Gut 2013;62(1):102–11.

26. Miller FH, Keppke AL, Dalal K, et al. MRI of pancreatitis and its complications: part 1, acute pancreatitis. AJR Am J Roentgenol 2004;183(6):1637–44.

27. Thomas S, Kayhan A, Lakadamyali H, et al. Diffusion MRI of acute pancreatitis and comparison with normal individuals using ADC values. Emerg Radiol 2012;19(1):5–9.

28. Islim F, Salik AE, Bayramoglu S, et al. Non-invasive detection of infection in acute pancreatic and acute necrotic collections with diffusion-weighted magnetic resonance imaging: preliminary findings. Abdom Imaging 2014;39(3):472–81.

29. Erturk SM, Ichikawa T, Motosugi U, et al. Diffusion-weighted MR imaging in the evaluation of pancreatic exocrine function before and after secretin stimulation. Am J Gastroenterol 2006;101(1):133–6.

30. Miller FH, Keppke AL, Wadhwa A, et al. MRI of pancreatitis and its complications: part 2, chronic pancreatitis. AJR Am J Roentgenol 2004;183(6):1645–52.

31. Wathle GK, Tjora E, Ersland L, et al. Assessment of exocrine pancreatic function by secretin-stimulated magnetic resonance cholangiopancreatography and diffusion-weighted imaging in healthy controls. J Magn Reson Imaging 2014;39(2):448–54.

32. Hamano H, Kawa S, Horiuchi A, et al. High serum IgG4 concentrations in patients with sclerosing pancreatitis. N Engl J Med 2001;344(10):732–8.

33. Omiyale AO. Autoimmune pancreatitis. Gland Surg 2016;5(3):318–26.

34. Hur BY, Lee JM, Lee JE, et al. Magnetic resonance imaging findings of the mass-forming type of autoimmune pancreatitis: comparison with pancreatic adenocarcinoma. J Magn Reson Imaging 2012;36(1):188–97.

35. Muhi A, Ichikawa T, Motosugi U, et al. Mass-forming autoimmune pancreatitis and pancreatic carcinoma: differential diagnosis on the basis of computed tomography and magnetic resonance cholangiopancreatography, and diffusion-weighted imaging findings. J Magn Reson Imaging 2012;35(4):827–36.

36. Oki H, Hayashida Y, Oki H, et al. DWI findings of autoimmune pancreatitis: comparison between symptomatic and asymptomatic patients. J Magn Reson Imaging 2015;41(1):125–31.

37. Ichikawa T, Haradome H, Hachiya J, et al. Pancreatic ductal adenocarcinoma: preoperative assessment with helical CT versus dynamic MR imaging. Radiology 1997;202(3):655–62.

38. Wang Y, Miller FH, Chen ZE, et al. Diffusion-weighted MR imaging of solid and cystic lesions of the pancreas. Radiographics 2011;31(3):E47–64.

39. Kartalis N, Lindholm TL, Aspelin P, et al. Diffusion-weighted magnetic resonance imaging of pancreas tumours. Eur Radiol 2009;19(8):1981–90.

40. Ichikawa T, Erturk SM, Motosugi U, et al. High-b value diffusion-weighted MRI for detecting pancreatic adenocarcinoma: preliminary results. AJR Am J Roentgenol 2007;188(2):409–14.

41. Wagner M, Doblas S, Daire JL, et al. Diffusion-weighted MR imaging for the regional characterization of liver tumors. Radiology 2012;264(2):464–72.

42. Rosenkrantz AB, Matza BW, Sabach A, et al. Pancreatic cancer: lack of association between apparent diffusion coefficient values and adverse pathological features. Clin Radiol 2013;68(4):e191–7.

43. Wang Y, Chen ZE, Nikolaidis P, et al. Diffusion-weighted magnetic resonance imaging of pancreatic adenocarcinomas: association with histopathology and tumor grade. J Magn Reson Imaging 2011;33(1):136–42.

44. Yao XZ, Yun H, Zeng MS, et al. Evaluation of ADC measurements among solid pancreatic masses by respiratory-triggered diffusion-weighted MR imaging with inversion-recovery fat-suppression technique at 3.0T. Magn Reson Imaging 2013;31(4):524–8.

45. Klauss M, Lemke A, Grunberg K, et al. Intravoxel incoherent motion MRI for the differentiation between mass forming chronic pancreatitis and pancreatic carcinoma. Invest Radiol 2011;46(1):57–63.

46. Ehehalt F, Saeger HD, Schmidt CM, et al. Neuroendocrine tumors of the pancreas. Oncologist 2009;14(5):456–67.

47. Herwick S, Miller FH, Keppke AL. MRI of islet cell tumors of the pancreas. AJR Am J Roentgenol 2006;187(5):W472–80.

48. Wang Y, Chen ZE, Yaghmai V, et al. Diffusion-weighted MR imaging in pancreatic endocrine tumors correlated with histopathologic characteristics. J Magn Reson Imaging 2011;33(5):1071–9.

49. Lotfalizadeh E, Ronot M, Wagner M, et al. Prediction of pancreatic neuroendocrine tumour grade with MR imaging features: added value of diffusion-weighted imaging. Eur Radiol 2017;27(4):1748–59.

50. De Robertis R, Tinazzi Martini P, Demozzi E, et al. Diffusion-weighted imaging of pancreatic cancer. World J Radiol 2015;7(10):319–28.

51. Klimstra DS, Pitman MB, Hruban RH. An algorithmic approach to the diagnosis of pancreatic neoplasms. Arch Pathol Lab Med 2009;133(3):454–64.

52. Kang BK, Kim JH, Byun JH, et al. Diffusion-weighted MRI: usefulness for differentiating intrapancreatic accessory spleen and small hypervascular neuroendocrine tumor of the pancreas. Acta Radiol 2014;55(10):1157–65.

53. Mottola JC, Sahni VA, Erturk SM, et al. Diffusion-weighted MRI of focal cystic pancreatic lesions at 3.0-Tesla: preliminary results. Abdom Imaging 2012;37(1):110–7.

54. Inan N, Arslan A, Akansel G, et al. Diffusion-weighted imaging in the differential diagnosis of cystic lesions of the pancreas. AJR Am J Roentgenol 2008;191(4):1115–21.

55. Fatima Z, Ichikawa T, Motosugi U, et al. Magnetic resonance diffusion-weighted imaging in the characterization of pancreatic mucinous cystic lesions. Clin Radiol 2011;66(2):108–11.

56. Manfredi R, Pozzi Mucelli R. Secretin-enhanced MR Imaging of the Pancreas. Radiology 2016;279(1):29–43.

57. Boraschi P, Donati F, Cervelli R, et al. Secretin-stimulated MR cholangiopancreatography: spectrum of findings in pancreatic diseases. Insights Imaging 2016;7(6):819–29.

58. Sugiyama M, Haradome H, Atomi Y. Magnetic resonance imaging for diagnosing chronic pancreatitis. J Gastroenterol 2007;42(Suppl 17):108–12.

59. Wang DB, Yu J, Fulcher AS, et al. Pancreatitis in patients with pancreas divisum: imaging features at MRI and MRCP. World J Gastroenterol 2013;19(30):4907–16.

60. Rustagi T, Njei B. Magnetic resonance cholangiopancreatography in the diagnosis of pancreas divisum: a systematic review and meta-analysis. Pancreas 2014;43(6):823–8.

61. Manfredi R, Costamagna G, Brizi MG, et al. Pancreas divisum and "santorinicele": diagnosis with dynamic MR cholangiopancreatography with secretin stimulation. Radiology 2000;217(2):403–8.

62. Matos C, Metens T, Deviere J, et al. Pancreas divisum: evaluation with secretin-enhanced magnetic resonance cholangiopancreatography. Gastrointest Endosc 2001;53(7):728–33.

63. Sugiyama M, Atomi Y, Kuroda A. Pancreatic disorders associated with anomalous pancreaticobiliary junction. Surgery 1999;126(3):492–7.

64. Komi N, Tamura T, Miyoshi Y, et al. Nationwide survey of cases of choledochal cyst. Analysis of coexistent anomalies, complications and surgical treatment in 645 cases. Surg Gastroenterol 1984;3(2):69–73.

65. Hosoki T, Hasuike Y, Takeda Y, et al. Visualization of pancreaticobiliary reflux in anomalous pancreaticobiliary junction by secretin-stimulated dynamic magnetic resonance cholangiopancreatography. Acta Radiol 2004;45(4):375–82.

66. Cappeliez O, Delhaye M, Deviere J, et al. Chronic pancreatitis: evaluation of pancreatic exocrine function with MR pancreatography after secretin stimulation. Radiology 2000;215(2):358–64.

67. Manfredi R, Perandini S, Mantovani W, et al. Quantitative MRCP assessment of pancreatic exocrine reserve and its correlation with faecal elastase-1 in patients with chronic pancreatitis. Radiol Med 2012;117(2):282–92.

68. O'Neill E, Hammond N, Miller FH. MR imaging of the pancreas. Radiol Clin North Am 2014;52(4):757–77.

69. Matos C, Metens T, Deviere J, et al. Pancreatic duct: morphologic and functional evaluation with dynamic MR pancreatography after secretin stimulation. Radiology 1997;203(2):435–41.

70. Gillams AR, Lees WR. Quantitative secretin MRCP (MRCPQ): results in 215 patients with known or suspected pancreatic pathology. Eur Radiol 2007;17(11):2984–90.

71. Fernandez-del Castillo C, Targarona J, Thayer SP, et al. Incidental pancreatic cysts: clinicopathologic characteristics and comparison with symptomatic patients. Arch Surg 2003;138(4):427–33 [discussion: 433–4].

72. Schmidt CM, White PB, Waters JA, et al. Intraductal papillary mucinous neoplasms: predictors of malignant and invasive pathology. Ann Surg 2007;246(4):644–51 [discussion: 651–4].

73. Prokesch RW, Chow LC, Beaulieu CF, et al. Isoattenuating pancreatic adenocarcinoma at multidetector row CT: secondary signs. Radiology 2002;224(3):764–8.

74. Manfredi R, Bonatti M, Mantovani W, et al. Non-hyperfunctioning neuroendocrine tumours of the pancreas: MR imaging appearance and correlation with their biological behaviour. Eur Radiol 2013;23(11):3029–39.

75. Ichikawa T, Sou H, Araki T, et al. Duct-penetrating sign at MRCP: usefulness for differentiating inflammatory pancreatic mass from pancreatic carcinomas. Radiology 2001;221(1):107–16.

76. Monill J, Pernas J, Clavero J, et al. Pancreatic duct after pancreatoduodenectomy: morphologic and functional evaluation with secretin-stimulated MR pancreatography. AJR Am J Roentgenol 2004;183(5):1267–74.

77. Schraml C, Schwenzer NF, Martirosian P, et al. Perfusion imaging of the pancreas using an arterial spin labeling technique. J Magn Reson Imaging 2008;28(6):1459–65.

78. Hirshberg B, Qiu M, Cali AM, et al. Pancreatic perfusion of healthy individuals and type 1 diabetic patients as assessed by magnetic resonance perfusion imaging. Diabetologia 2009;52(8):1561–5.

79. Niwa T, Ueno M, Shinya N, et al. Dynamic susceptibility contrast MRI in advanced pancreatic cancer: semi-automated analysis to predict response to chemotherapy. NMR Biomed 2010;23(4):347–52.

80. Essig M, Shiroishi MS, Nguyen TB, et al. Perfusion MRI: the five most frequently asked technical questions. AJR Am J Roentgenol 2013;200(1):24–34.

81. Cox EF, Smith JK, Chowdhury AH, et al. Temporal assessment of pancreatic blood flow and perfusion

following secretin stimulation using noninvasive MRI. J Magn Reson Imaging 2015;42(5):1233–40.

82. Yu CW, Shih TT, Hsu CY, et al. Correlation between pancreatic microcirculation and type 2 diabetes in patients with coronary artery disease: dynamic contrast-enhanced MR imaging. Radiology 2009; 252(3):704–11.

83. Ma W, Li N, Zhao W, et al. Apparent diffusion coefficient and dynamic contrast-enhanced magnetic resonance imaging in pancreatic cancer: characteristics and correlation with histopathologic parameters. J Comput Assist Tomogr 2016;40(5):709–16.

84. Akisik MF, Sandrasegaran K, Bu G, et al. Pancreatic cancer: utility of dynamic contrast-enhanced MR imaging in assessment of antiangiogenic therapy. Radiology 2010;256(2):441–9.

85. Kim JH, Lee JM, Park JH, et al. Solid pancreatic lesions: characterization by using timing bolus dynamic contrast-enhanced MR imaging assessment–a preliminary study. Radiology 2013;266(1):185–96.

86. Krebs TL, Daly B, Wong-You-Cheong JJ, et al. Acute pancreatic transplant rejection: evaluation with dynamic contrast-enhanced MR imaging compared with histopathologic analysis. Radiology 1999; 210(2):437–42.

87. Heverhagen JT, Wagner HJ, Ebel H, et al. Pancreatic transplants: noninvasive evaluation with secretin-augmented MR pancreatography and MR perfusion measurements–preliminary results. Radiology 2004; 233(1):273–80.

88. Watanabe H, Kanematsu M, Tanaka K, et al. Fibrosis and postoperative fistula of the pancreas: correlation with MR imaging findings–preliminary results. Radiology 2014;270(3):791–9.

89. Balci NC, Smith A, Momtahen AJ, et al. MRI and S-MRCP findings in patients with suspected chronic pancreatitis: correlation with endoscopic pancreatic function testing (ePFT). J Magn Reson Imaging 2010;31(3):601–6.

90. Shi Y, Glaser KJ, Venkatesh SK, et al. Feasibility of using 3D MR elastography to determine pancreatic stiffness in healthy volunteers. J Magn Reson Imaging 2015;41(2):369–75.

91. An H, Shi Y, Guo Q, et al. Test-retest reliability of 3D EPI MR elastography of the pancreas. Clin Radiol 2016;71(10):1068.e7-12.

PET/MR Imaging of the Pancreas

Nadine Mallak, MD[a], Thomas A. Hope, MD[b], Alexander R. Guimaraes, MD, PhD[a],*

KEYWORDS

• PET/MR imaging • Pancreas • Neuroendocrine tumor • DOTATATE

KEY POINTS

• PET/MR imaging is a robust quantitative imaging method that allows for high-resolution, multiparametric imaging of the pancreas.
• PET/MR imaging attenuation correction is based on tissue classification derived from MR imaging pulse sequences.
• PET/MR imaging of neuroendocrine tumors can be performed using somatostatin-sensitive imaging agents.

PET and MR imaging are provide complementary anatomic, physiologic, and functional information. PET is a robust, quantitative imaging modality that provides exceptionally sensitive assays of a wide range of biological processes. PET does, however, have lower spatial resolution, and in most cases limited anatomic information. PET involves ionizing radiation relative to MR imaging and other tomographic imaging approaches. MR imaging can provide high-resolution anatomic information with an array of different contrast mechanisms that are sensitive to metabolism, water, water mobility, and oxygenation state. However, its sensitivity is poor relative to PET, and it suffers from difficulty in quantification of these contrast mechanisms relative to PET.

Two fundamental technical advances have allowed for the advent of simultaneous PET/MR imaging possible in clinical use. On the PET side, the development of a new type of solid state photon detectors insensitive to magnetic fields (eg, avalanche photodiodes and silicon photomultiplier) in contrast to photomultiplier tubes. These devices have been demonstrated success in simultaneous PET and MR imaging data in vivo.[1,2] For MR imaging systems, the development of novel gradient designs functionally within large-bore systems facilitated the integration of this device. Yet, the significant constraints on the design of the PET system, ranging from limitations on the size of the crystals to the geometry of the whole detector ring, also caused delays in the integration.

ATTENUATION CORRECTION

Attenuation correction was the most difficult issue to address in quantitative MR-PET. Owing to engineering and size constraints available inside the MR scanner bore, the integrated scanners developed to date are not equipped with a transmission source. As a result, the development, implementation, and validation of an MR-based attenuation correction method became a necessity. The methods of how this is performed are challenging.

Whole body applications offer unique problems. Imaging the lungs with conventional MR sequences

Disclosure: Dr T.A. Hope has received grant support from GE Healthcare; Dr A.R. Guimaraes is affiliated with Siemens Speaker's Bureau, AGFA Imaging, Merck Pharmaceuticals, Inc; Dr N. Mallak has nothing to disclose.
[a] Department of Diagnostic Radiology, Oregon Health & Sciences University, 3181 Southwest Sam Jackson Park Road, Portland, OR 97239, USA; [b] Department of Radiology and Biomedical Imaging, University of California, San Francisco, 505 Parnassus Avenue, M391, San Francisco, CA 94158, USA
* Corresponding author.
E-mail address: guimaraa@ohsu.edu

Magn Reson Imaging Clin N Am 26 (2018) 345–362
https://doi.org/10.1016/j.mric.2018.03.003
1064-9689/18/© 2018 Elsevier Inc. All rights reserved.

offers unique challenges secondary to the varying attenuation properties in diseased versus normal respiration. Bone attenuation offers other unique challenges as well in most of the body regions, except perhaps the head and neck area, and the spine and pelvis. Within these regions it is assumed that it is not critical, and soft tissue linear attenuation coefficients can probably be assigned to these voxels. As a result, the attenuation correction solution is to segment the body into 4 compartments (ie, water, fat, lung, and air) and to neglect the bone. This is also likely secondary to the difficulty to accurately image bone density with MR imaging. Good quality images were obtained using this method, but the quantitative properties of these data still have to be evaluated. A second important issue when scanning the patients with their arms down or in the case of large patients is that the MR field of view is usually smaller than that of PET, and this factor can lead to truncation artifacts. One method for reconstructing the attenuation and the emission data in the same time using iterative techniques has been proposed, and implemented on the Siemens Biograph mMR scanner (Munich, Germany).[3]

PET/MR IMAGING HARDWARE CONSIDERATIONS

The probability of annihilation photons reaching the PET detectors depends on the total attenuation along each particular line of response. As a result, the attenuation of the radiofrequency coils being used for MR acquisition have to be incorporated into the attenuation correction algorithm as well. As a rule, the radiofrequency coils have to be carefully designed to the fulfill minimum attenuation requirements and are, therefore, not interchangeable with nonsimultaneous devices, because large underestimations could be introduced in the data if the coil attenuation map is ignored.

REGISTRATION

Misregistration between the emission data and the attenuation map is a common source of errors in PET imaging in general. This is often a result of subject motion, which theoretically on PET/MR scanners may be reduced as a result of allowing the MR imaging signal to track the motion of the subject through various established techniques and to integrate that information either prospectively or retrospectively into the PET acquisition. PET acquisitions, being lengthy, lead to voluntary and involuntary subject motion. This directly translates to degradation (blurring) of PET images and

to severe artifacts when motion has large amplitude. By motion tracking in the background, these data can be retrospectively woven into the PET reconstruction, or prospectively used for acquisition (eg, gating). These types of motion can be characterized as either rigid body and nonrigid problems. In the case or rigid body motion, the displacements of a limited number of points completely characterize the motion of the whole volume. However, no assumption can be made regarding the motion during the scan. In the case of non–rigid body cardiac and respiratory motion, the displacement of each voxels in the field of view has to be characterized but assumptions can and have to be made regarding the periodicity of the motion. An even more challenging problem is the nonperiodic non–rigid body motion, but potential solutions have already been suggested. Work in this arena is ongoing, but PET/MR imaging has the potential to solve this large problem in the upper abdomen.[4]

As a result of the emphasis on MR imaging examples and details for pancreatic illness throughout this issue, we emphasize and focus our efforts on PET applications within the pancreas. The following is a brief description of the PET radiotracers most commonly used in pancreatic imaging. Other radiotracers used for imaging of neuroendocrine tumors and noninvasive imaging of β-cell islets will be discussed below as well in the respective sections.

PET Metabolic Imaging: 18F-Fluorodeoxyglucose

Workhorse of PET oncology imaging; 18F-Fluorodeoxyglucose (^{18}F-FDG) is an analog of glucose, gets transported into cells via glucose transporter proteins (primarily GLUT-1 and GLUT-3) and subsequently undergoes phosphorylation by the rate-limiting key enzyme hexokinase 1 into ^{18}F-FDG monophosphate. Unlike glucose, after phosphorylation, ^{18}F-FDG monophosphate cannot undergo glycolysis and gets trapped within the cells.

Tumors usually show increased glucose metabolism, and this is primarily owing to inefficient mechanism of adenosine triphosphate (ATP) production compared with normal cells, also known as the Warburg effect, which consists of aerobic glycolysis with lactate production (generating only 2 ATPs per 1 molecule of glucose) rather than oxidative phosphorylation (which generates up to 36 ATPs per 1 molecule of glucose). This allowed ^{18}F-FDG to become the radiotracer most widely used for oncologic PET imaging.

Blood glucose should be stabilized before ^{18}F-FDG injection to reduce competition for glucose transporters. This measure is usually achieved by fasting for 4 to 6 hours before injection. The uptake period is generally 60 minutes.

It is very important to be aware of the pitfalls that might occur during ^{18}F-FDG PET interpretation. False negatives can be seen with small lesion size (<6 mm), low metabolic rate (such as well-differentiated neuroendocrine tumors and mucinous adenocarcinomas), high blood glucose levels, interfering cytotoxic treatment, and high background organ activity that might mask hypermetabolic lesions (such as physiologic activity in the brain, heart, and urinary system).

In contrast, FDG is not a specific radiotracer, and false positives can occur in the setting of infectious or inflammatory processes, postsurgical changes, and postradiation changes.

PET Cellular Proliferation Imaging: 3'-Deoxy-3'[18F]-Fluorothymidine

3'-Deoxy-3'[18F]-fluorothymidine (^{18}F-FLT) is a clinically practical PET thymidine analogue, an ^{18}F-labeled nucleoside that gets transported across the cell membrane by facilitated diffusion via nucleoside carrier proteins and is subsequently monophosphorylated by thymidine kinase 1. Unlike thymidine, monophosphorylated ^{18}F-FLT cannot get incorporated into DNA; it becomes trapped and accumulates within the cells instead.[5,6]

In many tissues, thymidine kinase 1 activity closely correlates with the DNA synthesis phase of proliferating cells (typically late G1-S), and is diminished in quiescent, nonproliferating cells. As a substrate for thymidine kinase, ^{18}F-FLT has been shown to accumulate in proliferating cells, with variable degrees of correlation with Ki-67.[7,8] Given that at any time more cancer cells are metabolically active and much less are proliferating, more uptake with higher standardized uptake values (SUVs) is expected to be seen with [18]FDG compared with [18]FLT.

However, an alternative pathway for thymidine utilization, the de novo pathway, which uses the enzyme thymidylate synthase instead to provide thymidine for DNA synthesis, and could lead to an underestimation of tumor proliferation by ^{18}F-FLT PET. However, more studies are needed to assess for potential implications in clinical settings.[9]

Another potential pitfall in oncologic imaging with ^{18}F-FLT is the high physiologic uptake in the liver and bone marrow, which might mask metastatic lesions.

PET Somatostatin Receptor Imaging: [68]Gallium-labeled Somatostatin Analogues

Targeting somatostatin receptors (SSTRs) for imaging of neuroendocrine tumors is an old concept that started in the 1980s with ^{111}In-octreotide scintigraphy; however, the recently developed PET radiotracers that target the same receptors were shown to be much superior and are quickly replacing ^{111}In-octreotide scintigraphy.

PET somatostatin analogues are short peptides linked to the positron emitter ^{68}Ga by 1,4,7,10-tetraazacyclododecane-1,4,7,10-tetraacetic acid (DOTA). They have a higher affinity to SSTRs, and they take advantage of PET technology (higher spatial resolution and ability of quantification) to provide higher accuracy compared with ^{111}In-octreotide and to conventional imaging. In addition to their higher performance, they allow lower patient dose owing to the 68-minute half-life of ^{68}Ga compared with the 2.8 days' half-life of ^{111}In, and they are more convenient to patients because imaging is performed at 45 to 60 minutes after injection compared with imaging at 4 and 24 hours for ^{111}In-octreotide. And last, the synthesis of ^{68}Ga-DOTA peptides is relatively easy and more cost effective.[10]

Three major ^{68}Ga-DOTA peptides are currently available for imaging: ^{68}Ga-DOTA-Phe^1-Tyr^3-octreotide, ^{68}Ga-DOTA-Nal^3-octreotide, and ^{68}Ga-DOTA-Tyr^3-octreotate. The main difference among them is their variable affinity to SSTR subtypes. All of them can bind to SSTR2 and SSTR5, whereas only DOTA-^{68}Ga-DOTA-Nal^3-octreotide shows good affinity for SSTR3. However, there is currently no evidence to support that these differences have a clinical impact, and the 3 agents are considered to be clinically equal.[11] An example of PET/MR imaging of ^{68}Ga-DOTA-^{68}Ga-DOTA-Tyr^3-octreotate imaging is demonstrated in **Fig. 1**.

PET Hypoxia Imaging: Such as ^{18}F-Fluoromisonidazole, ^{18}F-Fluoroazomycin Arabinoside, and ^{18}F-Flortanidazole

Tumor hypoxia is known to play a major role in cancer treatment response and prognosis; it has been linked to radiation resistance and to more aggressive tumor behavior. Thus, the noninvasive identification, quantification, and mapping of tumor hypoxia can potentially play a pivotal role in radiotherapy planning.[12–14]

Several 2-nitroimidazoles labeled with ^{18}F have already been used to identify hypoxia. The most familiar is ^{18}F-MISO, which is a very lipophilic molecule that enters the cells via passive diffusion; intracellularly, it gets reduced by nitroreductase enzymes. In normally oxygenated cells, reoxidation occurs and the molecule clears from the cell; however, with low oxygen levels, it becomes trapped in its reduced form, and accumulates within the cell, leading to increased uptake on PET imaging.[15,16]

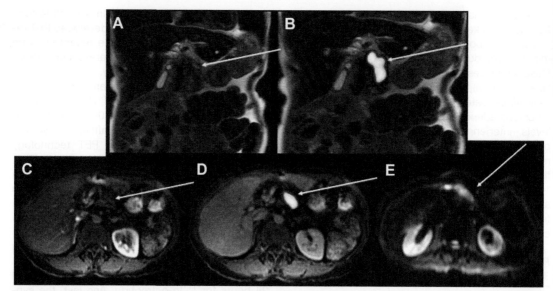

Fig. 1. PET-MR images of a patient with a pancreatic neuroendocrine tumor (*yellow arrows*). (*A*) T2-weighted coronal images demonstrate an irregular lesion within the body/tail of the pancreas demonstrating avidity on ^{68}Ga-DOTATATE PET-MR imaging (*B, D*) and demonstrating mild enhancement on after gadolinium-enhanced imaging (*C*), superimposed on postcontrast images (*D*). Diffusion-weighted imaging demonstrating mild restricted diffusion (*E*).

The main disadvantage of ^{18}F-MISO is its slow accumulation in hypoxic tissues and delayed clearance from normally oxygenated tissues, which necessitates long uptake periods (approximately 3 hours), and leads to low tumor to background contrast.[16] Therefore, alternative tracers have been developed with improved pharmacokinetic properties (more hydrophilic molecules with quicker clearance) such as ^{18}F-AZA and ^{18}F-HX4.[12,16]

APPLICATIONS IN PANCREATIC DISEASE
Pancreatic Ductal Adenocarcinoma

Pancreatic ductal adenocarcinoma (PDA) accounts for 80% of pancreatic malignancies, often presents at a late stage, and has a poor prognosis being the fourth-leading cause of cancer-related death in the United States with a 5-year survival rate of less than 8%. Complete resection is the only cure, but it is only possible in 15% to 30% of patients at presentation. Local tumor spread or distant metastases are contraindications for resection in most patients, which makes imaging crucial for early diagnosis, local staging, and assessment for metastatic disease.

Multidetector triple phase computed tomography (MDCT) with intravenous (IV) contrast is the most widely used and most validated modality for diagnosis and local staging of PDA; however, several studies showed that MR imaging is equivalent or even superior to MDCT in this setting,

because it provides a superior contrast resolution, which allows for the detection of smaller cancers and of cancers that are isodense to background pancreatic parenchyma on CT.[17–19] This is true also for noncontrast MR imaging, owing to the good evaluation of morphologic features of the tumor on unenhanced T1- and T2-weighted images, high signal of the tumor on diffusion-weighted imaging (DWI), and abrupt main pancreatic duct (MPD) or common bile duct narrowing or dilatation on MR cholangiopancreatography.[20,21]

The bright signal of the tumor on DWI makes it more conspicuous and easier to depict. Although several studies suggest that apparent diffusion coefficient (ADC) values can be helpful in lesion characterization to differentiate PDA from benign entities (primarily mass-forming pancreatitis),[22,23] no consensus exists so far, with significant overlap.[24]

Concerning local staging, it has been shown that MR imaging is equivalent to MDCT in evaluating for local extension, vascular invasion, and nodal involvement.[25,26] A major advantage of MR imaging, however, is its higher sensitivity for detection of small metastatic liver lesions,[18] and specificity in characterizing the indeterminate liver lesions seen on CT, which can potentially impact patient management.

In contrast, FDG PET/CT has shown promise in preoperative evaluation of PDA. In addition to its ability to detect smaller lesions (<2 cm) compared with MDCT,[27] multiple studies suggest that maximum SUV (SUV_{max}) values may help to differentiate mass-forming pancreatitis from PDA, with low-level uptake in pancreatitis compared with PDA (a suggested SUV_{max} cutoff of 2.5).[28–30]

One advantage of FDG PET/CT in the preoperative setting is its superiority in detecting metastatic disease, which makes the primary lesion unresectable. Some studies show change in management in up to 11% of patients in whom unnecessary surgery was avoided owing to detection of occult metastases on PET/CT.[31] Additionally, high SUV values on pretreatment FDG PET/CT scans were shown to correlate with a worse prognosis and decreased progression-free survival in patients with unresectable pancreatic cancer.[32]

However, FDG PET/CT suffers from multiple limitations. False negatives can be seen with mucinous tumors (owing to tissue hypocellularity), necrotic tumors, and metastatic lesions smaller than 1 cm. False positive cases, in contrast, may occur with acute inflammation (most commonly pancreatitis flare up), recent radiation therapy, or recent procedure (biopsy or common bile duct placement). Overall, data are contradictory about the cost effectiveness of including FDG PET/CT in the routine management of patients with PDA, and no consensus exists to date.

Given the advantages that MR imaging and PET/CT can offer separately, it would be expected that integrated PET/MR imaging can potentially be superior to each modality alone, taking advantage of the high soft tissue contrast for MR imaging and metabolic information from PET. Early studies performed with fusion of MR imaging with PET images acquired as part of FDG PET/CT studies show better performance of the fused images; Ruf and colleagues[33] showed that, in patients with pancreatic cancer, PET/MR imaging image fusion improves anatomic assignment and interpretation of foci of FDG uptake compared with side-by-side analysis; Donati and colleagues[34] found that, for hepatic metastases, FDG PET/MR imaging fused images from MR imaging with hepatospecific IV contrast had a sensitivity of 93% versus a sensitivity of 91% for MR imaging alone, and of 76% for PET alone. Few studies have been published using integrated PET/MR imaging in the setting of PDA. In a study including 37 patients with pancreatic cancer, Joo and colleagues[35] show that diagnostic performance of FDG PET/MR imaging is similar to that of PET/CT plus contrast-enhanced MDCT. Other studies show that, in addition to being a "one-stop-shop" as described by Joo and colleagues for the diagnosis, local staging, and assessment of metastatic disease, PET/MR imaging provides numerous useful imaging biomarkers to assess tumor characteristics. An inverse correlation between high SUV values on PET/CT and ADC values on MR imaging has been demonstrated in pancreatic cancer, similar to several other cancer types, which helps in the assessment of tumor aggressiveness and prognostication.[36] In this setting Bang-Bin and associates[37] showed that, compared with metabolic tumor volume or minimum ADC alone, the metabolic tumor volume/minimum ADC ratio demonstrated the highest predictive ability for determining the clinical TNM stage, and after treatment this ratio was an independent predictor of progression-free survival.

Prognosis, response to therapy, recurrence, and subsequent management

After neoadjuvant therapy, postradiation changes decrease the sensitivity of anatomic imaging to evaluate for treatment response and tumor resectability; PET imaging has been found very helpful in this setting because a decrease in FDG uptake may precede morphologic changes, and can be used to estimate response to treatment, supporting subsequent surgical intervention or continuing the current treatment regimen. This applies as well in postoperative setting, where surgical scarring limits evaluation of tumor recurrence on anatomic imaging.[38–40]

Other radiotracers that show promise in pancreatic ductal adenocarcinoma

Proliferation imaging Studies comparing ^{18}F-FDG PET/CT with ^{18}F-FLT PET/CT in the characterization of pancreatic masses show higher specificity of ^{18}F-FLT in detecting malignant tumors; in a series of 41 patients, Herrmann and colleagues[41] showed a specificity of 75% for ^{18}F-FLT versus 50% for ^{18}F-FDG with a suggested SUV_{max} cutoff of 2 for ^{18}F-FLT and 3.5 for ^{18}F-FDG.[42]

In some cancer types (mainly breast, lung, and brain tumors), ^{18}F-FLT has been shown to be a useful noninvasive method for early assessment of tumor response to treatment, which allows for the early identification of responders versus nonresponders in the aim of minimizing exposure to potentially toxic treatment regimens in nonresponders.[43] In a series of 25 patients, Challapalli and colleagues[44] demonstrated that, especially with the additional use of a kinetic spatial filter (a filter to remove physiologic hepatic and pancreatic FLT uptake and to enable visualization of specific uptake in malignant lesions), FLT PET/CT was a very promising predictive biomarker of response in patients with advanced pancreatic cancer; an increase in the SUV_{max} at 60 minutes of 12% or more after 1 cycle of chemotherapy was indicative of disease progression with a positive predictive value of 100%.

Hypoxia imaging Few studies have been published about hypoxia PET imaging in pancreatic adenocarcinoma with variable results. One study showed striking associations between hypoxia and the aggressive features of rapid growth and high metastatic potential in a series of orthotopically grown primary pancreatic cancer xenografts using the 2-nitroimidazole probe EF5, predicting that targeting hypoxic tumor by incorporating hypoxia-targeted agents into existing adjuvant or neoadjuvant treatment protocols might potentially improve patient outcome.[45]

A study with ^{18}F-FAZA shows significant interpatient variation in tumor hypoxic fraction in PDA; potentially, knowing the extent and distribution of hypoxia might play a role in radiation planning and in identifying patients who might benefit from radiation sensitizers, however more studies are needed to confirm this theory.[46]

^{18}F-HX4 is another hypoxia agent that could be used in pancreatic cancer, with 1 study showing feasibility and repeatability in vivo, but more work is needed to evaluate this agent for potential clinical use.[47]

Intraductal Papillary Mucinous Neoplasms and Mucinous Cystic Neoplasms

Serous cystic neoplasms and solid pseudopapillary neoplasms are not included in this section given their low malignant potential.

Intraductal papillary mucinous neoplasms (IMPNs) and mucinous cystic neoplasms (MCNs), in contrast, are considered premalignant lesions. The first classification to recognize them as separate entities was made in 1996 by World Health Organization (WHO), where they were called intraductal papillary mucinous tumor and mucinous cystic tumor, then renamed in 2000 as IPMNs and MCNs. Although both have malignant potential, IPMN is the entity that has been studied the most, especially with FDG PET, probably owing to the much higher prevalence of the disease; data for FDG PET performance with MCNs remains lacking.

Histologically, MCNs are characterized by 2 distinct histologic components: an inner epithelial layer composed of tall mucin-secreting cells (which distinguishes them form serous cystic neoplasms), and a dense cellular ovarian-type stroma (specific criterion to distinguish them from IPMNs). They are usually large, septated, thick-walled mucinous cysts that lack communication with the ductal system, and occur almost exclusively in the pancreatic body and tail of middle-aged women.

IPMNs are characterized by the papillary growth of the ductal epithelium with rich mucin production, which is responsible for cystic segmental or diffuse dilatation of the MPD and/or its branches. Based on the ductal involvement they are classified into main duct type (MPD of >5 mm, without other causes of obstruction), branch duct type (cystic lesion in continuity with MPD), and mixed type IPMN. Based on the degree of dysplasia of the ductal epithelium they are further classified into mild, intermediate, or high-grade dysplasia to invasive carcinoma (papillary mucinous carcinoma, according to last 2010 WHO classification).[48]

Main duct IPMNs are associated with a greater risk for malignant transformation (about 60%) compared with branch duct IPMNs (about 25%). International guidelines (according to the 2012 FUKUOKA consensus conference) consider "worrisome stigmata" to be MPD size of 5 to 9 mm, cyst greater than 3 cm, nonenhancing mural nodule, abrupt change in duct caliber with distal atrophy, acute pancreatitis, adjacent lymphadenopathy, and thickened enhancing cyst wall; and high-risk stigmata to be MDP size of greater than 10 mm, enhancing mural nodule, and pancreatic head cyst with obstructive jaundice.[49]

These lesions are usually found on CT or ultrasound imaging, either incidentally or during workup for vague abdominal symptoms; however, neither CT nor ultrasound imaging are the best modalities to make a definite diagnosis or assess for worrisome features; they can show the size and location of the cysts and the size of the pancreatic duct, and may show the presence of concerning features such as thickened walls or mural nodules. However, to confirm the diagnosis and demonstrate the communication with MPD, MR imaging or endoscopic ultrasound imaging are needed.

MR imaging/MR cholangiopancreatography and endoscopic ultrasound imaging are shown to be equivalent in confirming the diagnosis; MR imaging has the advantage of being noninvasive; however, endoscopic ultrasound imaging allows to perform fine needle aspiration if needed. MR cholangiopancreatography allows excellent evaluation of the MPD (size and focal vs diffuse dilatation), and of the communication between the pancreatic cysts and the MDP.[50] Contrast-enhanced sequences permit evaluation for enhancing mural nodules, and adding DWI has also been shown to improve diagnostic accuracy and specificity for differentiating benign from malignant IPMNs (IPMNs with high-grade dysplasia or with an associated invasive carcinoma).[51,52]

The role of ^{18}F-FDG PET/CT is still debated in the assessment of IPMNs. However, multiple studies so far demonstrate that increased FDG uptake is highly specific to differentiate between benign and invasive IPMNs with a suggested SUV_{max} cutoff value of 2.3.[53–56] Roch and colleagues[54] showed that the addition of FDG uptake to 2012 international consensus guidelines criteria improved significantly the identification of malignant IPMNS; with a sensitivity of 78% (vs 92% for the guidelines criteria alone and 62% for PET alone) and a specificity of 100% (vs 27% for the guidelines criteria alone and 95% for PET alone). One of the largest trial was published in 2011 by Pedrazzoli and colleagues[55] and shows a higher accuracy of FDG PET/CT in differentiating malignant from benign IPMN compared with 2006 international consensus guidelines with a sensitivity of 83%, specificity of 100%, and accuracy of 91% (vs 93%, 22%, and 61%, respectively, for the 2006 International Consensus Guidelines).

To our knowledge, no studies are published so far about PET/MR imaging in the assessment of IPMNs or MCNs, except for a single case report where ^{18}F-FDG PET/CT showed uptake in a pancreatic lesion without being able to further evaluate the location of the uptake, which was shown later to localize to the wall of a cystic lesion on ^{18}F-FDG PET/MR imaging; the lesion was proven to be IPMN with high-grade dysplasia on pathology.[57] Further studies are needed to look for a potential role and for the cost effectiveness of ^{18}F-FDG PET/MR imaging in the evaluation of IPMN.

Pancreatic Neuroendocrine Tumors

Neuroendocrine tumors are a heterogeneous group of neoplasms sharing a common origin from endocrine progenitor cells. A characteristic property shared by these tumors is staining with neuroendocrine immunohistochemical markers CgA and synaptophysin; approximately 80% of them express the SSTR2, which allows targeting with synthetic somatostatin for diagnostic and therapeutic purposes.[58]

PNETs are usually combined in 1 category with small bowel neuroendocrine tumors under the umbrella of gastroenteropancreatic neuroendocrine tumors; they are classified according to the WHO 2010 classification based to their mitotic count and Ki-67 proliferation index into low grade (G1) if they have a mitotic count less than 2 per 10 high-power fields and/or a Ki-67 index of less

than 2%; intermediate grade (G2) if they have a mitotic count of 2 to 20 per 10 high-power fields and/or a Ki-67 index of 3% to 20%, and high grade (G3) or neuroendocrine carcinoma if they have a mitotic count of greater than 20 per 10 high-power fields and/or a Ki-67 index of greater than 20%. The main changes that the new WHO 2017 classification is bringing are first raising the Ki-67 cutoff between G1 and G2 tumors from 2% to 3% (to include Ki-67 between 2% and 3% within the G1 group) and dividing G3 tumors based on morphologic changes into well-differentiated neuroendocrine tumors with high mitotic rate (Ki-67 >20%, usually 40%–50%) and poorly differentiated neuroendocrine carcinomas (small cell and large cell types; Ki-67% has to be >20%, usually >55%) with no definite Ki-67 cutoff between the 2 groups.

PNETs are much less common than exocrine pancreatic tumors, constituting less than 3% of primary pancreatic neoplasms. Currently, it is believed that most PNETs are nonfunctional (nonhormone producing), with a wide range of reported numbers ranging from 68% to 90% of cases; owing to the lack of symptoms, these tumors are often advanced at diagnosis (larger in size and often metastatic). In contrast, functional PNETs (hormone-producing PNETs) reveal themselves earlier, and with the exception of gastrinoma, most of them are benign. The most common functional PNET is insulinoma (17%) followed by gastrinoma (15%), VIPoma (2%), glucagonoma (1%), somatostatinoma (1%), and other exceedingly rare neoplasms.[59]

CT is usually the first study ordered in the evaluation of a suspected gastroenteropancreatic neuroendocrine tumors; it should always be obtained with IV contrast triple phase because primary pancreatic tumors and their metastases (primarily hepatic) are typically hypervascular and enhance on the arterial phase; portal venous and delayed phases, however, allow for the detection of hypovascular lesions.[60,61]

CT has a reported sensitivity of 70% for detection of PNETS overall, and this increases to 80% to 100% when the primary is greater than 2 cm. It also has a sensitivity of approximately 35% for the detection of unknown primaries.[58]

MR imaging is superior to CT in detecting hepatic metastases.[62,63] It should be performed with IV contrast triple phase as well and, as with CT, most neuroendocrine lesions are hypervascular and enhance on the arterial phase. Two very helpful tools for the detection of hepatic metastases on MR imaging are DWI and delayed postcontrast phase using gadoxetic acid as a contrast agent. Most hepatic metastases demonstrate a high signal on DWI, which makes them more conspicuous and easier to identify; this is especially helpful in patients with severe renal failure where IV gadolinium is contraindicated. In contrast, gadoxetic acid is a hepatospecific paramagnetic gadolinium-based contrast agent that shows uptake in hepatocytes but not in metastatic lesions, creating a high lesion to background contrast on the delayed phase (20 minutes after injection); it has been demonstrated that delayed postcontrast phase with gadoxetic acid has the highest sensitivity for detection of metastatic lesions compared with other gadolinium based agents, DWI, triple phase CT, and even SSTR PET imaging (which is discussed elsewhere in this article).[64–67]

Guo and colleagues[68] showed that common features of high-grade G3 tumors are ill-defined borders, larger size, necrosis, low to moderate enhancement, pancreatic duct dilatation, presence of metastases, and high DWI signal. Additionally, several studies confirm that ADC values inversely correlate with histopathologic factors, including mitotic count and Ki-67 proliferation index, which determine tumor grade; and increased tumor cellularity and cell density with higher tumor grade (with possible component of fibrosis) causes restriction of motion of water molecules, which leads to a decrease in ADC values. A significant difference in ADC values was observed between G1 and G2 tumors and between G1/G2 and G3 tumors, with suggested cutoff ADC values of less than 0.95×10^{-3} to $1.19 \text{ mm}^2/\text{s}$ for high-grade G3 tumors.[68–72]

From a functional approach, SSTR scintigraphy has been the gold standard for NET functional imaging for the last few decades using pentetreotide (In-111–labeled octreotide with DTPA as a chelator), which targets SSTR types 2 and 5. To perform this scan, less than 10 μg of the radiotracer is injected intravenously; a standard protocol consists of planar whole body images acquired at 4 and 24 hours after injection in addition to single photon emission CT (SPECT)/CT at 24 hours. Some institutions perform in addition to the standard protocol a SPECT only (without CT) of the abdomen at 4 hours, given that the physiologic bowel uptake at 4 hours is much less prominent than at 24 hours. This early SPECT can help to differentiate a pathologic form of physiologic uptake within the abdomen in case of equivocal findings on the 24 hours SPECT/CT images. Delayed imaging at 48 to 72 hours may be performed to help differentiate pathologic from physiologic bowel uptake if needed, although SPECT/CT often obviates the need for that. The 2 major limitations for SSTR scintigraphy are the intrinsic low resolution of γ ray scintigraphy (spatial resolution of about 1 cm) and the inability to quantify the uptake (although improved technology that allows quantification with SPECT/CT is being developed and might be incorporated into clinical use in the near future).

To overcome the limitations of SSTR scintigraphy, ^{68}Ga-labeled SSTR agonist PET radiotracers have been developed recently and they quickly became the new gold standard for staging and restaging of neuroendocrine tumors and to select patients who are candidate for therapy with radiolabeled somatostatin analogs (peptide receptor radionuclide therapy). SSTR hybrid imaging with PET/CT (SSTR PET/CT) has been proven to be significantly superior to conventional imaging including triple phase CT, MR imaging, and SSTR scintigraphy. As discussed, this modality takes advantages of a higher affinity of the radiotracers (largely owing to the use of DOTA as a chelator rather than DTPA), higher performance of PET compared with SPECT with a spatial resolution of 3 to 6 mm, the short half-life of the radiotracer (which reduces significantly the patient dose), the ability to complete the study within a couple of hours because images are acquired in 1 session at 60 minutes after injection, and finally the lower cost of ^{68}Ga compared with [111]In.

The superiority of the 3 SSTR PET radiotracers available currently (DOTATATE, DOTATOC, and DOTANOC) has been clearly demonstrated compared with other imaging modalities for diagnosis and staging of neuroendocrine tumors.[73–75]

A metaanalysis of 22 studies that included more than 2000 patients showed high performance of SSTR PET/CT using ^{68}Ga-DOTATATE with a sensitivity of 93% and a specificity of 95%, which is significantly higher than conventional imaging and SSTR scintigraphy.[76]

The impact of SSTR PET on patient management has been also clearly shown.[74,75] The largest single study evaluating the impact of ^{68}Ga-DOTATATE-PET/CT on patient management was retrospective, it included 728 patients and showed high sensitivity of 97% and specificity of 95.1%, and it changed management in 40.9% of patients.[73]

A metaanalysis of 14 studies evaluating the impact of SSTR PET/CT shows a change in the management in 44% of patients. Management was also changed in 39% of those patients who had undergone a previous octreoscan.[77]

SSTR PET imaging, however, has certain limitations that the interpreting physician needs to be aware of to avoid pitfalls. Among the most common causes of false positives is the physiologic uptake within the uncinate process of the pancreas, which might be diffuse or focal; in this setting, correlation with anatomic imaging is crucial to avoid overcall. A second common scenario is intense physiologic uptake in an accessory spleen or a splenule near the pancreatic tail, which might be easily confused with a NET lesion, especially if a splenule is increasing in size on anatomic imaging after splenectomy, which is often performed along with distal pancreatectomy for pancreatic tail neuroendocrine tumors. Other common sources of false positives are inflammation or infection, radiation pneumonitis, and recent postsurgical changes.

False negatives are most commonly related to dedifferentiated tumor, small lesion size (smaller than 5–7 mm), recent analog therapy, and high physiologic uptake of background organ parenchyma, which can mask small pathologic SSTR2 expression. Along these lines, it has been shown that small SSTR-positive hepatic lesions might be masked by physiologic liver uptake on SSTR PET and are better demonstrated by triple phase MDCT or MR imaging.[78,79]

PET/MR imaging seems to be a promising tool for evaluation of gastroenteropancreatic neuroendocrine tumors, combining the high accuracy of SSTR PET agents and the high soft tissue contrast of MR imaging. The first small pilot study including 8 patients with histopathologically proven NET using a dedicated whole body contrast-enhanced PET/MR imaging protocol shows that all lesions that were considered as NET manifestations in PET/CT could be visualized with PET/MR imaging; additionally, PET/MR imaging showed 1 hepatic lesion that was not seen on PET/CT. In contrast, limitations of PET/MR imaging were primarily in the detection of lung lesions and hypersclerotic bone lesions.[80]

A second study including 10 patients with a total of 101 metastatic liver lesions compared ^{68}Ga DOTATOC PET/CT with ^{68}Ga DOTATOC PET/MR imaging, the CT portion of PET/CT was performed with IV contrast in the portal phase and the MR imaging portion of PET/MR imaging using a hepato-specific IV contrast agent; the study found a higher sensitivity of postcontrast MR imaging in the hepatobiliary phase (99%) compared with CT (46%) and PET (64%) for the detection of liver lesions.[81]

Increased uptake on SSTR PET/CT has been shown to be a good prognostic factor and a good predictor to tumor response to peptide receptor radionuclide therapy. In contrast, although well-differentiated neuroendocrine tumors do not show significant uptake on ^{18}F-FDG PET, it is well-demonstrated that FDG uptake correlates with higher tumor grade and poor prognosis.[82–84] A study including 51 patients with neuroendocrine tumors of unknown primary demonstrates that as

MIB-1/Ki-67 index (proliferation index) increased and ^{68}Ga-DOTATATE uptake decreased in metastatic and primary lesions, whereas ^{18}F-FDG uptake showed a gradual increase; the group suggested that a combined dual tracer PET/CT would help with the assessment of tumor biology.[82] One study found increased FDG uptake to have the strongest prognostic value in terms of overall survival, exceeding the prognostic value of traditional markers such as Ki67, chromogranin A, and liver metastases.[83]

Recently, in a retrospective study of 62 patients with metastatic neuroendocrine tumors, Chan and colleagues[85] proposed a grading system they called the "NETPET grade," which consists of identifying the NET lesion with most FDG uptake compared with SSTR uptake because it is more likely to represent the most aggressive tumor phenotype, then assessing the tumor burden based on the behavior of the remaining NET lesions with both radiotracers; the classification is on a categorical scale from 0 to 5 with a grade of P0 being a normal scan with both radiotracers; then grades P1 to P5 from P1 indicating SSTR-positive disease with no FDG uptake in any lesion to P5 indicating the presence of significant FDG-positive SSTR-negative disease. Patients with lower grade disease were more likely to respond to peptide receptor radionuclide therapy. A higher NETPET grade, in contrast, correlated with a more aggressive histologic grade and, interestingly, was more predictive of outcome. This is likely due to the whole body coverage with PET, which can identify the most aggressive lesions based on the relative FDG/SSTR uptake, whereas histologic grade might be inaccurate owing to intrasubject heterogeneity; the evaluation of lesion uptake with both radiotracers may lead to better selection of biopsy site at diagnosis or during follow-up to identify the highest grade disease.[85,86]

A possible pitfall that one should be aware of while interpreting FDG PET for neuroendocrine tumors is that some well-differentiated tumors with a proliferation index of less than 2% might show FDG uptake (SUV$_{max}$ of >2), which a very recent study by Bucau and colleagues[87] suggests that this might be due to sporadic VHL gene inactivation.

As it became clear today, the integration of anatomic and functional imaging with both SSTR and FGD PET in management of neuroendocrine tumors is crucial given the dynamic process of the disease and the large intersubject and intrasubject heterogeneity. In a posttreatment setting, the interpretation of SSTR PET might be challenging; the significance of an increase or decrease in the uptake level after treatment with no significant changes on anatomic imaging is not well-understood. An increase in lesion size after treatment can be secondary to necrotic changes within the lesion and should not be interpreted automatically as disease progression; an increase in solid components or the appearance of new lesions, in contrast, is a red flag; at this point, if the lesions lack SSTR expression, evaluation with FDG PET would be very helpful, because it can identify more aggressive/less differentiated disease. SSTR PET/MR imaging might be a very helpful tool in staging and therapy monitoring; as it has been shown, MR imaging has the highest sensitivity for detection of liver metastases, and might identify progressing disease earlier than other imaging modalities. Additionally, lower ADC values may help to identify dedifferentiated lesions with more aggressive potential. More studies are needed to identify patient groups that would benefit more from this technology.

Other radiotracers have been used to image neuroendocrine tumors. The most widely studied radiotracer is ^{18}F-DOPA, which is a tracer of the catecholamine metabolic pathway. The mechanism of uptake of ^{18}F-DOPA is favored to be related to the increased activity of L-DOPA decarboxylase, which is characteristic of neuroendocrine tumors.[88] The radiotracer is transported across the membrane by an amino acid transporter, and is decarboxylated afterward into ^{18}F-fluorodopamine and stored in vesicles. Many papers in literature report the high accuracy of ^{18}F-DOPA for imaging of well-differentiated neuroendocrine tumors ($\geq$90%), compared with conventional imaging and SSTR scintigraphy. Particularly, several groups have reported successful imaging of insulinomas and β-cell hyperplasia.[89,90] It has been suggested to preadminister carbidopa to lower background pancreatic uptake, which allows better lesion to background contrast.[91] Currently, the potential role of ^{18}F-DOPA in the imaging of neuroendocrine tumors in general is in tumors with low or variable SSTR expression where it may be helpful, especially in identifying new lesions to define disease progression; however, the limited availability and high synthesis cost makes it less suitable for routine clinical use.[92–94]

A very promising development in SSTR targeting is the recent introduction of SSTR antagonists. Despite poor internalization rates, preclinical and early clinical studies show that SSTR antagonists have favorable pharmacokinetics, high tumor to background contrast, and label more sites than agonists allowing better tumor visualization.[95,96] The majority of these antagonists target primarily SSTR type 2, the first of which to be developed

was SST2-ANT or BASS developed by Bass and colleagues,[97] and several other followed such as LM3 (p-Cl-Phe-cyclo (D-Cys-Tyr-D-Aph(Cbm)-Lys-Thr-Cys)D-Tyr-NH$_2$), JR10 (p-NO$_2$-Phe-c[D-Cys-Tyr- D-Aph(Cbm)-Lys-Thr-Cys]-D-Tyr-NH$_2$), and JR11 (Cpa-c[D-Cys- Aph(Hor)-D-Aph(Cbm)-Lys-Thr-Cys]-D-Tyr-NH$_2$). These molecules were studied in combination with 3 chelators (DOTA, NODAGA (1,4,7-triazacyclononane,1-glutaric acid-4,7-acetic acid), and CB-TE2A (4,11-bis (carboxymethyl)-1,4,8,11-tetraazabicyclo[6.6.2]hexadecane)) and were labeled primarily with 2 radiometals (^{64}Cu and ^{68}Ga). Of these antagonists JR11 performed the best in preclinical settings and has been selected for clinical translation. Interestingly, the use of NODAGA as a chelator instead of DOTA substantially increases the binding affinity of these radiotracers, allowing even a low-affinity antagonist to be superior to a high-affinity agonist.[98,99]

A small pilot study with 4 patients shows promising results of peptide receptor radionuclide therapy using ^{177}Lu-DOTA-JR11 which showed higher tumor dose than ^{177}Lu-DOTATATE and at the same time higher tumor-to-kidney and tumor-to-bone marrow dose ratio.[100] Early clinical studies suggest that the diagnostic–therapeutic pair ^{68}Ga-NODAGA-JR11 and ^{177}Lu-DOTA-JR11 seems to be promising; further evaluation is warranted.

Finally, ^{11}C-5-Hydroxytryptophane (^{11}C-5-HTP), a serotonin precursor, is also being used for imaging of neuroendocrine tumors. ^{11}C-5-HTP is taken up by the large amino acid transporter (LAT) and metabolized by the DOPA decarboxylase to ^{11}C-serotonin, which is trapped intracellularly. Several studies show its superiority compared with anatomic imaging, however, it is much less used clinically compared with SSTR agents.[101–103]

A summary of the ligands that are used most often clinically for oncologic or potentially premalignant indications is shown in **Table 1**.

Noninvasive β-Cell Imaging

β-Cells constitute approximately 1% to 2% of the pancreatic mass (approximately 65%–80% of the endocrine cells of the islets of Langerhans). They are involved in the control of blood glucose levels in the body through insulin secretion. Loss of β-cell mass or function is a central player in most forms of diabetes; less commonly, β-cell hyperfunction leads to hyperinsulinemia and hypoglycemia.

The standard tests used currently to diagnose type 1 and type 2 diabetes (either plasma glucose or glycated hemoglobin levels) change only after the loss of more than 80% of the β-cells function

Table 1
Ligands that are used most often for oncologic or potentially premalignant indications

Pathology	PET Radiotracers and Potential Role	Additional Role of MR Imaging
Pancreatic ductal carcinoma	^{18}F-FDG (metabolic imaging): • Diagnosis: Questionable role in differentiating malignancy from focal pancreatitis (high rate of false positives and false negatives). • Local staging: No definite added value. • Detection of metastatic disease: Superiority in detecting distant metastases. • Treatment response: Very helpful in evaluating for treatment response and tumor resectability after radiotherapy and in evaluating for tumor recurrence after surgery. ^{18}F-FLT (proliferation imaging) • Higher accuracy than ^{18}F-FDG in differentiating malignancy from benign etiologies. • Potential role in early assessment of tumor response to treatment, more studies are needed. Hypoxia imaging • Might play a role in radiation planning, more studies are needed.	• Diagnosis and local staging: comparable and might be slightly superior to MDCT. • Detection of metastatic disease: Higher detection rate of liver metastases.
IPMN	^{18}F-FDG: • Differentiation between benign and invasive IPMNs.	• High accuracy in diagnosis and detection of high risk stigmata.

(continued on next page)

Table 1
(continued)

Pathology	PET Radiotracers and Potential Role	Additional Role of MR Imaging
Pancreatic neuroendocrine tumors	⁶⁸Ga labeled SSTR analogs: • New gold standard for staging and restaging of well-differentiated neuroendocrine tumors and to select patients for peptide receptor radionuclide therapy. • Highest accuracy in detection of primary site and metastatic lesions compared with SSTR scintigraphy and conventional imaging. • Degree of uptake decreases in high grade tumors. ¹⁸F-FDG: • No significant role in well-differentiated neuroendocrine tumors (G1 and majority of G2). • Important role in high grade tumors that show low SSTR expression. • Uptake correlates with poor prognosis. ¹⁸F-DOPA (tracer of the catecholamine metabolic pathway) • High accuracy for imaging of well-differentiated neuroendocrine tumors, compared with conventional imaging and SSTR scintigraphy. • Currently, the potential role is in tumors with low or variable SSTR expression SSTR antagonists • Very promising agents, still investigational.	• Highest sensitivity for detection of hepatic metastases (slightly higher than SSTR PET/CT). • Some features on MR imaging are predictive of higher grade tumors (such as ill-defined borders, larger size, necrosis, low to moderate enhancement, pancreatic duct dilatation, and high DWI signal). • Absence of ionizing radiation is a big advantage in this group of patients with long survival and repetitive imaging.

Abbreviations: CT, computed tomography; DWI, diffusion-weighted imaging; ¹⁸F-DOPA, 18F-fluorodihydroxyphenylalanine; ¹⁸F-FDG, fludeoxyglucose F 18; ¹⁸F-FLT, fluorothymidine; ⁶⁸Ga, ⁶⁸gallium; IPMN, intraductal papillary mucinous neoplasm; MDCT, multidetector computed tomography; NET, neuroendocrine tumor; SSTR, somatostatin receptor.

has already occurred. Noninvasive β-cell imaging would allow a better understanding of the pathogenesis of diabetes, early diagnosis, and potentially early intervention before the loss of β-cell mass is irreversible, but this development faces significant biological and technological problems owing primarily to the small size of the β-cell islets, which are dispersed throughout the pancreas, and to background pancreatic uptake with most radiotracers that have been developed. No hybrid PET/MR imaging work has been done so far in this setting; however, each modality alone has been studied using multiple agents mainly in preclinical setting, with variable degrees of success, which raises the question of whether integrated PET/MR imaging could be of added value.

Several approaches have been used in MR imaging, such as imaging with Zink (Zn^{2+})-responsive T1 contrast agent and using manganese (Mn^{2+}) as a contrast agent. The theory behind Zn^{2+}-responsive T1 contrast agent is that insulin is packaged as a Zn^{2+}/insulin complex in β-cell granules, so that the extracellular concentration of Zn^{2+} increases after the glucose-dependent release of insulin; a study conducted in mice shows increased uptake of the radiotracer in healthy mice after glucose administration, although no uptake is seen in diabetic mice or in healthy mice who didn't receive glucose.[104] Mn^{2+} in contrast mimics the behavior of Ca^{2+}, which is an essential regulator of insulin secretion; Mn^{2+} enter β-cells through voltage-gated Ca^{2+} channels resulting in a specific glucose-dependent signal. Several preclinical and clinical studies so far show decreased Mn^{2+} accumulation with a loss of β-cell mass.[105–107]

Another approach is the use of ferromagnetic cobalt or iron nanoparticles functionalized with a β-cell–specific single-chain antibody as a contrast agent; the concept here is to bind the nanoparticles (which will be responsible for the MR imaging signal) to an antibody that targets specifically pancreatic β-cells. The most promising target is glucagon-like peptide 1 receptor (GLP-1r), which is highly expressed in β-cells and is currently an important target in the treatment of type 2 diabetes.[108]

The endogenous peptide GLP-1 (ligand of GLP-1r) induces the release of insulin in a glucose-dependent manner and promotes β-cell proliferation; however, it has a very short plasma half-life, which makes it unsuitable as a tracer. For this purpose, exendin-4, a GLP1 long-acting analog has been developed.[108,109] Multiple preclinical studies in mice and rats have used exendin labeled with variable radiotracers to quantify β-cell mass with promising results; however, the main

challenge is the uptake in the background pancreas and the physiologic intersubject variability of the β-cell mass.[108]

The same challenges face molecular imaging in terms of quantification of β-cell mass. Several probes have been used so far, with targeting of GLP-1r being the most promising. Several preclinical studies using radiolabeled exendin for SPECT and PET imaging show decreased tracer uptake in the pancreas with loss of β-cells, suggesting that a noninvasive quantification of GLP-1r is feasible. Clinical studies, however, were conducted primarily to localize insulinomas and β-cell hyperplasia and to label transplanted islets; these are easier to visualize because they consist of clustered cells.[110–112]

Among the other targets that have been studied to image β-cell mass are the vesicular monoamine transporter 2, which is a membrane protein responsible for the transport of neurotransmitters and is widely expressed in the neuroendocrine systems, and the sulfonylurea receptor 1, which is a subunit of ATP-dependent potassium channels involved in the insulin secretion from β-cells. Both techniques face a high nonspecific pancreatic uptake with a low specific signal in comparison with the background.[108]

In conclusion, the clinical application of β-cell imaging so far is in the visualization of insulinomas and β-cell hyperplasia, and the assessment of transplanted islets. The assessment of β-cell mass in diabetic patients and its changes during the course of the disease is still facing multiple challenges that are secondary mainly to the small number of β-cells dispersed in the pancreas and the high interindividual differences in β-cell mass in individuals without diabetes.

SUMMARY

PET/MR imaging has the potential to markedly alter pancreatic care in both the malignant and premalignant states, with the ability to perform robust, high-resolution quantitative molecular imaging. The ability of PET/MR imaging to monitor the disease process, potentially correct for motion in the upper abdomen, and provide novel biomarkers that may be a combination of MR imaging and PET biomarkers, offers a unique, precise interrogation of the pancreatic milieu going forward.

REFERENCES

1. Pichler B, Lorenz E, Mirzoyan R, et al. Performance test of a LSO-APD PET module in a 9.4 Tesla magnet. Conference Record of the 1998 IEEE Nuclear

Science Symposium and Medical Imaging Conference. Piscataway (NJ): IEEE; 1998. p. 1237–9.

2. Catana C, Procissi D, Wu Y, et al. Simultaneous in vivo positron emission tomography and magnetic resonance imaging. Proc Natl Acad Sci U S A 2008;105:3705–10.

3. Drzezga A, Souvatzoglou M, Eiber M, et al. First clinical experience with integrated whole-body PET/MR: comparison to PET/CT in patients with oncologic diagnoses. J Nucl Med 2012;53:845–55.

4. Catana C, Guimaraes AR, Rosen BR. PET and MR imaging: the odd couple or a match made in heaven? J Nucl Med 2013;54:815–24.

5. Schwartz JL, Tamura Y, Jordan R, et al. Monitoring tumor cell proliferation by targeting DNA synthetic processes with thymidine and thymidine analogs. J Nucl Med 2003;44:2027–32.

6. Rasey JS, Grierson JR, Wiens L, et al. Validation of FLT uptake as a measure of thymidine kinase-1 activity in A549 carcinoma cells. J Nucl Med 2002;43:1210–7.

7. Kim SJ, Lee JS, Im KC, et al. Kinetic modeling of 3'-deoxy-3'-18F-fluorothymidine for quantitative cell proliferation imaging in subcutaneous tumor models in mice. J Nucl Med 2008;49:2057–66.

8. Plotnik DA, Asher C, Chu SK, et al. Levels of human equilibrative nucleoside transporter-1 are higher in proliferating regions of A549 tumor cells grown as tumor xenografts in vivo. Nucl Med Biol 2012;39:1161–6.

9. Arnes ES, Eriksson S. Mammalian deoxyribonucleoside kinases. Pharmacol Ther 1995;67:155–86.

10. Hofman MS, Lau WF, Hicks RJ. Somatostatin receptor imaging with 68Ga DOTATATE PET/CT: clinical utility, normal patterns, pearls, and pitfalls in interpretation. Radiographics 2015;35:500–16.

11. Kabasakal L, Demirci E, Ocak M, et al. Comparison of 68Ga-DOTATATE and 68Ga-DOTANOC PET/CT imaging in the same patient group with neuroendocrine tumors. Eur J Nucl Med Mol Imaging 2012;39:1271–7.

12. Van Elmpt W, Zegers CM, Das M, et al. Imaging techniques for tumour delineation and heterogeneity quantification of lung cancer: overview of current possibilities. J Thorac Dis 2014;6:319–27.

13. Rajendran JG, Schwartz DL, O'Sullivan J, et al. Tumor hypoxia imaging with [F-18] fluoromisonidazole positron emission tomography in head and neck cancer. Clin Cancer Res 2006;12:5435–41.

14. Tachibana I, Nishimura Y, Shibata T, et al. A prospective clinical trial of tumor hypoxia imaging with 18F-fluoromisonidazole positron emission tomography and computed tomography (F-MISO PET/CT) before and during radiation therapy. J Radiat Res 2013;54:1078–84.

15. Chapman JD, Baer K, Lee J. Characteristics of the metabolism-induced binding of misonidazole to hypoxic mammalian cells. Cancer Res 1983;43:1523–8.

16. Mees G, Dierckx R, Vangestel C, et al. Molecular imaging of hypoxia with radiolabelled agents. Eur J Nucl Med Mol Imaging 2009;36:1674–86.

17. Koelblinger C, Ba-Ssalamah A, Goetzinger P, et al. Gadobenate dimeglumine-enhanced 3.0-T MR imaging versus multiphasic 64-detector row CT: prospective evaluation in patients suspected of having pancreatic cancer. Radiology 2011;259:757–66.

18. Motosugi U, Ichikawa T, Morisaka H, et al. Detection of pancreatic carcinoma and liver metastases with gadoxetic acid–enhanced MR imaging: comparison with contrast-enhanced multi–detector row CT. Radiology 2011;260:446–53.

19. Schima W, Ba-Ssalamah A, Goetzinger P, et al. State-of-the-art magnetic resonance imaging of pancreatic cancer. Top Magn Reson Imaging 2007;18:421–9.

20. Park HJ, Jang KM, Song KD, et al. Value of unenhanced MRI with diffusion-weighted imaging for detection of primary small (20 mm) solid pancreatic tumours and prediction of pancreatic ductal adenocarcinoma. Clin Radiol 2017;72(12):1076–84.

21. Park HS, Lee JM, Choi HK, et al. Preoperative evaluation of pancreatic cancer: comparison of gadolinium-enhanced dynamic MRI with MR cholangiopancreatography versus MDCT. J Magn Reson Imaging 2009;30:586–95.

22. Muraoka N, Uematsu H, Kimura H, et al. Apparent diffusion coefficient in pancreatic cancer: characterization and histopathological correlations. J Magn Reson Imaging 2008;27:1302–8.

23. Hayano K, Miura F, Amano H, et al. Correlation of apparent diffusion coefficient measured by diffusion- weighted MRI and clinicopathologic features in pancreatic cancer patients. J Hepatobiliary Pancreat Sci 2013;20:243–8.

24. Sandrasegaran K, Nutakki K, Tahir B, et al. Use of diffusion-weighted MRI to differentiate chronic pancreatitis from pancreatic cancer. AJR Am J Roentgenol 2013;201:1002–8.

25. Zhang Y, Huang J, Chen M, et al. Preoperative vascular evaluation with computed tomography and magnetic resonance imaging for pancreatic cancer: a meta-analysis. Pancreatology 2012;12:227–33.

26. Chen FM, Ni JM, Zhang ZY, et al. Presurgical evaluation of pancreatic cancer: a comprehensive imaging comparison of CT versus MRI. AJR Am J Roentgenol 2016;206:526–35.

27. Okano K, Kakinoki K, Akamoto S, et al. 18F-fluorodeoxyglucose positron emission tomography in the diagnosis of small pancreatic cancer. World J Gastroenterol 2011;17:231–5.

28. VanKouwen MC, Jansen JB, van Goor H, et al. FDG-PET is able to detect pancreatic carcinoma in chronic pancreatitis. Eur J Nucl Med Mol Imaging 2005;32:399–404.

29. Other article about SUV being helpful Sánchez-Bueno F, García-Pérez R, Claver Valderas MA, et al. Utility of 18 fludeoxyglucose in preoperative positron-emission tomography-computed tomography (PET-CT) in the early diagnosis of exocrine pancreatic cancer: a study of 139 resected cases. Cir Esp 2016;94:511–7.

30. Yoshioka M, Uchinami H, Watanabe G, et al. F-18 fluorodeoxyglucose positron emission tomography for differential diagnosis of pancreatic tumors. Springerplus 2015;4:154.

31. Kim R, Prithviraj G, Kothari N, et al. PET/CT fusion scan prevents futile laparotomy in early stage pancreatic cancer. Clin Nucl Med 2015;40:501–5.

32. Schellenberg D, Quon A, Minn AY, et al. 18Fluorodeoxyglucose PET is prognostic of progression-free and overall survival in locally advanced pancreas cancer treated with stereotactic radiotherapy. Int J Radiat Oncol Biol Phys 2010;77:1420–5.

33. Ruf J, Lopez Hanninen E, Bohmig M, et al. Impact of FDG-PET/MRI image fusion on the detection of pancreatic cancer. Pancreatology 2006;6:512–9.

34. Donati OF, Hany TF, Reiner CS, et al. Value of retrospective fusion of PET and MR images in detection of hepatic metastases: comparison with 18F-FDG PET/CT and Gd-EOB-DTPA-enhanced MRI. J Nucl Med 2010;51:692–9.

35. Joo I, Lee JM, Lee DH, et al. Preoperative assessment of pancreatic cancer with FDG PET/MR imaging versus FDG PET/CT plus contrast-enhanced multidetector CT: a prospective preliminary study. Radiology 2017;282:149–59.

36. Sakane M, Tatsumi M, Kim T, et al. Correlation between apparent diffusion coefficients on diffusion-weighted MRI and standardized uptake value on FDG- PET/CT in pancreatic adenocarcinoma. Acta Radiol 2015;56:1034–41.

37. Chen BB, Tien YW, Chang MC, et al. PET/MRI in pancreatic and periampullary cancer: correlating diffusion-weighted imaging, MR spectroscopy and glucose metabolic activity with clinical stage and prognosis. Eur J Nucl Med Mol Imaging 2016;43(10):1753–64.

38. Kuwatani M, Kawakami H, Eto K, et al. Modalities for evaluating chemotherapeutic efficacy and survival time in patients with advanced pancreatic cancer: comparison between FDG-PET, CT, and serum tumor markers. Intern Med 2009;48:867–75.

39. Bang S, Chung HW, Park SW, et al. The clinical usefulness of 18- fluorodeoxyglucose positron emission tomography in the differential diagnosis, staging, and response evaluation after concurrent chemo-radiotherapy for pancreatic cancer. J Clin Gastroenterol 2006;40:923–9.

40. Pery C, Meurette G, Ansquer C, et al. Role and limitations of 18F-FDG positron emission tomography (PET) in the management of patients with pancreatic lesions. Gastroenterol Clin Biol 2010;34: 465–74.

41. Herrmann K, Eckel F, Schmidt S, et al. In vivo characterization of proliferation for discriminating cancer from pancreatic pseudotumors. J Nucl Med 2008;49:1437–44.

42. Herrmann K, Erkan M, Dobritz M, et al. Comparison of 3'-deoxy-3'-[(18)F]fluorothymidine positron emission tomography (FLT PET) and FDG PET/CT for the detection and characterization of pancreatic tumours. Eur J Nucl Med Mol Imaging 2012;39: 846–51.

43. Weber WA. Monitoring tumor response to therapy with 18F-FLT PET. J Nucl Med 2010;51:841–4.

44. Challapalli A, Barwick T, Pearson R, et al. 3'-Deoxy-3'-18F-fluorothymidine positron emission tomography as an early predictor of disease progression in patients with advanced and metastatic pancreatic cancer. Eur J Nucl Med Mol Imaging 2015; 42:831–40.

45. Chang Q, Jurisica I, Do T, et al. Hypoxia predicts aggressive growth and spontaneous metastasis formation from orthotopically grown primary xenografts of human pancreatic cancer. J Nucl Med 2016;57:361–6.

46. Metran-Nascente C, Yeung I, Vines D, et al. Measurement of tumor hypoxia in patients with advanced pancreatic cancer based on 18F-Fluoroazomyin arabinoside uptake. J Nucl Med 2016; 57:361–6.

47. Klaassen R, Bennink RJ, van Tienhoven G, et al. Feasibility and repeatability of PET with the hypoxia tracer [18F]HX4 in oesophageal and pancreatic cancer. Radiother Oncol 2015;116:94–9.

48. Pagliari D, Saviano A, Serricchio ML. Uptodate in the assessment and management of intraductal papillary mucinous neoplasms of the pancreas. Eur Rev Med Pharmacol Sci 2017;21:2858–74.

49. Tanaka M, CasTillo CF, Adsay V, et al. International consensus guideline 2012 for the management of IPMN and MCN of the pancreas. Pancreatology 2012;12:183–97.

50. Kim JH, Eun HW, Park HJ, et al. Diagnostic performance of MRI and EUS in the differentiation of benign from malignant pancreatic cyst and cyst communication with the main duct. Eur J Radiol 2012;81:2927–35.

51. Hoffman DH, Ream JM, Hajdu CH, et al. Utility of whole-lesion ADC histogram metrics for assessing the malignant potential of pancreatic intraductal papillary mucinous neoplasms (IPMNs). Abdom Radiol (NY) 2017;42:1222–8.

52. Ogawa T, Horaguchi J, Fujita N, et al. Diffusion-weighted magnetic resonance imaging for evaluating the histological degree of malignancy in patients with intraductal papillary mucinous neoplasm. J Hepatobiliary Pancreat Sci 2014;21: 801–8.

53. Baiocchi GL, Bretagna F, Gheza F, et al. Searching for indicators of malignancy in pancreatic IPMN; the value of (18) FDG-PET confirmed. Ann Surg Oncol 2012;19:3574–80.

54. Roch A, Barron M, Tann M, et al. Does PET with CT have clinical utility in the management of patients with intraductal papillary mucinous neoplasm? J Am Coll Surg 2015;221:48–56.

55. Pedrazzoli S, Sperti C, Pasquali C, et al. Comparison of international consensus guidelines versus 18-FDG PET in detecting malignancy of intraductal papillary mucinous neoplasm of the pancreas. Ann Surg 2011;254:171–6.

56. Sperti C, Bissoli S, Pasquali C, et al. 18-fluorodeoxyglucose positron emission tomography enhances computed tomography diagnosis of malignant intraductal papillary mucinous neoplasms of the pancreas. Ann Surg 2007;246:932–7.

57. Huo L, Feng F, Liao Q, et al. Intraductal papillary mucinous neoplasm of the pancreas with high malignant potential on FDG PET/MRI. Clin Nucl Med 2016;41:989–90.

58. Maxwell J, O'Dorisio T, Howe J. Biochemical diagnosis and preoperative imaging of gastroenteropancreatic neuroendocrine tumors. Surg Oncol Clin N Am 2016;25:171–94.

59. Ehehalt F, Saeger HD, Schmidt CM, et al. Neuroendocrine tumors of the pancreas. Oncologist 2009; 14:456–67.

60. Bushnell DL, Baum RP. Standard imaging techniques for neuroendocrine tumors. Endocrinol Metab Clin North Am 2011;40:153–62.

61. Sahani DV, Bonaffini PA, Fernandez-Del Castillo C, et al. Gastroenteropancreatic neuroendocrine tumors: role of imaging in diagnosis and management. Radiology 2013;266:38–61.

62. Dromain C, de Baere T, Lumbroso J, et al. Detection of liver metastases from endocrine tumors: a prospective comparison of somatostatin receptor scintigraphy, computed tomography, and magnetic resonance imaging. J Clin Oncol 2005;23: 70–8.

63. Yu R, Wachsman A. Imaging of neuroendocrine tumors: indications, interpretations, limits, and pitfalls. Endocrinol Metab Clin North Am 2017;46: 795–814.

64. Ba-Ssalamah A, Uffmann M, Saini S, et al. Clinical value of MRI liver-specific contrast agents: a tailored examination for a confident non-invasive diagnosis of focal liver lesions. Eur Radiol 2009; 19:342–57.

65. Shimada K, Isoda H, Hirokawa Y, et al. Comparison of gadolinium-EOB-DTPA-enhanced and diffusion-weighted liver MRI for detection of small hepatic metastases. Eur Radiol 2010;20:2690–8.

66. Qian HF, Zhu YM, Wu X, et al. Comparison of enhanced magnetic resonance and diffusion-weighted imaging for detection of hepatic metastases. Zhongguo Yi Xue Ke Xue Yuan Xue Bao 2012; 34:621–4.

67. Giesel FL, Kratochwil C, Mehndiratta A, et al. Comparison of neuroendocrine tumour detection and characterization using DOTATOC-PET in correlation with contrast enhanced CT and delayed contrast enhanced MRI. Eur J Radiol 2012;81: 2820–5.

68. Guo C, Chen X, Xiao W, et al. Pancreatic neuroendocrine neoplasms at magnetic resonance imaging: comparison between grade 3 and grade 1/2 tumors. Onco Targets Ther 2017;10:1465–74.

69. Lotfalizadeh E, Ronot M, Wagner M, et al. Prediction of pancreatic neuroendocrine tumour grade with MR imaging features: added value of diffusion-weighted imaging. Eur Radiol 2017;27: 1748–59.

70. Besa C, Ward S, Cui Y, et al. Neuroendocrine liver metastases: value of apparent diffusion coefficient and enhancement ratios for characterization of histopathologic grade. J Magn Reson Imaging 2016; 44:1432–41.

71. Kim M, Kang TW, Kim YK, et al. Pancreatic neuroendocrine tumour: correlation of apparent diffusion coefficient or WHO classification with recurrence-free survival. Eur J Radiol 2016;85:680–7.

72. Guo C, Zhuge X, Chen X, et al. Value of diffusion-weighted magnetic resonance imaging in predicting World Health Organization grade in G1/G2 pancreatic neuroendocrine tumors. Oncol Lett 2017;13:4141–6.

73. Skoura E, Michopoulou S, Mohmaduvesh M, et al. The impact of 68Ga-DOTATATE PET/CT imaging on management of patients with neuroendocrine tumors: experience from a national referral center in the United Kingdom. J Nucl Med 2016;57:34–40.

74. Naswa N, Sharma P, Kumar A, et al. Gallium-68-DOTA-NOC PET/CT of patients with gastroenteropancreatic neuroendocrine tumors: a prospective single-center study. AJR Am J Roentgenol 2011; 197:1221–8.

75. Sadowski SM, Neychev V, Millo C, et al. Prospective study of 68Ga-DOTATATE positron emission tomography/computed tomography for detecting gastro-entero-pancreatic neuroendocrine tumors and unknown primary sites. J Clin Oncol 2016;34: 588–96.

76. Geijer H, Breimer LH. Somatostatin receptor PET/CT in neuroendocrine tumours: update on

systematic review and meta-analysis. Eur J Nucl Med Mol Imaging 2013;40:1770–80.

77. Barrio M, Czernin J, Fanti S, et al. The impact of somatostatin receptor-directed PET/CT on the management of patients with neuroendocrine tumor: a systematic review and meta-analysis. J Nucl Med 2017;58:756–61.

78. Bodei L, Ambrosini V, Herrmann K, et al. Current concepts in 68Ga-DOTATATE imaging of neuroendocrine neoplasms: interpretation, biodistribution, dosimetry, and molecular strategies. J Nucl Med 2017. https://doi.org/10.2967/jnumed.116.186361.

79. Ruf J, Schiefer J, Furth C, et al. 68Ga-DOTATOC PET/CT of neuroendocrine tumors: spotlight on the CT phases of a triple-phase protocol. J Nucl Med 2011;52:697–704.

80. Beiderwellen KJ, Poeppel TD, Hartung-Knemeyer V, et al. Simultaneous 68Ga-DOTATOC PET/MRI in patients with gastroenteropancreatic neuroendocrine tumors: initial results. Invest Radiol 2013;48:273–9.

81. Hope TA, Pampaloni MH, Nakakura E, et al. Simultaneous (68)Ga-DOTA-TOC PET/MRI with gadoxetate disodium in patients with neuroendocrine tumor. Abdom Imaging 2015;40:1432–40.

82. Sampathirao N, Basu S. MIB-1 index-stratified assessment of dual-tracer PET/CT with ^{68}Ga-DOTATATE and ^{18}F-FDG and multimodality anatomic imaging in metastatic neuroendocrine tumors of unknown primary in a PRRT workup setting. J Nucl Med Technol 2017;45:34–41.

83. Binderup T, Knigge U, Loft A, et al. 18F-fluorodeoxyglucose positron emission tomography predicts survival of patients with neuroendocrine tumors. Clin Cancer Res 2010;16:978–85.

84. Garin E, Le Jeune F, Devillers A, et al. Predictive value of 18F-FDG PET and somatostatin receptor scintigraphy in patients with metastatic endocrine tumors. J Nucl Med 2009;50:858–64.

85. Chan DL, Pavlakis N, Schembri GP, et al. Dual somatostatin receptor/FDG PET/CT imaging in metastatic neuroendocrine tumours: proposal for a novel grading scheme with prognostic significance. Theranostics 2017;7:1149–58.

86. Hindié E. The NETPET score: combining FDG and somatostatin receptor imaging for optimal management of patients with metastatic well-differentiated neuroendocrine tumors. Theranostics 2017;7:1159–63.

87. Bucau M, Laurent-Bellue A, Poté N, et al. 18F-FDG uptake in well-differentiated neuroendocrine tumors correlates with both Ki-67 and VHL pathway inactivation. Neuroendocrinology 2017. https://doi.org/10.1159/000480239.

88. Gazdar AF, Helman LJ, Israel MA, et al. Expression of neuroendocrine cell markers L-dopa decarboxylase, chromogranin A, and dense core granules in human tumors of endocrine and nonendocrine origin. Cancer Res 1988;48:4078–82.

89. Gopal-Kothandapani JS, Hussain K. Congenital hyperinsulinism: role of fluorine-18L-3, 4 hydroxy-phenylalanine positron emission tomography scanning. World J Radiol 2014;6:252–60.

90. Kauhanen S, Seppänen M, Minn H, et al. Clinical PET imaging of insulinoma and beta-cell hyperplasia. Curr Pharm Des 2010;16:1550–60.

91. Imperiale A, Sebag F, Vix M, et al. 18F-FDOPA PET/CT imaging of insulinoma revisited. Eur J Nucl Med Mol Imaging 2015;42:409–18.

92. Zanzi I, Studentsova Y, Bjelke D, et al. Fluorine-18-fluorodihydroxyphenylalanine positron-emission tomography scans of neuroendocrine tumors (carcinoids and pheochromocytomas). J Clin Imaging Sci 2017;7:20.

93. Bozkurt MF, Virgolini I, Balogova S, et al. Guideline for PET/CT imaging of neuroendocrine neoplasms with 68Ga-DOTA-conjugated somatostatin receptor targeting peptides and 18F-DOPA. Eur J Nucl Med Mol Imaging 2017;44:1588–601.

94. Kauhanen S, Seppänen M, Ovaska J, et al. The clinical value of [18F]fluoro-dihydroxyphenylalanine positron emission tomography in primary diagnosis, staging, and restaging of neuroendocrine tumors. Endocr Relat Cancer 2009;16:255–65.

95. Ginj M, Zhang H, Waser B, et al. Radiolabeled somatostatin receptor antagonists are preferable to agonists for in vivo peptide receptor targeting of tumors. Proc Natl Acad Sci U S A 2006;103:16436–41.

96. Fani M, Nicolas GP, Wild D. Somatostatin receptor antagonists for imaging and therapy. J Nucl Med 2017;58:61S–6S.

97. Bass RT, Buckwalter BL, Patel BP, et al. Identification and characterization of novel somatostatin antagonists. Mol Pharmacol 1996;50(4):709–15.

98. Fani M, Braun F, Waser B, et al. Unexpected sensitivity of sst2 antagonists to N-terminal radiometal modifications. J Nucl Med 2012;53:1481–9.

99. Fani M, Del Pozzo L, Abiraj K, et al. PET of somatostatin receptor–positive tumors using 64Cu- and 68Ga-somatostatin antagonists: the chelate makes the difference. J Nucl Med 2011;52:1110–8.

100. Wild D, Fani M, Fischer R, et al. Comparison of somatostatin receptor agonist and antagonist for peptide receptor radionuclide therapy: a pilot study. J Nucl Med 2014;55:1248–52.

101. Nikolaou A, Thomas D, Kampanellou C, et al. The value of 11C-5-hydroxy-tryptophan positron emission tomography in neuroendocrine tumor diagnosis and management: experience from one center. J Endocrinol Invest 2010;33:794–9.

102. Orlefors H, Sundin A, Ahlström H, et al. Positron emission tomography with 5-hydroxytryprophan in

neuroendocrine tumors. J Clin Oncol 1998;16: 2534–41.

103. Sundin A, Eriksson B, Bergström M, et al. Demonstration of [11C] 5-hydroxy-L-tryptophan uptake and decarboxylation in carcinoid tumors by specific positioning labeling in positron emission tomography. Nucl Med Biol 2000;27: 33–41.

104. Lubag AJ, De Leon-Rodriguez LM, Burgess SC, et al. Noninvasive MRI of β-cell function using a Zn^{2+}-responsive contrast agent. Proc Natl Acad Sci U S A 2011;108:18400–5.

105. Antkowiak PF, Vandsburger MH, Epstein FH. Quantitative pancreatic β cell MRI using manganese-enhanced look-locker imaging and two-site water exchange analysis. Magn Reson Med 2011;67: 1730–9.

106. Dhyani AH, Fan X, Leoni L, et al. Empirical mathematical model for dynamic manganese-enhanced MRI of the murine pancreas for assessment of β-cell function. Magn Reson Imaging 2013;31: 508–14.

107. Botsikas D, Terraz S, Vinet L, et al. Pancreatic magnetic resonance imaging after manganese injection distinguishes type 2 diabetic and normoglycemic patients. Islets 2012;4:243–8.

108. Jodal A, Schibli R, Béhé M. Targets and probes for non-invasive imaging of β-cells. Eur J Nucl Med Mol Imaging 2017;44:712–27.

109. Wild D, Béhé M, Wicki A, et al. [Lys⁴⁰ (Ahx-DTPA-¹¹¹In)NH₂]-exendin-4, a very promising ligand for glucagon-like peptide-1 (GLP-1) receptor targeting. J Nucl Med 2006;47:2025–33.

110. Christ E, Wild D, Ederer S, et al. Glucagon-like peptide-1 receptor imaging for the localisation of insulinomas: a prospective multicentre imaging study. Lancet Diabetes Endocrinol 2013;1: 115–22.

111. Sowa-Staszczak A, Pach D, Mikołajczak R, et al. Glucagon-like peptide-1 receptor imaging with [Lys⁴⁰ (Ahx-HYNIC- ⁹⁹ᵐTc/EDDA)NH2]-exendin- 4 for the detection of insulinoma. Eur J Nucl Med Mol Imaging 2013;40:524–31.

112. Wu Z, Todorov I, Li L, et al. In vivo imaging of transplanted islets with ⁶⁴Cu-DO3A-VS-Cys⁴⁰- exendin-4 by targeting GLP-1 receptor. Bioconjug Chem 2011;22:1587–94.

The Role of MR Imaging in Pancreatic Cancer

Priyanka Jha, MD[a], Benjamin M. Yeh, MD[a], Ronald Zagoria, MD[a], Eric Collisson, MD[b], Zhen J. Wang, MD[a],*

KEYWORDS

• Pancreas • Adenocarcinoma • Pancreatic neoplasm • MR imaging • Staging • Diagnosis

KEY POINTS

• The superior soft tissue contrast of MR imaging facilitates the detection of small, non–contour-deforming pancreas tumors that are suspected but remain occult on CT.
• MR imaging can serve as a problem-solving tool for characterizing indeterminate findings in the pancreas at CT.
• MR imaging can improve the detection and characterization of liver lesions in patients with pancreatic ductal adenocarcinoma, thereby improving the selection of appropriate surgical candidates.

INTRODUCTION

Pancreatic ductal adenocarcinoma (PDAC) is the third leading cause of cancer-related deaths in the United States and is anticipated to become second by 2030.[1] Accurate diagnosis and staging are pivotal for guiding treatment planning and potentially for improving outcome for patients with this malignancy. PDAC is particularly challenging to image, and meticulous technique is imperative to diagnose and stage this often subtle and infiltrative tumor. Although computed tomography (CT) is the established and most widely used modality for imaging PDAC, MR imaging can play an important role. This article reviews the MR imaging appearance of PDAC and its mimics, and the role of MR imaging in the diagnosis and staging of this disease.

MR IMAGING TECHNIQUES FOR IMAGING PANCREATIC DUCTAL ADENOCARCINOMA

A complete MR imaging evaluation of the pancreatic parenchyma and the pancreaticobiliary ductal system should include the following sequences: (1) T1-weighted dual-echo; (2) T2-weighted fast spin-echo or single-shot fast spin-echo; (3) 3-D magnetic resonance cholangiopancreatography (MRCP); and (4) T1-weighted fat suppressed 3D gradient-echo acquisition before and dynamically after intravenous administration of gadolinium-based contrast material. Additionally, diffusion-weighted imaging (DWI) is an increasingly used optional sequence that may improve the detection and characterization of pancreatic lesions. A suggested protocol for pancreas MR imaging is included in **Table 1**.

The characteristic MR imaging appearance of PDAC includes a hypoenhancing infiltrative pancreatic mass, abrupt ductal cutoff at the site of the mass, pancreatic ductal obstruction, and pancreatic atrophy (**Fig. 1**). The classic double duct sign may be seen in up to 77% cases of pancreatic head masses, which causes obstruction of both the pancreatic and bile ducts.[2] Masses in the uncinate process may present with no or minimal ductal dilation, and the uncinate process

Disclosure Statement: The authors have nothing to disclose.
[a] Department of Radiology and Biomedical Imaging, University of California, San Francisco, 505 Parnassus Avenue, San Francisco, CA 94143, USA; [b] Department of Medicine, University of California, San Francisco, 1825 4th Street, San Francisco, CA 94158, USA
* Corresponding author.
E-mail address: Zhen.Wang@ucsf.edu

Table 1
Suggested pancreatic MR imaging protocol

Sequences	Plane	Slice Thickness/Gap	Comments
2-D T2-weighted single-shot fast spin-echo	Axial and/or coronal	4–5 mm/no gap	Alternative: 2-D axial T2-weighted fast spin-echo
2-D T1-weighted gradient-echo in/opposed phase	Axial	5–6 mm/0.5–1 mm	Alternative: 3-D Dixon technique for in/opposed phase
3-D MRCP	Coronal	1.5 mm/no gap	
3-D T1-weighted SPGR with fat saturation, precontrast	Axial and coronal	3–4 mm/no gap	
3D T1-weighted SPGR with fat saturation, dynamic postcontrast	Axial and coronal	3–4 mm/no gap	Dynamic timing[a]: Axial: 20 s, 45 s, 90 s, 120 s Coronal: 300 s
DWI	Axial	5–6 mm/no gap	Suggested b-values: 0–50 s/mm^2, 400–500 s/mm^2, 800–1000 s/mm^2

Abbreviation: SPGR, spoiled gradient.
[a] If hepatobiliary contrast material such as gadoxetate disodium is used, further delayed imaging at hepatobiliary phase (15–20 min) would be added.

should always be carefully evaluated at imaging for presence of any subtle abnormalities.

One of the biggest strengths of MR imaging is the superior soft tissue contrast compared with other modalities, such as CT. This can be particularly useful when a patient is unable to get iodine-based CT contrast. MR imaging without gadolinium contrast can still provide important information on the abdominal organs including pancreas and liver. Normal pancreas has high signal on T1-weighted fat-suppressed images prior to contrast administration. The hyperintense signal has been attributed to aqueous proteinaceous contents of the gland; high content of paramagnetic ions, such as manganese; and high amounts of endoplasmic reticulum within the glandular tissue.[3,4] In contrast, PDAC is usually hypointense against the background of hyperintense parenchyma on T1-weighted sequences, thereby facilitating its visualization. Pancreatic duct obstruction by tumors can lead to pancreatitis in the obstructed gland, which may become hypointense relative to the unobstructed glandular tissue on T1-weighted images. On T2-weighted images,

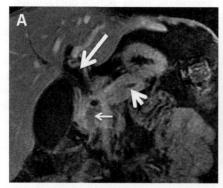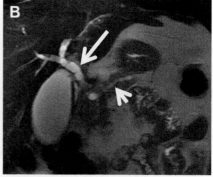

Fig. 1. Classic imaging appearance of PDAC in a 45-year-old man. (*A*) Coronal gadolinium-enhanced T1-weighted image shows a hypoenhancing mass (*thin arrow*) in the head of the pancreas with pancreatic duct dilatation (*short thick arrow*) and bile duct dilatation (*long thick arrow*). (*B*) Coronal T2-weighted single-shot fast spin-echo image shows the pancreatic duct dilatation (*short thick arrow*) and bile duct dilatation (*long thick arrow*), caused by the obstructing mass, to better advantage.

the obstructed portions of the gland may become relatively hyperintense due to edema from the underlying pancreatitis.

Dynamic contrast-enhanced imaging is an important component of a pancreas MR imaging. It provides detailed delineation of the vasculature and its relationship to the tumor; this is critical for determining resectability in PDAC and is discussed later. Dynamic imaging also allows optimal visualization of the primary tumors and liver metastases. The primary PDAC is most conspicuous during the pancreatic parenchymal phase of enhancement, at 45 seconds to 60 seconds after the start of the contrast injection, when the hypovascular PDAC appears as a hypointense mass in contrast to the avidly enhancing normal pancreatic parenchyma. PDACs usually remain hypoenhancing on the portal venous phase (approximately 70–100 seconds). Hepatic metastases, when present, are hypovascular and are best detected in the portal venous phase. Given the desmoplastic nature of PDAC, the tumors may demonstrate delayed enhancement at several minutes after contrast administration due to the delayed enhancement of the stromal fibrosis.[5] Although not specifically evaluated for MR imaging, a prior study reported that 3-minute delayed-phase CT imaging improved visualization of PDACs that are isoattenuating at pancreatic parenchymal phase.[6]

Highly T2-weighted MRCP images facilitate the delineation of ductal anatomy.[7] The site of abrupt cutoff and upstream pancreatic ductal dilatation can be easily visualized, and this area of duct transition should be scrutinized for obstructing lesions.[2,7,8] Lack of ductal cutoff and duct dilatation in the presence of a visible pancreatic mass should point to alternate diagnoses, such as pancreatic neuroendocrine tumors or lymphoma, which usually cause less mass effect than PDAC. By providing an accurate depiction of pancreaticobiliary obstruction, MRCP images also provide depiction of duct anatomy for stent placement and/or external biliary drainage.[7]

DWI has shown promise for the evaluation of PDAC. PDACs commonly restrict diffusion and appear hyperintense relative to adjacent parenchyma on DWI sequences. A prior study has shown that high b-value DWI provided a sensitivity and specificity of 96% and 99%, respectively, for the diagnosis of PDAC.[9] Another study has also reported high diagnostic performance of DWI for detection of PDACs, and DWI with a b-value of 500 s/mm^2 was equivalent to gadolinium-enhanced MR imaging for PDAC diagnosis.[10] Additionally, the addition of DWI findings to contrast-enhanced MR imaging may improve the detection of small liver metastases[11,12] and potentially improve the selection of patients with resectable tumors.

ROLE OF MR IMAGING IN PANCREATIC DUCTAL ADENOCARCINOMA DIAGNOSIS
Detection of Small, Non–Contour-Deforming Tumors Occult on Computed Tomography

Although CT is the most commonly used modality for the diagnosis of PDAC, MR imaging can play an important role. The superior soft tissue contrast of conventional MR imaging as well as DWI facilitates the detection of small, non–contour-deforming tumors, which may be occult on CT, as illustrated in **Figs. 2** and **3**. A recent study has reported that the addition of DWI to conventional MR imaging improves the sensitivity for small PDAC detection.[13] Some PDACs are poorly visualized, however,

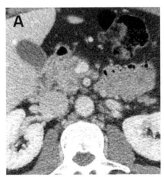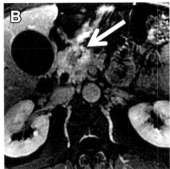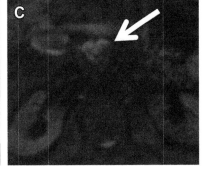

Fig. 2. CT occult tumor demonstrated on MR imaging in a 54-year-old woman with PDAC. (*A*) Axial contrast-enhanced CT shows no visible mass in the pancreatic head, although there is pancreatic duct dilation in the body and tail (not shown). (*B*) Axial gadolinium-enhanced T1-weighted MR imaging shows a small hypoenhancing mass (*arrow*) in the pancreatic head that was proven to be PDAC at surgery. (*C*) Axial DWI (b-value of 800 s/mm^2) shows the mass (*arrow*) to be hyperintense, consistent with diffusion restriction.

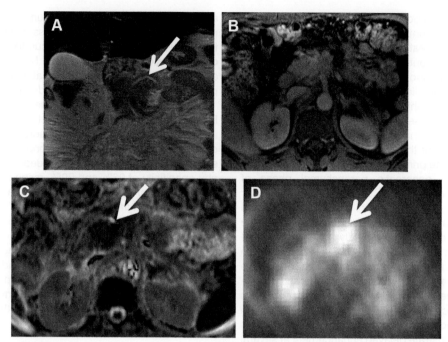

Fig. 3. PDAC demonstrated by restricted diffusion in a 53-year-old man with abdominal pain and weight loss. (*A*) Coronal T2-weighted image shows pancreatic duct dilatation (*arrow*) in the body and tail. (*B*) Axial gadolinium-enhanced T1-weighted image shows no visible tumors in the pancreatic head. (*C*) Axial ADC map derived from DWI shows low ADC lesion (*arrow*) in the pancreatic head, consistent with restricted diffusion from a pancreatic head PDAC that was subsequently biopsy proved. (*D*) ^{18}F-FDG–PET shows increased ^{18}F-FDG uptake (*arrow*) in the pancreatic head, again consistent with a PDAC.

despite optimal MR imaging techniques. In some cases, the only findings are pancreatic ductal dilation with abrupt cutoff of the dilated duct, which may be better seen on the heavily T2-weighted MRCP than CT. Isolated obstruction of the pancreatic duct, even in the absence of a visible mass, should be viewed with great suspicion for the possibility of an underlying tumor.[14] Such cases mandate close surveillance and potentially endoscopic ultrasound.

Characterizing Indeterminate Pancreatic Findings at Computed Tomography

MR imaging can serve as a problem-solving tool in cases of indeterminate findings in the pancreas at CT. For example, focal fatty infiltration of the pancreas can occasionally mimic PDAC on CT due to its hypodense appearance. On MR imaging, fatty filtration manifests as decreased signal intensity with fat suppression and signal drop on opposed-phased images (**Fig. 4**). These features

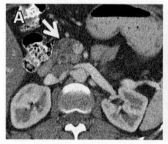 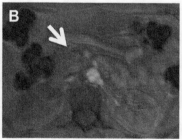 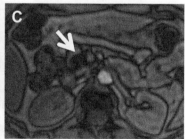

Fig. 4. MR imaging diagnosis of focal fat infiltration that mimicked PDAC on CT in a 40-year-old woman with abdominal pain. (*A*) Axial contrast-enhanced CT shows a subtle focal area of low density in the pancreatic head (*arrow*) that can mimic a PDAC. Axial T1-weighted in-phase (*B*) and opposed-phase (*C*) images show signal drop in the pancreatic head on the opposed-phase MR imaging relative to the in-phase MR imaging (*arrow*), confirming that the low-density area on CT represents fatty infiltration.

allow a confident diagnosis of fatty infiltration and distinguish it from cancer.

Differentiation from Other Mimics of Pancreatic Ductal Adenocarcinoma

Focal chronic pancreatitis can mimic PDACs. Several findings on MR imaging have been suggested to aid in the differentiation between the 2. For example, the duct penetrating sign and the icicle sign at MRCP have been reported to support a diagnosis of focal pancreatitis.[15,16] The duct penetrating sign refers to a nonobstructed main pancreatic duct penetrating an apparent pancreatic mass. The icicle sign describes a smooth tapered narrowing of the pancreatic duct upstream from a pancreatic mass. In contrast, an abrupt cutoff of a dilated pancreatic duct by a mass favors a PDAC. Homogenous enhancement after gadolinium contrast administration, and low apparent diffusion coefficient (ADC) values have also been reported to favor focal chronic pancreatitis over PDAC.[17–19] Reliable differentiation between the 2 remains difficult, however, given the overlapping imaging features. Furthermore, chronic pancreatitis is a known risk factor for developing PDAC. Therefore, despite best imaging techniques, biopsy may be necessary for a definitive diagnosis.

Pancreatic neuroendocrine tumors can occasionally mimic PDACs when they do not demonstrate typical arterial enhancement. Useful MR imaging features that may distinguish nonhypervascular pancreatic neuroendocrine tumors from PDACs include a well-defined margin and portal hyperenhancement or isoenhancement[20] (Fig. 5). In contrast, PDACs are usually infiltrative and remain hypoenhancing on the portovenous phase (Fig. 6).

With known extrapancreatic malignancy, pancreatic metastases should be considered in the differential of a pancreatic mass. Metastases are usually T2 hyperintense, and metastases from hypervascular primary tumors, such as renal cell carcinoma and melanoma, are typically hypervascular,[21] distinctly different from the hypovascular appearance of PDACs. Primary pancreatic lymphoma is uncommon.[22] Focal lymphomatous involvement of the gland presents as a homogeneously T1-hypointense mass, which mildly enhances after contrast administration. Ductal dilation, if present, is usually mild.[23]

Screening of Patients at High Risk for Pancreatic Ductal Adenocarcinoma

There is increasing interest in screening for PDAC because of the recognition of various high-risk patient groups and the relatively favorable prognosis of small asymptomatic tumors.[24–29] Most of the screening programs have focused on patients with a familial or genetic predisposition to PDAC,

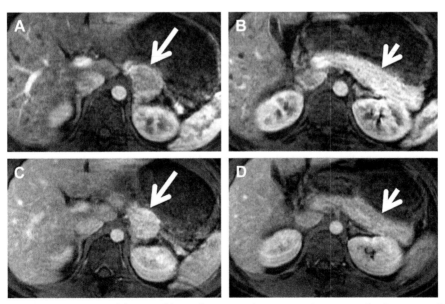

Fig. 5. MR imaging in a 24-year-old man with nonhypervascular pancreatic neuroendocrine tumor. (*A*, *B*) Axial T1-weighted MR imaging obtained during the arterial phase shows a well-defined exophytic pancreatic tumor that is hypoenhancing (*arrow* [*A*]) relative to the normal pancreas (*arrow* [*B*]). (*C*, *D*) Axial T1-weighted MR imaging obtained during the portovenous phase shows the tumor to be hyperenhancing (*arrow* [*C*]) relative to the normal pancreas (*arrow* [*D*]).

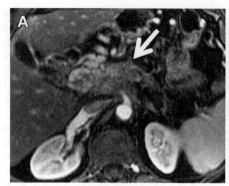 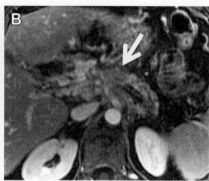

Fig. 6. Classic hypovascular infiltrative PDAC in a 63-year-old woman. (*A*) Axial gadolinium-enhanced T1-weighted MR obtained during arterial phase shows infiltrative hypoenhancing pancreatic body tumor (*arrow*) with tumor encasement of the celiac artery. (*B*) Axial gadolinium-enhanced T1-weighted MR obtained during portovenous phase shows persistent hypoenhancement of the tumor (*arrow*).

including those with familial pancreatic cancer, Peutz-Jeghers syndrome, familial atypical multiple mole melanoma, and hereditary breast and ovarian cancer. The target lesions for screening include both precursor lesions, such as intraductal papillary mucinous tumor and small solid pancreatic lesions. MR imaging is a key imaging modality for screening for these lesions in high-risk patients. In an MR imaging–based screening trial of 40 high-risk patients with a median follow-up of approximately 1 year, the overall rate of MR imaging–detected early cancer was 7.5%.[30] In another study, MR imaging with MRCP was used for screening of 79 high-risk patients; imaging detected early cancer in 9% of patients during a median 4 year follow-up.[31] Comparative studies have suggested that MR imaging and endoscopic ultrasound have a complementary role in pancreatic cancer screening,[28] and both are superior to CT for screening high-risk patients.[32]

ROLE OF MR IMAGING IN PANCREATIC DUCTAL ADENOCARCINOMA STAGING

Although surgery remains the only potential cure for patients with PDAC, only 15% to 20% of them have potentially resectable disease at the time of diagnosis.[33] Patients with margin-positive resection (either residual microscopic or macroscopic disease) have similar prognosis compared with patients with metastatic disease and, therefore, would not benefit from surgery.[34] Therefore, accurate staging is critical in identifying potentially resectable patients and preventing others from undergoing unnecessary surgery.

CT is the most commonly used modality for PDAC staging. Studies have shown, however, that MR imaging and multidetector CT have similar performance in the local staging of PDACs.[35,36]

MR imaging improves detection of hepatic metastases and characterization of CT-indeterminate liver lesions,[37,38] which in turn improves the determination of resectability. A recent study showed that in patients with potentially resectable PDAC, preoperative MR imaging detected hepatic metastases in 5% of the patients who did not have any liver lesions seen CT and in 32% of patients with indeterminate liver lesions at CT.[37] MR imaging with hepatobiliary contrast may further improve the detection of small liver metastases compared with CT.[38] Hepatobiliary contrast agents, such as gadoxetate disodium (Eovist), can increase the conspicuity of liver metastases by increasing the contrast between normal liver that is enhanced by the uptake of the hepatobiliary contrast and the hypointense liver metastases. The reported sensitivity of Eovist-enhanced liver MR imaging is 85% for detecting liver metastasis from PDAC, which is significantly higher compared with that of contrast-enhanced CT (69%).[38] Another study showed that Eovist-enhanced liver MR imaging was useful in detecting tiny PDAC liver metastases that were missed by CT.[39]

Factors that influence the resectability of PDAC include arterial and venous vascular invasion, locoregional spread, and distant metastases. The criteria for resectability are reviewed elsewhere.[40–42] In the absence of metastatic disease, PDACs are classified into 3 main groups: resectable, borderline-resectable, and locally advanced. Assessment of vascular involvement by the tumor is key in the local tumor staging and determination of resectability. Standardization of the reporting of PDAC staging at imaging is also critical in the care of these patients. A consensus statement on a standardized reporting template for imaging in PDAC was published recently.[43]

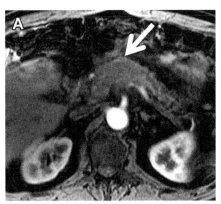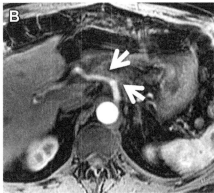

Fig. 7. Vascular involvement in a 63-year-old man with PDAC. (*A*) Gadolinium-enhanced T1-weighted MR image shows hypovascular tumor (*arrow*) in the pancreatic body with pancreatic duct dilatation and atrophy in the pancreatic tail. (*B*) Gadolinium-enhanced T1-weighted MR image at a slightly superior location shows tumor abutting the distal celiac artery and proximal common hepatic artery (*arrows*).

Vascular Involvement

Although institutional variations in criteria for resectability exist, encasement (>180° tumor contact) of celiac artery, common hepatic artery, or the superior mesenteric artery usually renders a tumor unresectable.[40] **Figs. 7** and **8** show examples of arterial involvement by PDAC on MR imaging. Variant arterial anatomy should also be noted to provide a road map for the surgeons. Among the multiple arterial variants, the presence of a replaced right hepatic artery arising from the superior mesenteric artery should be noted because this variant courses closely behind the pancreatic head and can be involved by tumor.

MR imaging features of venous involvement include occlusion, irregular vein contour, such as beaking, and more than 180° tumor contact of

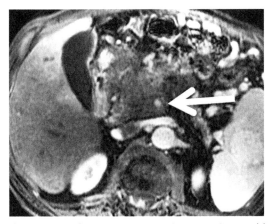

Fig. 8. Vascular encasement in a 76-year-old woman with advanced PDAC. Gadolinium-enhanced T1-weighted MR image shows complete encasement of the superior mesenteric artery by the tumor (*arrow*).

the vein. Venous involvement that would preclude resection in PDAC patients include portal vein (PV) or superior mesenteric vein (SMV) occlusion without the possibility of reconstruction.[44] For example, thrombosis of the PV and SMV with tumor extending to major branches of the SMV is considered unresectable. Multiple jejunal branches inserting high on the SMV near the PV may also preclude an adequate proximal surgical margin and vein reconstruction.

Locoregional Nodal Disease

Lymph nodes are commonly well seen on T2-weighted fat-suppressed images and DWI, with the nodes appearing hyperintense on both of these sequences. Determination of lymph node involvement, however, using conventional size criteria (1 cm as the threshold) have both high false-positive and false-negative rates with all imaging modalities, including MR imaging. The location of lymph node metastases affects resectability and prognosis for PDAC. The peripancreatic lymph nodes involved by PDAC are considered regional nodal disease and are typically dissected during PDAC resection. In contrast, identification of lymph nodes outside of the usual surgical field, such as in the para-aortic region, is usually considered distant nodal metastatic disease with poor prognosis.[45]

Metastatic Disease

After lymph nodes, liver is the second most common site for PDAC metastases. The detection of liver metastases is crucial for PDAC staging because the presence of liver metastases renders the tumor unresectable and prevents unnecessary surgery. With CT, small (<1cm) hypodense liver

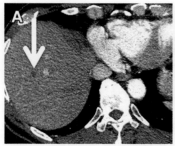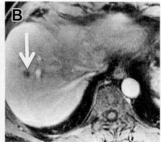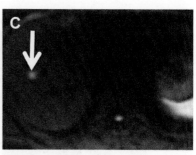

Fig. 9. A 68-year-old man with liver metastases from PDAC. (*A*) Staging contrast-enhanced CT shows a small and indeterminate hypodensity (*arrow*) in the liver dome. (*B*) Gadolinium-enhanced MR imaging obtained 3 days later shows a corresponding hypoenhancing lesion with thick rim enhancement (*arrow*), highly suspicious for metastasis from PDAC. Multiple other similar liver lesions were seen on the MR imaging that were not seen on the CT. (*C*) DWI (b-value of 800 s/mm^2) shows the lesion to be hyperintense (*arrow*), consistent with restricted diffusion and with metastases.

lesions are frequently difficult to characterize. In additional, small liver metastases can be inconspicuous and missed with CT.[37–39] MR imaging can aid in the detection and characterization of liver lesions as cysts, hemangiomas versus metastases (**Figs. 9 and 10**), thereby potentially altering patient management. Hepatic metastases from PDAC are usually hypointense on T1-weighted images and slightly hyperintense on T2-weighted images. They are hypovascular and typically show ring enhancement after gadolinium contrast administration. For extracellular gadolinium contrast agents, the portal venous phase is the ideal phase for detecting the hypovascular metastases. For hepatobiliary contrast agents, the additional delayed hepatobiliary phase may further improve the conspicuity of liver metastases.[46]

Peritoneal metastases from PDAC can occur with advanced disease and this area should be carefully evaluated in all cases. Peritoneal disease can manifest as multifocal peritoneal nodules or diffuse peritoneal thickening. Bowel motion and susceptibility caused by bowel gas can make the detection of peritoneal disease a challenge at MR imaging. The addition of DWI and gadolinium-enhanced MR imaging has been shown to improve the sensitivity and specificity for depicting peritoneal disease.[47] **Fig. 11** shows an example of peritoneal metastases from PDAC at MR imaging.

ROLE OF MR IMAGING IN PANCREATIC DUCTAL ADENOCARCINOMA RESPONSE MONITORING

Treatment response in PDAC is commonly assessed by evaluating tumor size with anatomic imaging using CT or MR imaging. Change in tumor size is a relatively late endpoint in PDAC treatment response, however. Several studies have

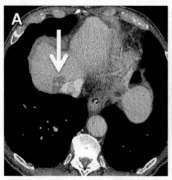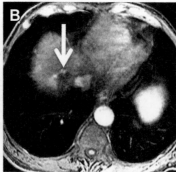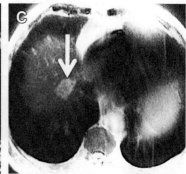

Fig. 10. Improved liver mass characterization with MRI in a 77-year-old man with locally advanced PDAC. (*A*) Staging contrast-enhanced CT shows a predominantly low-density lesion (*arrow*) in the liver dome, with questionable peripheral nodular enhancement, that is indeterminate on this staging CT. (*B*) Subsequent gadolinium-enhanced MR imaging shows the lesion (*arrow*) with peripheral discontinuous nodular enhancement to better advantage. (*C*) T2-weighted MR image shows the lesion to be significantly T2 hyperintense (*arrow*). The combinations of the MR imaging findings are diagnostic of a benign hepatic hemangioma.

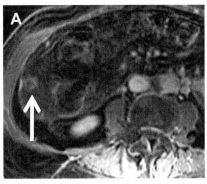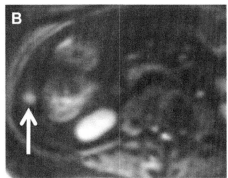

Fig. 11. Peritoneal metastasis in a 76-year-old woman with PDAC. (*A*) Gadolinium-enhanced MR image shows enhancing nodule along the right peritoneum (*arrow*), consistent with a peritoneal implant. (*B*) DWI (b-value of 800 s/mm^2) shows the nodule to be hyperintense (*arrow*), consistent with diffusion restriction.

suggested a role of DWI for response assessment in PDAC. ADC changes obtained from DWI have been reported to be potentially predictive of early progression in patients with nonresectable PDAC,[48] and low tumor ADC values at baseline may predict poor response to chemo-radiation in a small pilot study.[49] More recently, ADCs have been shown to predict progression-free survival and overall survival in patients with unresectable PDAC.[50] Although not currently standard clinical practice, these initial studies show the possibility of adding functional imaging to anatomic MR imaging for treatment response evaluation in PDAC. If validated in larger series, multiparametric MR imaging has the potential to minimize the toxicities of ineffective treatment and allow earlier adaptation of management for PDAC patients.

FUTURE DIRECTIONS

The integrated PET–MR imaging is a promising hybrid imaging technology that combines the metabolic information obtained from PET with superior soft tissue contrast and other functional information from MR imaging. It has generated much interest in the imaging community, especially for oncological imaging. In the case of PDAC, a recent study has shown that fluorodeoxyglucose (^{18}F-FDG) PET–MR imaging is feasible and has similar diagnostic performance compared with ^{18}F-FDG–PET plus contrast-enhanced multidetector CT for preoperative staging and evaluation of resectability.[51] Another recent study showed that the integrated PET–MR imaging may predict clinical stage and progression-free survival in patients with PDAC or periampullary cancer.[52] Given the multiple prior studies that have reported on the value of ^{18}F-FDG–PET and DWI in PDAC prognosis and response monitoring,[48–50,53–55] the integrated PET–MR imaging

has the potential to allow earlier and more effective therapy-response assessment for this disease. Additional potential applications for PDAC that take advantage of the integrated PET–MR imaging include the detection of recurrent and metastatic disease. Many more studies are needed to evaluate such potential benefits of this hybrid technology in the context of PDAC.

SUMMARY

Given the wide availability and the rapid image acquisition, CT is likely to remain the main modality in the imaging evaluation of PDAC. MR imaging plays an important and complementary role in this disease, however, for example, in patients who cannot receive iodinated contrast, for visualizing small primary tumors that are suspected but remain occult on CT and for the detection and characterization of liver lesions. The recent advances in hybrid imaging that combines MR imaging with PET have the potential to provide prognostic and predictive biomarkers that can further improve the oncological care in patients with PDAC.

REFERENCES

1. Rahib L, Smith BD, Aizenberg R, et al. Projecting cancer incidence and deaths to 2030: the unexpected burden of thyroid, liver, and pancreas cancers in the United States. Cancer Res 2014;74: 2913–21.
2. Ahualli J. The double duct sign. Radiology 2007; 244:314–5.
3. Ly JN, Miller FH. MR imaging of the pancreas: a practical approach. Radiol Clin North Am 2002;40: 1289–306.
4. Semelka RC, Ascher SM. MR imaging of the pancreas. Radiology 1993;188:593–602.

5. Hata H, Mori H, Matsumoto S, et al. Fibrous stroma and vascularity of pancreatic carcinoma: correlation with enhancement patterns on CT. Abdom Imaging 2010;35:172–80.

6. Ishigami K, Yoshimitsu K, Irie H, et al. Diagnostic value of the delayed phase image for iso-attenuating pancreatic carcinomas in the pancreatic parenchymal phase on multidetector computed tomography. Eur J Radiol 2009;69:139–46.

7. Schindera ST, Merkle EM. MR cholangiopancreatography: 1.5T versus 3T. Magn Reson Imaging Clin N Am 2007;15:355–64, vi–vii.

8. Lopez Hänninen E, Amthauer H, Hosten N, et al. Prospective evaluation of pancreatic tumors: accuracy of MR imaging with MR cholangiopancreatography and MR angiography. Radiology 2002;224:34–41.

9. Ichikawa T, Erturk SM, Motosugi U, et al. High-b value diffusion-weighted MRI for detecting pancreatic adenocarcinoma: preliminary results. AJR Am J Roentgenol 2007;188:409–14.

10. Kartalis N, Lindholm TL, Aspelin P, et al. Diffusion-weighted magnetic resonance imaging of pancreas tumours. Eur Radiol 2009;19:1981–90.

11. Kim YK, Lee MW, Lee WJ, et al. Diagnostic accuracy and sensitivity of diffusion-weighted and of gadoxetic acid-enhanced 3-T MR imaging alone or in combination in the detection of small liver metastasis (≤1.5 cm in diameter). Invest Radiol 2012;47:159–66.

12. Nasu K, Kuroki Y, Nawano S, et al. Hepatic metastases: diffusion-weighted sensitivity-encoding versus SPIO-enhanced MR imaging. Radiology 2006;239: 122–30.

13. Park MJ, Kim YK, Choi SY, et al. Preoperative detection of small pancreatic carcinoma: value of adding diffusion-weighted imaging to conventional MR imaging for improving confidence level. Radiology 2014;273:433–43.

14. Gangi S, Fletcher JG, Nathan MA, et al. Time interval between abnormalities seen on CT and the clinical diagnosis of pancreatic cancer: retrospective review of CT scans obtained before diagnosis. AJR Am J Roentgenol 2004;182:897–903.

15. Ichikawa T, Sou H, Araki T, et al. Duct-penetrating sign at MRCP: usefulness for differentiating inflammatory pancreatic mass from pancreatic carcinomas. Radiology 2001;221:107–16.

16. Kim HJ, Kim YK, Jeong WK, et al. Pancreatic duct "icicle sign" on MRI for distinguishing autoimmune pancreatitis from pancreatic ductal adenocarcinoma in the proximal pancreas. Eur Radiol 2015;25:1551–60.

17. Choi SY, Kim SH, Kang TW, et al. Differentiating mass-forming autoimmune pancreatitis from pancreatic ductal adenocarcinoma on the basis of contrast-enhanced MRI and DWI findings. AJR Am J Roentgenol 2016;206:291–300.

18. Lee SS, Byun JH, Park BJ, et al. Quantitative analysis of diffusion-weighted magnetic resonance imaging of the pancreas: usefulness in characterizing solid pancreatic masses. J Magn Reson Imaging 2008;28:928–36.

19. Fattahi R, Balci NC, Perman WH, et al. Pancreatic diffusion-weighted imaging (DWI): comparison between mass-forming focal pancreatitis (FP), pancreatic cancer (PC), and normal pancreas. J Magn Reson Imaging 2009;29:350–6.

20. Jeon SK, Lee JM, Joo I, et al. Nonhypervascular pancreatic neuroendocrine tumors: differential diagnosis from pancreatic ductal adenocarcinomas at MR imaging-retrospective cross-sectional study. Radiology 2017;284:77–87.

21. Palmowski M, Hacke N, Satzl S, et al. Metastasis to the pancreas: characterization by morphology and contrast enhancement features on CT and MRI. Pancreatology 2008;8:199–203.

22. Rad N, Khafaf A, Mohammad Alizadeh AH, et al. Primary pancreatic lymphoma: what we need to know. J Gastrointest Oncol 2017;8:749–57.

23. Anand D, Lall C, Bhosale P, et al. Current update on primary pancreatic lymphoma. Abdom Radiol (NY) 2016;41:347–55.

24. Wada K, Takaori K, Traverso LW. Screening for pancreatic cancer. Surg Clin North Am 2015;95: 1041–52.

25. Becker AE, Hernandez YG, Frucht H, et al. Pancreatic ductal adenocarcinoma: risk factors, screening, and early detection. World J Gastroenterol 2014;20: 11182–98.

26. Lu C, Xu CF, Wan XY, et al. Screening for pancreatic cancer in familial high-risk individuals: a systematic review. World J Gastroenterol 2015;21:8678–86.

27. Al-Sukhni W, Borgida A, Rothenmund H, et al. Screening for pancreatic cancer in a high-risk cohort: an eight-year experience. J Gastrointest Surg 2012;16:771–83.

28. Harinck F, Konings IC, Kluijt I, et al. A multicentre comparative prospective blinded analysis of EUS and MRI for screening of pancreatic cancer in high-risk individuals. Gut 2016;65:1505–13.

29. Verna EC, Hwang C, Stevens PD, et al. Pancreatic cancer screening in a prospective cohort of high-risk patients: a comprehensive strategy of imaging and genetics. Clin Cancer Res 2010;16: 5028–37.

30. Del Chiaro M, Verbeke CS, Kartalis N, et al. Short-term results of a magnetic resonance imaging-based swedish screening program for individuals at risk for pancreatic cancer. JAMA Surg 2015;150: 512–8.

31. Vasen HF, Wasser M, van Mil A, et al. Magnetic resonance imaging surveillance detects early-stage pancreatic cancer in carriers of a p16-Leiden mutation. Gastroenterology 2011;140:850–6.

32. Canto MI, Hruban RH, Fishman EK, et al. Frequent detection of pancreatic lesions in asymptomatic

high-risk individuals. Gastroenterology 2012;142: 796–804 [quiz: e14–5].

33. Conlon KC, Klimstra DS, Brennan MF. Long-term survival after curative resection for pancreatic ductal adenocarcinoma. Clinicopathologic analysis of 5-year survivors. Ann Surg 1996;223:273–9.

34. Han SS, Jang JY, Kim SW, et al. Analysis of long-term survivors after surgical resection for pancreatic cancer. Pancreas 2006;32:271–5.

35. Chen FM, Ni JM, Zhang ZY, et al. Presurgical evaluation of pancreatic cancer: a comprehensive imaging comparison of CT versus MRI. AJR Am J Roentgenol 2016;206:526–35.

36. Park HS, Lee JM, Choi HK, et al. Preoperative evaluation of pancreatic cancer: comparison of gadolinium-enhanced dynamic MRI with MR cholangiopancreatography versus MDCT. J Magn Reson Imaging 2009;30:586–95.

37. Kim HW, Lee JC, Paik KH, et al. Adjunctive role of preoperative liver magnetic resonance imaging for potentially resectable pancreatic cancer. Surgery 2017;161:1579–87.

38. Motosugi U, Ichikawa T, Morisaka H, et al. Detection of pancreatic carcinoma and liver metastases with gadoxetic acid-enhanced MR imaging: comparison with contrast-enhanced multi-detector row CT. Radiology 2011;260:446–53.

39. Ito T, Sugiura T, Okamura Y, et al. The diagnostic advantage of EOB-MR imaging over CT in the detection of liver metastasis in patients with potentially resectable pancreatic cancer. Pancreatology 2017;17:451–6.

40. Callery MP, Chang KJ, Fishman EK, et al. Pretreatment assessment of resectable and borderline resectable pancreatic cancer: expert consensus statement. Ann Surg Oncol 2009;16:1727–33.

41. Bockhorn M, Uzunoglu FG, Adham M, et al. Borderline resectable pancreatic cancer: a consensus statement by the International Study Group of Pancreatic Surgery (ISGPS). Surgery 2014;155: 977–88.

42. Tempero MA, Malafa MP, Al-Hawary M, et al. Pancreatic adenocarcinoma, version 2.2017, NCCN clinical practice guidelines in oncology. J Natl Compr Canc Netw 2017;15:1028–61.

43. Al-Hawary MM, Francis IR, Chari ST, et al. Pancreatic ductal adenocarcinoma radiology reporting template: consensus statement of the Society of Abdominal Radiology and the American Pancreatic Association. Radiology 2014;270:248–60.

44. Ly DL, Thipphavong S, Sreeharsha B. Pictorial review of vascular involvement and complex vascular reconstructions in borderline to minimally advanced pancreatic malignancies. Abdom Radiol (NY) 2017; 42(11):2675–85.

45. Agalianos C, Gouvas N, Papaparaskeva K, et al. Positive para-aortic lymph nodes following pancreatectomy for pancreatic cancer. Systematic review and meta-analysis of impact on short term survival and association with clinicopathologic features. HPB (Oxford) 2016;18:633–41.

46. Jeong HT, Kim MJ, Park MS, et al. Detection of liver metastases using gadoxetic-enhanced dynamic and 10- and 20-minute delayed phase MR imaging. J Magn Reson Imaging 2012;35:635–43.

47. Low RN, Sebrechts CP, Barone RM, et al. Diffusion-weighted MRI of peritoneal tumors: comparison with conventional MRI and surgical and histopathologic findings–a feasibility study. AJR Am J Roentgenol 2009;193:461–70.

48. Niwa T, Ueno M, Ohkawa S, et al. Advanced pancreatic cancer: the use of the apparent diffusion coefficient to predict response to chemotherapy. Br J Radiol 2009;82:28–34.

49. Cuneo KC, Chenevert TL, Ben-Josef E, et al. A pilot study of diffusion-weighted MRI in patients undergoing neoadjuvant chemoradiation for pancreatic cancer. Transl Oncol 2014;7:644–9.

50. Nishiofuku H, Tanaka T, Marugami N, et al. Increased tumour ADC value during chemotherapy predicts improved survival in unresectable pancreatic cancer. Eur Radiol 2016;26:1835–42.

51. Joo I, Lee JM, Lee DH, et al. Preoperative assessment of pancreatic cancer with FDG PET/MR imaging versus FDG PET/CT plus contrast-enhanced multidetector CT: a prospective preliminary study. Radiology 2017;282:149–59.

52. Chen BB, Tien YW, Chang MC, et al. PET/MRI in pancreatic and periampullary cancer: correlating diffusion-weighted imaging, MR spectroscopy and glucose metabolic activity with clinical stage and prognosis. Eur J Nucl Med Mol Imaging 2016;43: 1753–64.

53. Asagi A, Ohta K, Nasu J, et al. Utility of contrast-enhanced FDG-PET/CT in the clinical management of pancreatic cancer: impact on diagnosis, staging, evaluation of treatment response, and detection of recurrence. Pancreas 2013;42:11–9.

54. Kittaka H, Takahashi H, Ohigashi H, et al. Role of (18)F-fluorodeoxyglucose positron emission tomography/computed tomography in predicting the pathologic response to preoperative chemoradiation therapy in patients with resectable T3 pancreatic cancer. World J Surg 2013;37:169–78.

55. Chang JS, Choi SH, Lee Y, et al. Clinical usefulness of ^{18}F-fluorodeoxyglucose-positron emission tomography in patients with locally advanced pancreatic cancer planned to undergo concurrent chemoradiation therapy. Int J Radiat Oncol Biol Phys 2014;90: 126–33.

Genetics of Pancreatic Neoplasms and Role of Screening

Venkata S. Katabathina, MD[a], Omid Y. Rikhtehgar, MD[a],
Anil K. Dasyam, MD[b], Rohan Manickam, BS[c],
Srinivasa R. Prasad, MD[c],*

KEYWORDS

- Genomics • Pancreatic ductal adenocarcinoma • Neuroendocrine neoplasm
- Solid-pseudopapillary tumor • Serous cystadenoma • Screening

KEY POINTS

- A diverse group of histobiologically and genetically distinct tumors arise from the exocrine and endocrine components of the pancreas.
- Pancreatic adenocarcinoma, the most common and most lethal pancreatic malignancy, originates from microscopic and macroscopic precursors that are mainly characterized by *KRAS* mutations.
- Pancreatic neuroendocrine neoplasms are primarily characterized by germline or somatic mutations involving *MEN-1, TSC 1/2, ATRX,* and *DAXX* genes. Activating somatic mutations in *CTNNB1* occur in 95% of solid-pseudopapillary neoplasms.
- Detailed studies of hereditary pancreatic tumor syndromes have thrown fresh light on the frequency/relevance of genetic abnormalities, tumor pathways, tumor biology, and prognostic significance of the more common sporadic tumors.
- Current recommendations for screening of pancreatic neoplasms pertain to high-risk individuals, primarily patients with a familial and hereditary predisposition to early and frequent tumor development.

INTRODUCTION

The broad spectrum of pancreatic neoplasms may be classified based on the direction of cellular differentiation into exocrine and endocrine tumors. Pancreatic ductal adenocarcinoma (PDAC), the most lethal pancreatic cancer, comprises 90% of all malignant neoplasms. Pancreatic neuroendocrine tumors (PanNET) account for 5% of pancreatic tumors, and rarer solid pseudopapillary neoplasms (SPNs) and acinar cell carcinomas (ACC) constitute 1% to 2% of tumors. Although most tumors are sporadic in nature, up to 10% of tumors occur in the setting of hereditary syndromes that predispose to early onset development of characteristic tumor phenotypes. For example, although patients with Lynch syndrome (LS) show an increased propensity to develop the rare medullary variant of PDAC, PanNET tumors occur more frequently in patients with multiple endocrine neoplasia (MEN)-1 syndrome, von Hippel-Lindau (VHL) disease, type 1

[a] Department of Radiology, University of Texas Health Science Center at San Antonio, 7703 Floyd Curl Drive, San Antonio, TX 78229, USA; [b] Department of Radiology, University of Pittsburgh Medical Center, 200 Lothrop Street, Pittsburgh, PA 15213, USA; [c] Department of Radiology, The University of Texas MD Anderson Cancer Center, 1400 Pressler street, Unit 1473, Houston, TX 77030, USA
* Corresponding author. Department of Radiology, MD Anderson Cancer Center, 1400 Pressler Street, Unit 1473, Houston, TX 77030.
E-mail address: sprasad2@mdanderson.org

Magn Reson Imaging Clin N Am 26 (2018) 375–389
https://doi.org/10.1016/j.mric.2018.03.005

neurofibromatosis (NF-1), and tuberous sclerosis complex (TSC). Patients with VHL disease develop serous cystadenomas and PanNET tumors. This article provides a broad overview of the genetic landscape of a diverse spectrum of pancreatic tumors (**Table 1**), a synopsis of characteristic hereditary syndromes with specific pancreatic tumors (**Tables 2** and **3**), and current recommendations for screening in high-risk individuals (**Box 1**).

PANCREATIC DUCTAL ADENOCARCINOMA

PDAC, the most common pancreatic malignant neoplasm, is the most lethal pancreatic malignancy

Table 1
Summary of epidemiology and genomic landscape of pancreatic neoplasms

Tumor (Prevalence, Comments)	Gene (Prevalence)	Comments	Average Number (Mutations)
Ductal adenocarcinoma (90%; mean age, 66 y; M:F, 3:2)	*KRAS* (95%) *P16/CDKN2A* (95%) *TP53* (75%) *SMAD4/DPC4* (55%)	Marker of PanIN Marker of high-grade dysplasia Marker of high-grade dysplasia	26–63
IPMN (median age, 66 y; more common in men; 25%–50% of resected cystic pancreatic lesions; two-thirds of tumors in the head region)	*KRAS* (80%) *GNAS* (60%) *RNF43* (60%) *p16/CDKN2A* *TP53* *SMAD4/DPC4* *PIK3CA* (10%) *STK11/LKB1* (5%)	Intestinal type, colloid *p16* loss (10% noninvasive; 100% invasive) SMAD4 loss (one-third invasive)	26
Mucinous cystic neoplasm (perimenopausal women; 40–60 y; F:M, 20:1; 95% in pancreatic body/tail; low malignant potential in cyst <4 cm)	*KRAS* (80%) *RNF43* (40%) *p16/CDKN2A* *TP53* *SMAD4/DPC4*	Marker of late cancer Marker of late cancer	16
Serous cystadenoma (predominantly women, 75%; mean age, 62 y; 16% resected cystic tumors; 10% oligocystic/macrocystic)	*VHL* (50%: somatic mutations; LOH: 90%) Loss of *10q* (50%)		10
Solid-pseudopapillary tumor (1%–2%; mean age, 29 y; M:F, 9:1; low malignant potential; 8% with metastatic disease)	*CTNNB1* (95%)		3
Acinar cell carcinoma (1%–2%; mean age, 56 y; M:F, 2:1)	*SMAD4, JAK1, BRAF, RB1, TP53* (up to 30%) *RAF* rearrangements (25%)		131
Pancreatoblastoma (<1%; mean age, 5 y; M:F, 2:1)	*CTNNB1* (55%) *APC* (10%) *11p* loss (85%)		18
Neuroendocrine tumors (5%; mean age, 58 y; M:F, 3:2)	*MEN1, ATRX, DAXX, TSC2* (*KRAS* [30%] Rb [70%], p53 [60%] in NECs)	45% in *MEN1*, 45% in *ATRX/DAXX*, 15% *mTOR* pathway	16

Abbreviations: IPMN, intraductal papillary mucinous neoplasm; LOH, loss of heterozygosity; NEC, neuroendocrine carcinoma; PanIN, pancreatic intraepithelial neoplasia.

Table 2
Hereditary syndromes predisposing to PDAC

Syndrome	Gene Abnormalities	RR/(CLR by Age 70) for PDAC, Comments	Other Cancers/Tumors
Peutz-Jeghers	STK11/LKB1	132-fold (36%), IPMN	GI/GYN, breast cancers
Lynch, HNPCC	MLH1, MSH2, MSH6	9- to 11-fold (<5%), medullary variant of PDAC	Colon, endometrial cancers
Familial adenomatous polyposis	APC	5-fold (<5%)	Colon cancer, desmoid fibromatosis
Familial atypical multiple mole melanoma	CDKN2A	13- to 39-fold (17%)	Melanomas
Cystic fibrosis	CFTR	5-fold (<5%)	
Familial breast and ovarian	BRCA1, BRCA2	3- to 10-fold (3%–8%)	Breast, ovarian cancers
Li-Fraumeni	p53	7-fold (unknown)	Sarcomas, breast, brain, adrenal
Hereditary pancreatitis	PRSS1, SPINK1	50- to 80-fold (40%)	
Familial pancreatic cancer syndrome	BRCA2, PALB2, ATM (15%–20% of patients)	2 FDR: 8%–12% >3 FDR: 16%–38%	

Abbreviations: CLR, cumulative lifetime risk; FDR, first-degree relative; GI, gastrointestinal; GYN, gynecologic; HNPCC, hereditary nonpolyposis cancer syndrome; IPMN, intraductal papillary mucinous neoplasm; RR, relative risk.

with an overall 5-year-survival of 5%.[1] Although most patients present with advanced, inoperable, or metastatic disease at presentation, more than 70% of patients die within the first year of diagnosis.[2] The uniformly poor prognosis of PDAC is caused by several complex factors including an inability to detect cancer early, biologically aggressive behavior with early metastasis, and lack of effective therapy.[3]

Most PDACs originate from microscopic precursors referred to as pancreatic intraepithelial neoplasias (PanINs). A significant proportion of

PDACs develop from macroscopic precursors, such as mucinous cystic neoplasms (MCNs) and intraductal papillary mucinous neoplasms (IPMNs). It is now established that PDAC and its precursors are characterized by specific genetic abnormalities that predate microscopic disease. PDAC is a genetically heterogeneous cancer with an average of 26 to 63 gene mutations including those that affect several core signaling pathways.[4,5] Four key driver mutations involving KRAS, TP53, SMAD4, and CDKN2A genes characterize most PDACs (see **Table 1**).[2,3,6] Specific

Table 3
Hereditary syndromes with associated PanNETs

Syndrome (Comments)	Gene Abnormalities	Other Tumors	Frequency of Gene Mutations in Sporadic PanNETs
MEN-1 (30%–80% PanNETs)	MEN-1 (Menin)	Pituitary, parathyroid tumors	45%
VHL (10%–17% PanNETs)	VHL HIF pathway	CNS hemangioblastomas, clear cell RCCs, serous cystadenomas, pheochromocytomas	18%
Tuberous sclerosis (1% PanNETs)	TSC1, TSC2 mTOR pathway	Angiomyolipomas, lymphangioleimyomatosis	70% altered in mTOR pathway
Neurofibromatosis-1 (10% PanNETs)	NF-1 (Neurofibromin)	Neurofibromas	

Abbreviations: CNS, central nervous system; RCC, renal cell carcinoma.

Box 1
Candidates for screening for PDAC

- Individuals with greater than two FDRs with PDAC
- Individuals with Lynch syndrome with greater than one case of PDAC in FDR
- Individuals with Peutz-Jeghers syndrome
- Individuals with hereditary pancreatitis
- CDKN2A mutation carriers
- BRCA 1 or BRCA 2, PALB2 mutation carriers with at least one case of PDAC in FDR

Abbreviation: FDRs, first-degree relatives.

---

histologic subtypes of PDACs are associated with distinct genetic signatures.[2,3,6] Colloid carcinomas, histologically characterized by large stromal mucin pools and associated with intestinal-type of IPMN, display *GNAS* mutations.[7] Although LS is associated with development of medullary carcinomas characterized by a hallmark feature of microsatellite instability, frequent somatic mutations in *UPF1* are seen in adenosquamous variants of PDAC.[2,5,8] Evolving knowledge of the origin, pathogenesis, cytogenetics, and molecular biology of PDAC is paving the path for the development of novel techniques and biomarkers for early identification of PDAC and its precursors and targeted therapeutics that selectively act on tumor pathways to improve survival rates.

Approximately 10% of PDACs are secondary to inherited tumor predisposition syndromes.[9] The hereditary/familial risk of PDAC may be categorized into two groups: genetic syndromes with an increased risk of PDAC; and familial pancreatic cancer (FPC), a polygenic familial syndrome with at least two first-degree relatives (FDR) with PDACs.[10,11] Genetic data have suggested a long latent period (average of 17 years) for development of invasive malignancy from these precursors.[5] Thus identification of the precursor lesions or their biomarkers is important to detect PDAC early, potentially leading to improved surgical resectability and better prognosis. Given the low prevalence of PDAC, screening the general population is not cost effective. Thus, the current trend is toward identifying high-risk individuals that include family members of FPC and known genetic syndromes with significantly increased risk of PDAC and screening them appropriately for early cancer detection.[12]

Molecular Pathogenesis

Various complex genetic and epigenetic changes are involved in the initiation and progression of PDAC. Among them, there are four main driver gene mutations that characterize PDAC and its precursor lesions; these include one oncogene (*KRAS*) and three tumor suppressor genes (*p16/CDKN2A*, *TP53*, and *SMAD4*) (**Fig. 1**).[13,14]

KRAS

The *KRAS* gene (located on chromosome 12p) is an early and most commonly mutated oncogene with clustering of somatic mutations in select hotspot regions in greater than 95% of PDACs.[2,14,15] *KRAS* encodes a small GTPase that mediates downstream signaling for growth factor receptors. Point mutations of *KRAS* impairs intrinsic GTPase activity; thus, active GTPs continuously stimulate downstream signaling pathways, such as PI3K/AKT/mTOR and RAF/MAP Kinase, leading to uncontrolled cellular proliferation and PDAC development.[1,2,4,14,16] KRAS, however, remains an undruggable target given the failure of multiple attempts to block the activity of mutated KRAS protein.[2]

p16/CDKN2A

p16/CDKN2A gene (located on chromosome 9p) is somatically mutated in more than 95% of PDACs resulting in inactivation of P16 protein, which commonly functions as a mediator of RB signaling pathway.[1,2] *p16* inhibits CDK4/6 mediated phosphorylation of RB and blocks entry of cells from G1 to S phase (DNA synthesis) of cell cycle; loss of function of P16 results in the progression of the cell cycle through the G1/S checkpoint in an unrestricted manner, leading to accelerated cell proliferation.[3,14]

TP53

TP53 (located on chromosome 17p) is inactivated in up to 75% of PDACs by a somatic mutation coupled with the loss of the second allele.[2] P53 protein plays a central role in cellular homeostasis by activating target genes to induce proliferation arrest and apoptosis in response to cellular stress, such as DNA damage, hypoxia, and nutrient deprivation. Inactivated *TP53* results in unbridled cellular growth and failed apoptosis that leads to PDAC development.[1,13]

SMAD4

SMAD4 (chromosome 18q) is inactivated in 53% to 66% of PDACs either by deletion or intragenic mutation followed by loss of the second allele.[17,18] SMAD4 protein acts as a mediator of the transforming growth factor-β signaling pathway that transmits signals from the extracellular growth factors to the nucleus.[17] The loss of SMAD4 expression occurs late in PDAC progression and leads to development of metastatic disease.[1] Tumors

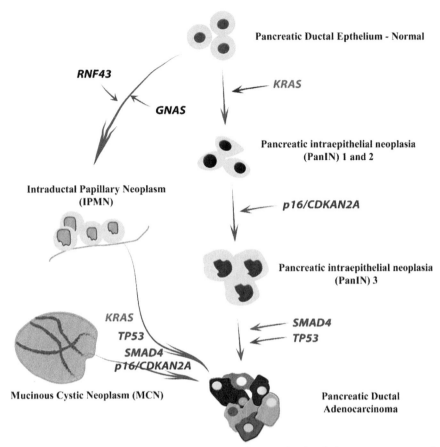

Fig. 1. Schematic diagram demonstrating the precursors and seminal role of driver mutations in the evolution and molecular pathogenesis of pancreatic ductal adenocarcinoma.

with loss of SMAD4 expression have higher rates of distant metastases and carry a grim prognosis.[18] Recently, an immunostain has been developed to identify SMAD4 protein on tissue samples that can help in prognostication.[2]

In addition, multiple other oncogenes (c-myc, p21-activated kinase 4 [PAK4], and HER2), tumor suppressor genes (PTEN, BRCA2, PALB2, and PRSS1), and DNA mismatch repair genes (MLH1, MSH2, MSH6, and PMS2) are also involved in the pathogenesis of sporadic and familial cases of PDACs.

Epigenetic Regulations

In addition to mutations/deletions, functional effects of the genes are altered by epigenetic mechanisms, such as methylation, acetylation, and regulation through micro-RNAs.[14] Among these events, micro-RNAs have been widely investigated in relation to PDAC progression; miR-34a has been shown to play a role in the TP53 expression and is often deleted in PDAC.[14]

Hereditary Syndromes Associated with Pancreatic Ductal Adenocarcinoma

Peutz-Jeghers syndrome

Peutz-Jeghers syndrome (PJS) is an autosomal-dominant syndrome secondary to germline mutation of the STK11/LKB1 gene (chromosome 19p) characterized by intestinal hamartomatous polyps and mucocutaneous pigmentation.[2] There is an estimated 11% to 32% lifetime risk of developing PDAC.[11,19] In addition, PJS with loss of heterozygosity of the wild-type STK11 allele has been reported to increase the risk of IPMN.[19]

Lynch syndrome

LS is an autosomal-dominant condition, characterized by a germline mutation in one of the four DNA mismatch repair genes: MLH1, MSH2, MSH6, and PMS2.[1,2,11] LS most commonly presents with colorectal and endometrial carcinomas.[2,19] There is a cumulative risk of 3.7% to develop PDAC by the age of 70 years.[1,11] PDACs in patients with LS have a characteristic medullary histology and show microsatellite instability, similar to that of colon cancers. These tumors do not respond to fluorouracil-based chemotherapy; new immunotherapy drugs, such as PD1 inhibitors, are being explored to treat these patients.[19]

Hereditary pancreatitis

Hereditary pancreatitis is an autosomal-dominant disorder caused by mutations in PRSS1 or SPINK1 genes that involve in production and activation of pancreatic enzyme trypsinogen and cause recurrent bouts of acute pancreatitis at a younger age.[4,11,13] Patients develop precursor lesions that likely progress to frank malignancy.[19] The relative risk of PDAC is 50- to 70-fold compared with general population; the risk is highest in smokers and those with diabetes.[19,20]

Hereditary breast and ovarian cancer syndrome

Hereditary breast and ovarian cancer syndrome is caused by mutations in BRCA1, BRCA2, and PALB2 genes, which encode for proteins responsible for DNA repair.[14] The relative risk of PDAC is 3- to 10-fold in patients with hereditary breast and ovarian cancer syndrome compared with the general population; BRCA-2 mutations carry a higher risk (**Fig. 2**).[11,14] PDACs with BRCA abnormalities may be more responsive to DNA cross-linking agents, such as mitomycin, oxaliplatin, and ADP-ribose polymerase (PARP) inhibitors.[11]

Familial pancreatic cancer

FPC is defined as an inherited syndrome with at least two FDRs in a family with a proven diagnosis of PDAC in the absence of known genetic cancer susceptible syndrome (**Fig. 3**).[10] FPC

accounts for approximately 90% of familial cases and constitutes 10% of all PDACs.[10] The risk of PDAC increases to 17- to 32-fold if three or more FDRs in an FPC.[11] Known genetic mutations have been identified in about 20% of the FPC cancers (BRCA1, BRCA2, P16/CDKN2A, PALB2, and ATM genes mutations); however, in most of the cases, the responsible genetic mutation is unknown.[5,10,11] BRCA2 mutations have been found in up to 17% of patients with FPC and mutations in the PALB2 gene is found in about 5%.[21,22]

Familial atypical multiple mole and melanoma syndrome

Familial atypical multiple mole melanoma syndrome is an autosomal-dominant syndrome characterized by multiple nevi, melanomas, and PDACs and is secondary to mutations in the p16/CDKN2A gene.[11] The relative risk of PDAC in familial atypical multiple mole melanoma syndrome carriers ranges from 13- to 65- fold.[1,11,21] A variant syndrome called familial atypical multiple mole melanoma syndrome–pancreatic carcinoma syndrome carries a cumulative risk of PDAC up to 17% by the age of 75.[11]

Precursors of Pancreatic Ductal Adenocarcinoma

Pancreatic intraepithelial neoplasia

PanIN, the main precursor of PDAC, refers to microscopic, intraductal proliferation of the mucin-producing epithelial cells. PanINs harbor genetic abnormalities similar to PDACs.[2,21,23] PanINs are microscopic lesions (by definition, <5 mm) and cannot be identified by current imaging methods. PanINs are classified into three categories based on the architectural and

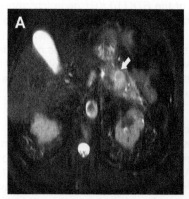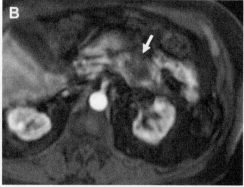

Fig. 2. Pancreatic ductal adenocarcinoma in a 74-year-old man with BRCA2 mutations and previous history of bilateral breast cancers and prostate cancer. Axial T2-weighted (A), and contrast-enhanced T1-weighted (B) MR images show a T2-intermediate signal intensity mass that is hypointense to the pancreas after contrast administration (arrows).

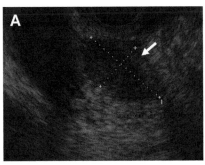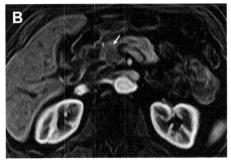

Fig. 3. PDAC in a 62-year-old man with FPC syndrome; his father died of pancreatic cancer at the age of 41. (A) Endoscopic ultrasound image shows a hypoechoic lesion (arrow). (B) Axial contrast-enhanced T1-weighted MR image demonstrates a hypovascular mass in head of the pancreas (arrow) consistent with PDAC.

cytonuclear abnormalities: low-grade (PanIN-1 and PanIN-2) and high-grade (PanIN-3) lesions.[1,2,4] Many low-grade PanINs are commonly seen in the normal pancreas after the age of 40; however, only high-grade PanINs transform into invasive lesions. Telomere shortening and KRAS mutations are the earliest genetic events in PanINs, occurring in greater than 90% of low-grade PanINs; the prevalence of the p16/CDKN2A mutations increase with PanIN grade.[2,14] SMAD4 and TP53 mutations occur more frequently in high-grade PanINs.[4,22]

Intraductal papillary mucinous neoplasms

IPMNs are larger cystic lesions that are characterized by intraductal growth of papillary tumors with abundant mucin secretion. They occur more commonly in elderly men (mean age, 65 years). Based on disease distribution, IPMNs may be classified into three types: main-duct IPMN, branch-duct IPMN, and the mixed-type (Fig. 4). Main duct and mixed types have been shown to develop invasive malignancy in 31% to 45.5% of cases.[24] Branch duct IPMNs show 2.9% to 15% risk of progression to invasive

pancreatic cancer. Although there may be overlap, a multitude of tumor epithelial subtypes (gastric, intestinal, pancreatobiliary, and oncocytic) with varying degrees of dysplasia and potential for malignant transformation have been described in patients with IPMN. Gastric subtype is seen more commonly in branch-duct type IPMNs. The colloid (associated with intestinal type) and oncocytic subtypes of malignant IPMNs show indolent behavior and better prognosis than tubular carcinomas associated with pancreatobiliary and gastric type epithelia.[25] KRAS mutations are frequent in IPMN occurring up to 80% of the lesions.[7] Loss of expression of p16 has been identified in 100% of invasive carcinomas associated with IPMNs. Similar to PanINs, mutations of TP53 and SMAD4 are more commonly seen in high-grade lesions.[1] In addition to the previously mentioned common driver gene mutations (KRAS, P16/CDKN2A/TP53, SMAD4), distinct mutations have been described in IPMNs. Although somatic mutations in the oncogenic hotspot of GNAS gene have been described in 60% of IPMNs (most frequently found in the intestinal subtype and absent

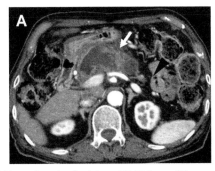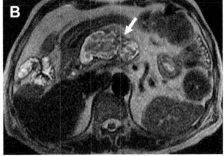

Fig. 4. Malignant main-duct type IPMN in an 86-year-old man. Axial contrast-enhanced computed tomography (A) and T2-weighted MR (B) images of the pancreas show diffusely dilated main pancreatic duct with heterogeneously enhancing, solid components (arrows) consistent with main-duct IPMN.

in oncocytic variant), recurrent inactivating mutations involving ubiquitin-dependent tumor pathways and specifically involving tumor suppressor gene, *RNF43*, have been described in 60% of IPMNs.[21] Mutant *GNAS* (that encodes the Gαs protein) causes constitutive activation of adenylyl cyclase leading to increased generation of the cyclic AMP with downstream effects on intracellular pathways. Interestingly, McCune-Albright syndrome, an autosomal-dominant syndrome with activating *GNAS* mutations, is characterized by increased risk of development of IPMNs.[25] *RNF43* is a transmembrane ubiquitin ligase protein that inhibits the canonical Wnt/β-catenin signaling pathway.

Mucinous cystic neoplasm

MCN, the least common macroscopic precursor of PDAC, occurs almost exclusively in perimenopausal women of 40 to 60 years. In contradistinction to IPMNs that are commonly multifocal and communicate with the ducts, MCNs are almost always solitary with most not communicating with the ductal system.[26] Up to 95% of MCNs are seen in the pancreatic body/tail regions. MCNs are histologically characterized by neoplastic epithelia of varying dysplasia and invasiveness and a classical ovarian-type stroma. They show an average of 16 nonsynonymous mutations and demonstrate lesser frequency of malignant degeneration than IPMNs.[3] Most common mutations seen on cyst fluid analysis in MCN are *KRAS* mutations, especially in MCNs with high-grade dysplasia.[27,28] GNAS mutation, which is common in IPMNs, is rarely positive in MCN.[6] MCNs typically transform to tubular variants of PDAC (**Fig. 5**). The prognosis of MCNs is usually favorable with excellent 5-year survival rates that vary from 100% in patients with noninvasive tumors to greater than 60% in patients with invasive cystadenocarcinomas.[29]

Screening

Although the benefits of PDAC screening remain unclear at this point of time, different imaging techniques and serum biomarkers are being used for this purpose.[9,30,31] Based on the improved understanding of PDAC molecular pathogenesis, researchers are working to develop novel biomarkers and imaging methods for early PDAC detection and effective therapeutic options that can improve overall prognosis.[32] Early detection of noninvasive/early invasive PDACs and precancerous lesions with high-grade dysplasia (PanINs, IPMNs, and MCNs) are the main goals for screening.[30] Screening should start with the identification of high-risk individuals, based on careful personal and family history of PDAC and patients with IPMNs and MCNs.[33,34] Currently, PDAC screening is recommended in certain patient cohorts (see **Box 1**).[9,33,34] Although there is no consensus about the age to start screening, a simplified approach is as follows. The screening begins at age 45 to 50 years, or 10 to 15 years younger than the youngest relative with pancreatic cancer. Screening for PDAC in PJS patients typically starts at 30 years, and in hereditary pancreatitis patients, screening should begin at the age of 40 years. Screening should begin earlier in people who have ever smoked, given that smokers from PDAC-prone families develop cancer on average a decade earlier than nonsmokers.[9,33,34]

Endoscopic ultrasound (EUS) and MR imaging/ magnetic resonance cholangiopancreatography (MRCP) are currently used to screen for pancreatic

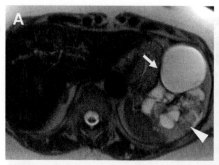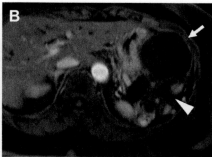

Fig. 5. Mucinous cystadenocarcinoma in an 84-year-old woman. Axial T2-weighted (*A*) and contrast-enhanced T1-weighted (*B*) MR images of the pancreas show a multiloculated, complex cystic mass in the pancreatic tail (*arrows*) with enhancing solid components (*arrowheads*) consistent with invasive mucinous cystadenocarcinoma.

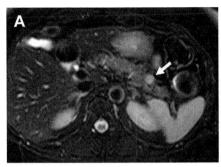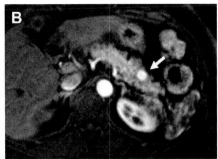

Fig. 6. Pancreatic neuroendocrine neoplasm in a 35-year-old woman with known MEN-1 syndrome. Axial T2-weighted (A) and contrast-enhanced T1-weighted (B) MR images of the pancreas show a small, T2-hyperintense pancreatic tail nodule (arrows) that shows uniform and intense contrast enhancement.

lesions in high-risk individuals.[30,31,34] Although EUS and MR imaging have sensitivity and specificity values greater than 95% in detecting PDACs/precursors, there is an advantage of obtaining tissue samples with EUS, whereas MR imaging carries the advantage of noninvasive nature.[31] If the pancreas is normal on the initial examination, repeat imaging can be performed every year, typically alternating MR imaging/MRCP and EUS.[34] Follow-up MR imaging EUS in 3 months is recommended for patients with a newly detected, small (<1 cm), indeterminate solid lesion, whereas solid lesions of size greater than 1 cm should be resected.[9,31,33,34] Repeat imaging should be performed within 3 months in patients with an indeterminate main pancreatic duct stricture.[34] The age to stop screening in these individuals should be individualized by life expectancy, preferences, and overall health.[9] MicroRNAs may provide information on the degree of malignant transformation and survival prediction in patients with PDAC.[31] However, they have yet to become a standard part of the PDAC management despite many individual experimental and clinical studies.[9,31,33]

The screening and surveillance guidelines regarding diagnosis and management of asymptomatic neoplastic pancreatic cysts have been evolving with the aim of early identification of the PDAC and avoiding unnecessary imaging tests and interventions. The American Gastroenterology Association guidelines are one of the widely used methods for this purpose.[35] All incidental pancreatic cysts should be evaluated with MR imaging/MRCP. EUS is recommended for cysts greater than 3 cm in size or cysts with suspicious features, such as dilated main pancreatic duct with diameter greater than 1 cm, enhancing septations/solid components, and wall thickening.[35] Surveillance MR imaging is performed after 1 year in individuals with unresected cysts, followed by every 2 years; the surveillance may be stopped on observing lesion stability for 5 years without the development of high-risk features.[35]

NEUROENDOCRINE TUMORS

PanNETs are distinct neoplasms with characteristic histomorphology, genetic changes, biologic behavior, and prognostic features.[20] The prognosis of PanNETs is better than PDAC with a 5-year survival of 42%. They comprise 5% of all pancreatic tumors and frequently occur in a sporadic setting. Approximately 10% of PanNETs may occur as part of hereditary syndromes, such as MEN-1, VHL syndrome, NF1, and TSC.[20,36,37] Although about 10% of PanNETs occur as a part of MEN1 syndrome, patients with this condition present with PanNETs in up to 80% of cases (Fig. 6).[36] Up to 17% of patients with VHL disease may develop PanNETs; they are usually incidental findings, and almost exclusively nonfunctional (Fig. 7).[38]

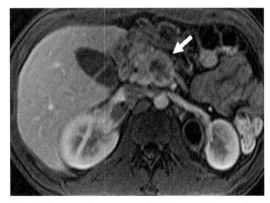

Fig. 7. Pancreatic neuroendocrine carcinoma in a 25-year-old man with VHL syndrome. Axial contrast-enhanced T1-weighted MR image of the pancreas depicts a heterogeneously enhancing mass in the head region (arrow) that was pathologically verified to be a pancreatic neuroendocrine carcinoma.

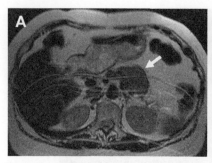
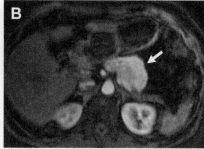
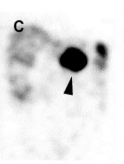

Fig. 8. Sporadic PanNET in a 77-year-old man. Axial T2-weighted (*A*) and contrast-enhanced T1-weighted (*B*) MR images of the pancreas show an isointense T2 lesion with intense and homogenous contrast enhancement (*arrows*). (*C*) Octreotide nuclear medicine scan demonstrates intense tracer uptake within the lesion consistent with a PanNET (*arrowhead*).

Based on World Health Organization classification schemata, PanNETs are classified into well-differentiated tumors and poorly differentiated NE carcinomas (small and large cell types; PanNECs). PanNETs are further classified into functional and nonfunctional based on hormone production and associated clinical findings. Although insulinomas and gastrinomas are the two most common functional PanNETs, characteristic syndromes have been described with the rarer VIPomas, glucagonomas, and somatostatinomas.[20] About 85% of all PanNETs are nonfunctional and carry worse prognosis compared with functional tumors (**Fig. 8**). It is shown that germline/somatic mutations in a broad spectrum of genes are responsible for variable tumor biology and prognosis of PanNETs and PanNECs. Although abnormalities of *MEN1* and *VHL* gene abnormalities are seen in distinct hereditary syndromes, mutations involving *DAXX* (death-domain-associated protein), *ATRX* (α-thalassemia/mental retardation syndrome X-linked), and mammalian target of rapamycin (*mTOR*) pathway genes (*PTEN*, *TSC2*, and *PIK3CA*) are commonly seen in sporadic PanNETs (**Fig. 9**).[3,39,40]

Molecular Pathogenesis

Genetic mutations with associated microenvironment changes that mimic glucose stimulation are the first events that may result in an uncontrolled proliferation of islet cells and subsequent tumor development of PanNETs.[41,42] In one study, mutations of *MEN1* (chromosome 11q13), *DAXX/ATRX* complex, and mTOR pathway genes were identified in 44%, 43%, and 15% of sporadic PanNETs, respectively.[39] These mutational abnormalities can cause aberrations of endothelial cell–independent islet cell survival, G1/S phase cell

cycle progression, and hypoxia signaling with associated angiogenesis resulting in PanNET development.[39,41] However, some investigators have proposed that PanNETs may originate from nonislet, pluripotent stem cells in the pancreatic ductal/acinar cells.[43] The common genetic mutations in PanNETs act in three different ways: (1) affect cell cycle regulation and cell growth, (2) disrupt cellular communication, and (3) promote angiogenesis.[41]

Mutations of *MEN1*, *PTEN*, *PIK3CA*, *TSC2*, *DAXX*, and *NF1* genes affect the PI3K/AKT/

Pancreatic islet cells - Normal

MEN1   *DAXX/ATRX*

VHL   *mTOR Pathway genes (PTEN, TSC2 & PIK3CA)*

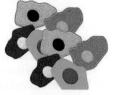

Fig. 9. Schematic diagram demonstrates the molecular pathogenesis of pancreatic neuroendocrine tumors.

mTOR pathway, which is one of the important intracellular signaling systems that play a crucial role in controlling cell cycle progression and cellular proliferation. Menin is the product MEN1 gene, which is ubiquitously expressed in normal pancreatic islet cells and is critical to homeostasis and glucose sensing. Menin suppresses cell proliferation and antiapoptosis and acts as a negative regulator of AKT kinase activity.[44] Loss of menin function in islet cells results in unrestricted S-phase progression, cell division, and tumor development.[41,45] About 14% of sporadic PanNETs show mutations in PTEN, PIK3CA, and TSC2 genes.[39] Mutations of PTEN or TSC2 cause uninhibited PI3KCA-mTOR signaling and increased cell proliferation; the loss of PTEN and TSC2 expression was correlated with reduced disease-free and overall survival in PanNETs.[46] The DAXX causes up-regulation of p53 expression in pancreatic endocrine cells leading to negative control on cell cycle progression. DAXX mutations in PanNETs lead to decreased p53 levels; impairment of p53-controlled G1/S progression results in tumor growth.[41,47]

DAXX and ATRX proteins function as chromatin remodeling dimers. Loss of DAXX/ATRX results in a phenotype known as alternative lengthening of telomeres, a telomerase-independent mechanism of telomere lengthening.[47] Mutations of these genes were observed in 43% of tumors in one series and are confirmed to occur in a mutually exclusive manner.[39] Also, alternative lengthening of telomeres stimulates mTOR pathway increasing the cell proliferation with PanNET development.[46] It has been shown that DAXX/ATRX is unique to PanNETs among other gastrointestinal neuroendocrine tumors.[48] The presence of alternative lengthening of telomeres phenotype has been proposed as a method to predict the site of origin of NE liver metastases with unknown primary.[49]

High degree of vascularity is one of the characteristic features of the PanNETs, primarily because of the close association between endocrine and endothelial cells within pancreatic islet cells. The capillary network is denser in islet cells compared with exocrine pancreas with significantly higher blood volumes.[50] The vascular endothelial growth factors (VEGFs) play a major role in the angiogenesis of PanNETs; others include platelet-derived growth factor, c-kit, and angiopoietin-1 and -2. Hypoxia-inducible factor-1 pathway is the main regulator of all these genes.[41] Sporadic and hereditary PanNETs show abnormalities of multiple genes involved in a hypoxia-inducible factor-1 pathway that can result in increased tumor vascularity.[37]

Activating mutations of KRAS and inactivating mutations of the RB1 and TP53 are seen in PanNECs, and these abnormalities are typically absent in well-differentiated PanNETs.[3]

Clinical Implications of Genetic Mutations

Sunitinib and everolimus are the most commonly used drugs for the treatment of metastatic/advanced PanNETs. Sunitinib is a multitarget, protein tyrosine kinase inhibitor that targets VEGF receptors, platelet-derived growth factor receptors, and c-kit, whereas everolimus is a mTOR inhibitor.[51,52] Bevacizumab, a monoclonal antibody to VEGF-A, has shown partial response in PanNETs when combined with everolimus.[41] Drugs that mimic menin activity (agonists) are being investigated for effective treatment in PanNETs, given the presence of MEN1 mutations in most sporadic PanNETs.[41]

PanNETs with mTOR mutations tend to carry poor prognosis; in this subset, everolimus and sunitinib may show good response rates and overall survival benefits if patients are screened for mutations before treatment. Loss of DAXX and ATRX genes in PanNETs is associated with chromosome instability and reduced survival and carries grim prognosis.[53] PanNETs with mutations in the DAXX or ATRX genes demonstrate imaging evidence of aggressive behavior, including vascular invasion, hepatic or osseous metastases, larger size, irregular contour, tumor calcification, and pancreatic ductal dilatation.[54]

Screening

Carriers of MEN1 and VHL gene mutations should be proactively screened for PanNETs for early diagnosis and treatment, which significantly improves the patient outcomes. Annual clinical examination of MEN1 carriers for identifying manifestations of the functional tumors is mandatory on initial diagnosis. Gadolinium-enhanced abdominal MR imaging for every 2 years starting at age 10 is recommended. Serum gastrin, insulin, and gut hormone profile should be recommended if there is evidence of pancreatic tumor on imaging.[1] Tumors of size greater than 2 cm or rapidly growing tumors should be treated, and others may be managed conservatively.[1] Screening for pancreatic lesions using contrast-enhanced pancreatic MR imaging every 2 to 3 years starting at age 12 has been recommended in all VHL gene carriers; computed tomography or MR imaging are used

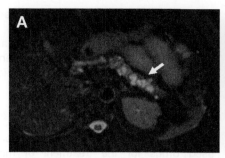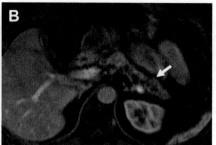

Fig. 10. Multiple serous cystadenomas in a 42-year-old man with known VHL syndrome. Axial T2-weighted (*A*) and contrast-enhanced T1-weighted (*B*) MR images of the pancreas show multiple cystic lesions with few, thin enhancing septations (*arrows*) consistent with serous cystadenomas.

after the age of 18 years.[8] Also, annual serum chromogranin levels are also to be considered based on the clinical assessment. The risk of malignancy is the key indicator for resection of PanNETs; tumors greater than 3 cm in the body and tail of the pancreas or greater than 2 cm in the head of the pancreas, or tumors with suspicious metastases to locoregional lymph nodes should be resected.[8] Tumors with advanced/metastatic disease may be treated with antiangiogenic therapies or palliative surgery. Given the rarity of PanNETs in NF1 and TSC, no specific screening guidelines have been proposed.

SEROUS CYSTADENOMA

Serous cystadenoma is a slow-growing, benign cystic neoplasm that develops in approximately 10% of patients with VHL disease (**Fig. 10**).[55] The tumor is composed of multiple small cysts lined by nonmucinous epithelium and may show a calcified central scar (**Fig. 11**).[4] Serous cystic neoplasms (SCNs) in patients with VHL demonstrate germline mutation of the tumor suppressor *VHL* gene (chromosome 3p25) coupled with somatic inactivation of second allele.[4] Up to 70% of sporadic SCNs also show somatic, inactivating mutations of *VHL* gene (point mutations and loss of heterozygosity).[2,4] SCNs lack genetic mutations that are commonly seen in PDACs, IPMNs, and MCNs, indicating distinctive pathogenesis of SCNs; this feature also assists in the differentiation of SCN from other cystic pancreatic lesions by cyst fluid mutational profile analysis.[2,4]

SOLID PSEUDOPAPILLARY NEOPLASM

SPN is a low-grade malignancy of young women with distinct molecular, histologic, and clinical characteristics.[16] SPN begins as a solid tumor that often undergoes extensive cystic

degeneration caused by hemorrhage and necrosis (**Fig. 12**).[3] Activating somatic mutations in the β-catenin gene (*CTNNB1*) on chromosome 3p occur in almost 100% of SPNs resulting in abnormal nuclear localization of the β-catenin protein that stimulates genes, such as *cyclin D1* and *c-myc* promoting neoplastic proliferation through Wnt/beta-catenin pathway.[2,6] Alterations of β-catenin protein also cause dysregulation of E-cadherin expression (a key regulator of cell-cell adhesions) leading to dyscohesive tumor cells.[6] SPNs lack gene mutations commonly seen in PDACs and other cystic neoplasms and demonstrate excellent prognosis after surgical resection, although

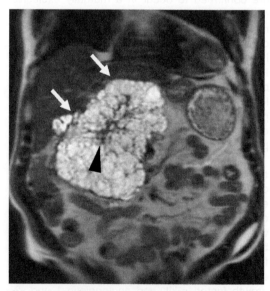

Fig. 11. Sporadic serous cystadenoma in a 73-year-old man. Coronal T2-weighted MR image of the pancreas shows a large cystic lesion containing multiple small cysts (*arrows*) and a central hypointense scar (*arrowhead*) consistent with a serous cystadenoma.

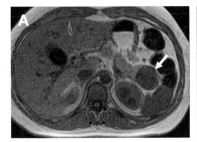 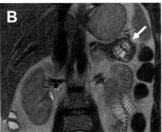 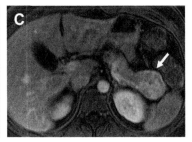

Fig. 12. Solid pseudopapillary neoplasm in a 29-year-old woman. Axial T1-weighted (*A*), coronal T2-weighted (*B*), and contrast-enhanced T1-weighted (*C*) MR images of the pancreas show a well-defined solid-cystic mass with mixed signal intensity on T2-weighted image and heterogeneous enhancement after contrast administration (*arrows*) consistent with a solid pseudopapillary neoplasm.

10% patients may present with distant metastases.[3]

ACINAR CELL CARCINOMA

ACC is a rare, solid malignant neoplasm that recapitulates the growth pattern, immunohistochemistry, and secretory products of nonneoplastic acini.[3] Some ACCs may release enzymes, such as lipase, into blood leading to characteristic syndrome; up to 15% of patients may present with metastatic fat necrosis, arthralgias, and peripheral eosinophilia from elevated lipase levels.[3,4] Although loss of chromosome 11p is seen in up to 50% of patients, ACC is a genetically heterogeneous and complex tumor (**Fig. 13**).[2,3] Somatic activating mutations in *CTNNB1* and inactivating mutations in *APC* genes with alterations of APC/β-catenin pathway are seen in 25% of ACCs.[4,6] Mutations of *BRCA1/2*, *TP53*, *SMAD4*, and *PALB2* genes are also identified in ACCs.[3,6]

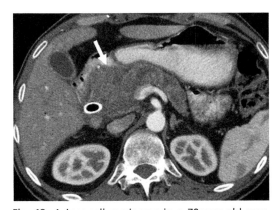

Fig. 13. Acinar cell carcinoma in a 79-year-old man. Axial contrast-enhanced computed tomography image of the abdomen shows a heterogeneously enhancing infiltrative pancreatic mass (*arrow*), which was proven to be an acinar cell carcinoma on pathologic examination.

SUMMARY

Pancreatic neoplasms are a heterogeneous group of tumors that demonstrate characteristic histogenesis, pathology, genetic abnormalities, and tumor pathways. Recent studies have clarified the distinct genomic signatures of tumors of the exocrine and endocrine pancreas. Evolving knowledge about tumor genomics and specific tumor pathways of pancreatic tumors may lead to the identification of novel biomarkers and development of targeted therapeutics to improve diagnosis and management. Current recommendations for screening strategies apply to high-risk individuals with a hereditary predisposition to pancreatic tumors.

REFERENCES

1. Bernard V, Fleming J, Maitra A. Molecular and genetic basis of pancreatic carcinogenesis: which concepts may be clinically relevant? Surg Oncol Clin N Am 2016;25(2):227–38.
2. Hosoda W, Wood LD. Molecular genetics of pancreatic neoplasms. Surg Pathol Clin 2016;9(4):685–703.
3. Hackeng WM, Hruban RH, Offerhaus GJ, et al. Surgical and molecular pathology of pancreatic neoplasms. Diagn Pathol 2016;11(1):47.
4. Wood LD, Hruban RH. Pathology and molecular genetics of pancreatic neoplasms. Cancer J 2012; 18(6):492–501.
5. Amundadottir LT. Pancreatic cancer genetics. Int J Biol Sci 2016;12(3):314–25.
6. Reid MD, Saka B, Balci S, et al. Molecular genetics of pancreatic neoplasms and their morphologic correlates: an update on recent advances and potential diagnostic applications. Am J Clin Pathol 2014; 141(2):168–80.
7. Amato E, Molin MD, Mafficini A, et al. Targeted next-generation sequencing of cancer genes dissects the molecular profiles of intraductal papillary neoplasms of the pancreas. J Pathol 2014;233(3): 217–27.

8. Keutgen XM, Hammel P, Choyke PL, et al. Evaluation and management of pancreatic lesions in patients with von Hippel-Lindau disease. Nat Rev Clin Oncol 2016;13(9):537–49.

9. Grover S, Jajoo K. Screening for pancreatic cancer in high-risk populations. Gastroenterol Clin North Am 2016;45(1):117–27.

10. Petersen GM. Familial pancreatic adenocarcinoma. Hematol Oncol Clin North Am 2015;29(4): 641–53.

11. Connor AA, Gallinger S. Hereditary pancreatic cancer syndromes. Surg Oncol Clin N Am 2015;24(4): 733–64.

12. Pandharipande PV, Heberle C, Dowling EC, et al. Targeted screening of individuals at high risk for pancreatic cancer: results of a simulation model. Radiology 2015;275(1):177–87.

13. Wood LD, Klimstra DS. Pathology and genetics of pancreatic neoplasms with acinar differentiation. Semin Diagn Pathol 2014;31(6):491–7.

14. Khan MA, Azim S, Zubair H, et al. Molecular drivers of pancreatic cancer pathogenesis: looking inward to move forward. Int J Mol Sci 2017;18(4) [pii:E779].

15. Eser S, Schnieke A, Schneider G, et al. Oncogenic KRAS signalling in pancreatic cancer. Br J Cancer 2014;111(5):817–22.

16. Shi C, Daniels JA, Hruban RH. Molecular characterization of pancreatic neoplasms. Adv Anat Pathol 2008;15(4):185–95.

17. Tascilar M, Skinner HG, Rosty C, et al. The SMAD4 protein and prognosis of pancreatic ductal adenocarcinoma. Clin Cancer Res 2001;7(12):4115–21.

18. Yamada S, Fujii T, Shimoyama Y, et al. SMAD4 expression predicts local spread and treatment failure in resected pancreatic cancer. Pancreas 2015; 44(4):660–4.

19. Pittman ME, Brosens LA, Wood LD. Genetic syndromes with pancreatic manifestations. Surg Pathol Clin 2016;9(4):705–15.

20. Halfdanarson TR, Rubin J, Farnell MB, et al. Pancreatic endocrine neoplasms: epidemiology and prognosis of pancreatic endocrine tumors. Endocr Relat Cancer 2008;15(2):409–27.

21. Wood LD, Hruban RH. Genomic landscapes of pancreatic neoplasia. J Pathol Transl Med 2015; 49(1):13–22.

22. Rishi A, Goggins M, Wood LD, et al. Pathological and molecular evaluation of pancreatic neoplasms. Semin Oncol 2015;42(1):28–39.

23. Fric P, Sedo A, Skrha J, et al. Early detection of sporadic pancreatic cancer: time for change. Eur J Gastroenterol Hepatol 2017;29(8):885–91.

24. Rezaee N, Barbon C, Zaki A, et al. Intraductal papillary mucinous neoplasm (IPMN) with high-grade dysplasia is a risk factor for the subsequent development of pancreatic ductal adenocarcinoma. HPB (Oxford) 2016;18(3):236–46.

25. Gaujoux S, Salenave S, Ronot M, et al. Hepatobiliary and pancreatic neoplasms in patients with McCune-Albright syndrome. J Clin Endocrinol Metab 2014; 99(1):E97–101.

26. Nilsson LN, Keane MG, Shamali A, et al. Nature and management of pancreatic mucinous cystic neoplasm (MCN): a systematic review of the literature. Pancreatology 2016;16(6):1028–36.

27. Theisen BK, Wald AI, Singhi AD. Molecular diagnostics in the evaluation of pancreatic cysts. Surg Pathol Clin 2016;9(3):441–56.

28. Jimenez RE, Warshaw AL, Z'Graggen K, et al. Sequential accumulation of K-ras mutations and p53 overexpression in the progression of pancreatic mucinous cystic neoplasms to malignancy. Ann Surg 1999;230(4):501–9 [discussion: 509–11].

29. Yamao K, Yanagisawa A, Takahashi K, et al. Clinicopathological features and prognosis of mucinous cystic neoplasm with ovarian-type stroma: a multi-institutional study of the Japan Pancreas Society. Pancreas 2011;40(1):67–71.

30. Lindquist CM, Miller FH, Hammond NA, et al. Pancreatic cancer screening. Abdom Radiol (NY) 2017;43(2):264–72.

31. Fric P, Skrha J, Sedo A, et al. Early detection of pancreatic cancer: impact of high-resolution imaging methods and biomarkers. Eur J Gastroenterol Hepatol 2016;28(12):e33–43.

32. Kim VM, Ahuja N. Early detection of pancreatic cancer. Chin J Cancer Res 2015;27(4):321–31.

33. Syngal S, Brand RE, Church JM, et al. ACG clinical guideline: genetic testing and management of hereditary gastrointestinal cancer syndromes. Am J Gastroenterol 2015;110(2):223–62 [quiz: 263].

34. Canto MI, Harinck F, Hruban RH, et al. International Cancer of the Pancreas Screening (CAPS) Consortium summit on the management of patients with increased risk for familial pancreatic cancer. Gut 2013;62(3):339–47.

35. Vege SS, Ziring B, Jain R, et al, Clinical Guidelines Committee, American Gastroenterology Association. American Gastroenterological Association Institute guideline on the diagnosis and management of asymptomatic neoplastic pancreatic cysts. Gastroenterology 2015;148(4):819–22 [quiz: e12–3].

36. Oberg K. Pancreatic endocrine tumors. Semin Oncol 2010;37(6):594–618.

37. Jensen RT, Berna MJ, Bingham DB, et al. Inherited pancreatic endocrine tumor syndromes: advances in molecular pathogenesis, diagnosis, management, and controversies. Cancer 2008;113(7 Suppl): 1807–43.

38. Cassol C, Mete O. Endocrine manifestations of von Hippel-Lindau disease. Arch Pathol Lab Med 2015; 139(2):263–8.

39. Jiao Y, Shi C, Edil BH, et al. DAXX/ATRX, MEN1, and mTOR pathway genes are frequently altered in

pancreatic neuroendocrine tumors. Science 2011; 331(6021):1199–203.

40. Ehehalt F, Franke E, Pilarsky C, et al. Molecular pathogenesis of pancreatic neuroendocrine tumors. Cancers (Basel) 2010;2(4):1901–10.

41. Zhang J, Francois R, Iyer R, et al. Current understanding of the molecular biology of pancreatic neuroendocrine tumors. J Natl Cancer Inst 2013; 105(14):1005–17.

42. Shi C, Klimstra DS. Pancreatic neuroendocrine tumors: pathologic and molecular characteristics. Semin Diagn Pathol 2014;31(6):498–511.

43. Vortmeyer AO, Huang S, Lubensky I, et al. Non-islet origin of pancreatic islet cell tumors. J Clin Endocrinol Metab 2004;89(4):1934–8.

44. Wang Y, Ozawa A, Zaman S, et al. The tumor suppressor protein menin inhibits AKT activation by regulating its cellular localization. Cancer Res 2011;71(2):371–82.

45. Milne TA, Hughes CM, Lloyd R, et al. Menin and MLL cooperatively regulate expression of cyclin-dependent kinase inhibitors. Proc Natl Acad Sci U S A 2005;102(3):749–54.

46. Missiaglia E, Dalai I, Barbi S, et al. Pancreatic endocrine tumors: expression profiling evidences a role for AKT-mTOR pathway. J Clin Oncol 2010;28(2): 245–55.

47. de Wilde RF, Heaphy CM, Maitra A, et al. Loss of ATRX or DAXX expression and concomitant acquisition of the alternative lengthening of telomeres phenotype are late events in a small subset of MEN-1 syndrome pancreatic neuroendocrine tumors. Mod Pathol 2012;25(7):1033–9.

48. McKenna LR, Edil BH. Update on pancreatic neuroendocrine tumors. Gland Surg 2014;3(4): 258–75.

49. Dogeas E, Karagkounis G, Heaphy CM, et al. Alternative lengthening of telomeres predicts site of origin in neuroendocrine tumor liver metastases. J Am Coll Surg 2014;218(4):628–35.

50. Jansson L, Carlsson PO. Graft vascular function after transplantation of pancreatic islets. Diabetologia 2002;45(6):749–63.

51. Capurso G, Festa S, Valente R, et al. Molecular pathology and genetics of pancreatic endocrine tumours. J Mol Endocrinol 2012;49(1):R37–50.

52. Ro C, Chai W, Yu VE, et al. Pancreatic neuroendocrine tumors: biology, diagnosis, and treatment. Chin J Cancer 2013;32(6):312–24.

53. Marinoni I, Kurrer AS, Vassella E, et al. Loss of DAXX and ATRX are associated with chromosome instability and reduced survival of patients with pancreatic neuroendocrine tumors. Gastroenterology 2014;146(2):453–460 e5.

54. McGovern J, Singhi A, Borhani A, et al. CT Radiogenomic characterization of ATRX and DAXX alterations in primary pancreatic neuroendocrine tumors. Radiological Society of North America 2016 Scientific Assembly and Annual Meeting, Chicago, IL, November 27–December 2, 2016. Available at: archive.rsna.org/2016/16010605.html. Accessed September 18, 2017.

55. Leung RS, Biswas SV, Duncan M, et al. Imaging features of von Hippel-Lindau disease. Radiographics 2008;28(1):65–79 [quiz: 323].

MR Imaging of Pancreatic Neuroendocrine Tumors

Grace C. Lo, MD[a], Avinash Kambadakone, MD, FRCR[b,*]

KEYWORDS

- Pancreatic neuroendocrine tumor • MR imaging • Tumor classification • Tumor grading and staging

KEY POINTS

- Pancreatic neuroendocrine tumors (PNETs) are uncommon pancreatic tumors that are potentially malignant neoplasms, with a World Health Organization classification system based on the proliferative rate to predict tumor aggressiveness.
- Tumor detection, localization, and staging with diagnostic imaging are crucial to determine treatment strategy. Although computed tomography (CT) is the mainstay for evaluation of PNETs, MR imaging continues to expand its role as an important tool in diagnostic imaging of these lesions.
- With superior soft tissue and contrast resolution, MR imaging offers improved detection of small tumors (<2 cm) and hepatic metastatic lesion detection over CT, particularly with the help of fat-saturated T2-weighted, diffusion-weighted, and arterial phase postcontrast imaging.
- MR imaging avoids radiation exposure in patients who will be undergoing repeated examinations for surveillance or screening, which often begins at a young age in patients with inherited familial syndromes.

INTRODUCTION

Neuroendocrine tumors are neoplasms that possess neuroendocrine differentiation. These tumors can be found throughout the body, including the lung, pancreas, and gastrointestinal tract; the focus of this review is on pancreatic neuroendocrine tumors (PNETs). PNETs have previously been called islet cell tumors, although this is a misnomer, because these tumors have since been shown to arise from ductal pluripotent cells rather than islets of Langerhans.[1,2] Imaging plays a crucial role in identifying and diagnosing PNETs as well as in treatment planning based on size, location, and extrapancreatic spread of the tumor. Imaging is also involved in tumor surveillance and evaluating treatment response to systemic therapies. Although computed tomography (CT) has been traditionally used for evaluation of neuroendocrine tumors, evolving techniques with MR imaging have broadened and strengthened its role as an important diagnostic tool in assessing PNETs.

EPIDEMIOLOGY

PNETs account for 1% to 5% of all pancreatic neoplasms, with a prevalence rate of less than 1 in 100,000.[1,3] PNETs do not have a significant age or gender predilection, although are most commonly encountered between the fourth and seventh decades of life.[3] PNETs that present earlier are often associated with a familial syndrome. The tumors are generally well-demarcated, round neoplasms, the majority ranging from 1 to 5 cm.[3] In rare cases, more

Disclosures: The authors have nothing to disclose.
[a] Department of Radiology, Weill Cornell Medical College, 525 East 68th Street, New York, NY 10065, USA;
[b] Department of Radiology, Massachusetts General Hospital, 55 Fruit Street, Boston, MA 02114, USA
* Corresponding author.
E-mail address: akambadakone@mgh.harvard.edu

mri.theclinics.com

than one tumor may be found within the pancreas; in these situations, the presence of an associated familial syndrome should be questioned.

Most PNETs are sporadic in nature, although the minority of PNETs are a part of inherited familial syndromes.[4] Common syndromes associated with PNETs include those with autosomal dominant inheritance, such as multiple endocrine neoplasia type 1 (MEN-1), von Hippel-Lindau (VHL) syndrome, neurofibromatosis type 1 (NF-1), and tuberous sclerosis complex (TSC). Patients with MEN-1 have the highest incidence of PNET, followed by VHL, NF-1, and then TSC.[5]

TUMOR CLASSIFICATION

PNETs can be classified as functioning or nonfunctioning tumors based on the presence or absence of associated clinical symptoms. Because of the associated clinical symptoms, functional tumors often present earlier when the tumors are small (often subcentimeter) in size, whereas nonfunctioning tumors often present when they are several centimeters in size, when they are exerting mass effect on surrounding structures, or when there is metastatic disease.[6] Specific hormone assays are required to establish the diagnosis of functioning PNETs.

Insulinomas are the most common type of functional PNET, accounting for 50% of functioning PNETs.[3,7–9] Diagnosis relies on supervised fasting with documentation of glucose and insulin levels at the time of symptoms.[10] Because of its dramatic clinical symptoms, insulinomas often present early when they are small, which may explain why insulinomas generally have the best prognosis of all PNETs, with only about 5% to 10% demonstrating malignant behavior.[9,11] There is an even distribution throughout the pancreas, and 90% of tumors are smaller than 2 cm in diameter and 40% are smaller than 1 cm.[12]

Gastrinomas are the second most common type of functioning PNET after insulinomas. More than 90% of patients with gastrinomas have peptic ulcer disease, and differentiation of gastrinomas from other PNETs is based solely on the presence of hypergastrinemia.[12] At the time of diagnosis, 50% to 60% of gastrinomas are malignant.[9] Gastrinomas are commonly found within the so-called gastrinoma triangle, which comprises the head of the pancreas, the duodenal sweep, and the porta hepatis.[3,13–15]

Other less common functioning PNETs include glucagonomas, VIPomas, and somatostatinomas. Glucagonomas and VIPomas are both usually large when discovered, in the distal part of the pancreas, and most often are malignant.[3,9] Somatostatinomas are also rather large when discovered, commonly in the pancreatic head, with 50% of them being malignant.[3,9] Rarely, functional PNETs can secrete other hormones, including adrenocorticotropic hormone, parathyroid hormone-related protein, calcitonin, luteinizing hormone, renin, or erythropoietin.[10]

The reported overall percentage of PNETs classified as nonfunctioning varies greatly in the literature, ranging from 10% to 70%.[9,10,12] This wide range can possibly be attributed to recent advances in imaging and the increased discovery of incidental nonfunctioning PNETs. Many of these nonfunctioning PNETs do also secrete hormones, although are not significant enough to cause a specific associated syndrome. Nonfunctioning PNETs are generally larger than functioning PNETs, and they are often large, solitary, and heterogeneous in appearance, with up to 60% to 80% with metastatic disease at the time of diagnosis.[3,9,12]

TUMOR GRADING AND STAGING

Management and prognostication of PNETs are based on both tumor grading and staging. All PNETs are potentially malignant neoplasms, although the rate of malignancy varies between tumor types. In general, these neoplasms are slow growing, with a survival period from the time of diagnosis ranging from 2 to 10 years.[3] The World Health Organization (WHO) classification system divides PNETs into well-differentiated and poorly differentiated categories related to their histologic grade, ranging from grade 1 to grade 3, with a higher grade correlating to increased biologic aggressiveness of the tumor.[16] Well-differentiated tumors are generally either low or intermediate grade and can be rather indolent, whereas poorly differentiated tumors are high-grade tumors that are highly aggressive[16] (**Figs. 1** and **2**). The proliferative rate, which is used to assign grade, has been shown to provide prognostic information about PNETs. The rate is assessed as the mitotic counts (number of mitoses per unit area of tumor, usually expressed as mitoses per 10 high-power microscopic fields or per 2 mm^2) or as the Ki67 labeling index (percentage of neoplastic cells immunolabeling for the proliferation marker Ki67).[16]

There are currently 2 staging systems available for PNETs proposed by the American Joint Committee on Cancer (AJCC) and European Neuroendocrine Tumor Society (ENETS), which are both highly prognostic for relapse-free and overall survival.[17–19] Neither system is widely accepted, although the AJCC system is more widely used in

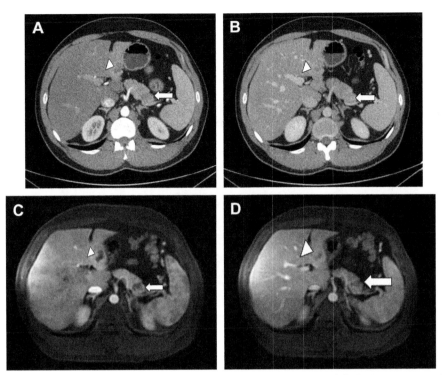

Fig. 1. A 33-year-old man with well-differentiated, intermediate grade PNET with hepatic metastases. On arterial phase CT (*A*), the pancreatic tail PNET (*arrow*) is peripherally enhancing, with a hepatic metastatic lesion (*arrowhead*) that demonstrates a similar arterial enhancement pattern. On portal venous phase of the CT (*B*), there is peripheral enhancement of the hepatic lesion (*arrowhead*), with less conspicuity of the pancreatic lesion (*arrow*) compared with the arterial phase. On MR imaging, the PNET (*arrow*) and hepatic metastatic lesion (*arrowhead*) are both more conspicuous on both arterial phase (*C*) and venous phase (*D*) imaging, with marked peripheral enhancement.

the United States, and the ENETS system is more commonly used in Europe.[20] A combined, modified classification system using both AJCC and ENETS classification has been proposed, which may provide better prognostication, using the T, N, and M definitions from ENETS and the staging definitions of AJCC.[20] With this combined system, termed the modified ENETS system, tumors are staged as following: T1 tumors are limited to the pancreas at less than 2 cm; T2 tumors are limited to the pancreas measuring 2 to 4 cm; T3 tumors are limited to the pancreas but are greater than 4 cm, or demonstrate invasion of the duodenum or common bile duct; and T4 tumors invade the adjacent structures.[20] N staging is based on the presence or absence of regional lymph node metastases, and M staging is based on the presence or absence of distant metastatic disease.

IMAGING TECHNIQUES

Anatomic and functional imaging techniques not only allow accurate detection and staging of PNETs but also facilitate assessment of extent of disease, biological behavior of these tumors, and response to therapy. CT is often used for initial evaluation of patients with abdominal pain or to identify suspected functioning tumors, as it is widely available, fast, and has excellent resolution. A range of sensitivities has been reported for CT, ranging from 30% to 80% for small tumors, with significantly higher sensitivities reaching up to 95% for larger lesions.[21–23]

The role of MR imaging in PNET evaluation is expanding. The superior soft tissue and contrast resolution of MR imaging allow improved detection of small tumors (<2 cm) with a sensitivity of 85%.[14,24–26] MR may also be superior in evaluation of hepatic metastatic disease and monitoring treatment response given its high sensitivity in lesion detection and characterization of tumor enhancement.[14] MR may also be preferred when radiation dose exposure is a concern, for example, in screening of high-risk patients and for patients undergoing surveillance or postoperative imaging.

Diagnostic imaging with endoscopic ultrasound (EUS) demonstrates a high sensitivity of 80% to 90% for detection of PNETs, particularly in patients with negative CT results (sensitivity

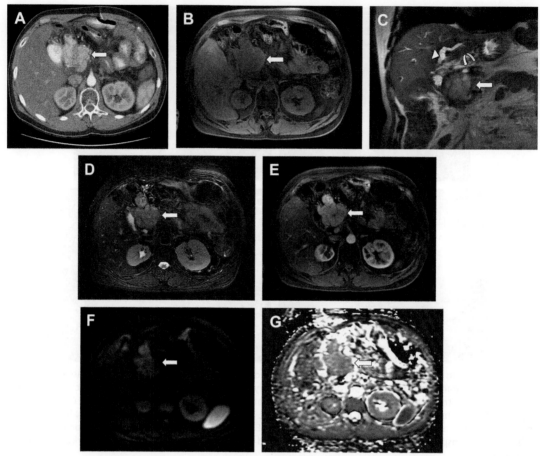

Fig. 2. A 64-year-old man with pathology-proven well-differentiated neuroendocrine tumor. At presentation on CT (*A*), the mass (*arrow*) was locally invasive into the mesenteric fat and was deemed unresectable. The patient underwent chemotherapy. Sixteen years later, the mass is largely unchanged in size. On MR imaging, the mass (*arrow*) is hypointense on axial T1-weighted imaging (*B*) and moderately hyperintense on coronal T2-weighted imaging (*C*), where there is also biliary ductal dilatation (*arrowhead*) and pancreatic ductal dilatation (*curved arrow*) secondary to mass effect. The mass (*arrow*) demonstrates mildly hyperintense signal on axial fat-saturated T2-weighted imaging (*D*), avid enhancement on arterial phase imaging (*E*), and hyperintensity on DWI (*F*) with corresponding low signal on the ADC map (*G*).

82%).[27–29] EUS allows improved visualization of morphologic features of lesions as well as clear spatial relationships between the tumor and bilio-pancreatic ductal anatomy; on occasion, nodal or hepatic metastases may be identified. A distinct advantage of EUS over other imaging techniques is the ability to sample the lesion with fine needle aspiration (FNA) or biopsy. Drawbacks of EUS include operator dependence with specialty training required, lower sensitivity of lesion detection in the tail of the pancreas, limited ability to interrogate the liver, and the invasive nature of the procedure. In general, CT and MR imaging are recommended for initial detection, characterization, and staging of PNETs, whereas EUS can be particularly helpful when aspiration or biopsy is needed for indeterminate findings.[30]

MR IMAGING PROTOCOLS

Dedicated MR imaging of the pancreas can be performed at 1.5 T or 3 T, although 3 T imaging is preferred given its improved signal-to-noise ratio and superior ability to perform parallel imaging.[31] Patients ideally fast for 4 to 6 hours before scanning, and negative oral contrast is administered before the examination. Some institutions prefer to use pineapple or blueberry juice, because the manganese content results in increased signal on T1-weighted images and reduced signal on T2-weighted images.[6,32–34]

The following sequences are generally included in a pancreatic protocol MR imaging: T2-weighted axial and coronal sequences; in-phase and opposed-phase T1-weighted sequences; fat-suppressed

T2-weighted sequence; diffusion-weighted images (DWI) sequence with corresponding apparent diffusion coefficient (ADC) map; T1-weighted gradient-echo sequence without contrast; T1-weighted gradient-echo sequence with dynamic contrast enhancement; and delayed fat-suppressed T1-weighted sequence. Two-dimensional and 3-dimensional (3D) MR cholangiopancreatography sequences can be optionally added to the pancreatic protocol, if assessment of the biliary and pancreatic ducts is desired. The protocol in its entirety can be completed within 30 minutes for most patients.

Fat-suppressed and DWI are particularly helpful when evaluating the pancreas. On T1-weighted images, fat suppression allows for superior depiction of the normal pancreas and enhances conspicuity of focal lesions. On T2-weighted images, fat suppression improves lesion detection, recognition of edema in the pancreas, and identification of hepatic metastases. DWI have been shown to be helpful in the diagnosis of PNETs, for primary tumors in the pancreas as well as for metastatic lesions in the liver, and the ADC values may be helpful in determining tumor aggressiveness, as discussed in detail later.[35–37]

Dynamic contrast administration is most commonly performed with 3D fat-suppressed spoiled gradient-echo sequences. Gadolinium is injected via a power injector at a rate of 2 mL/s, followed by a saline flush. Images are acquired in the arterial, venous, and equilibrium phases at 25 to 40, 45 to 65, and 180 to 300 seconds, respectively, and acquisition through the liver is usually performed to evaluate for hepatic involvement. When acquisition timing of the arterial phase is slightly off, the PNET may not be seen with its characteristic avid enhancement and may therefore be missed among the surrounding pancreas; other sequences such as fat-suppressed T2-weighted images and DWI will then be of crucial importance for lesion detection in these situations.[9,38–41] Similarly, in patients with contraindications to gadolinium administration, including severe allergy, pregnancy, and renal dysfunction with estimated glomerular filtration rate less than 30 mL/min/1.73 m^2, noncontrast MR imaging may be also helpful in PNET and metastatic lesion detection, although not characterization. The utility of fat-suppressed T2-weighted and diffusion-weighted sequences are discussed in more detail later.

IMAGING FINDINGS

On routine T1-weighted imaging, PNETs are usually relatively hypointense to the uniformly T1 hyperintense pancreatic parenchyma (**Box 1**). On

---

Box 1
Salient MR imaging features of pancreatic neuroendocrine tumors

Commonly solitary, although multiple lesions seen with syndromes

Low signal on T1-weighted images

Intermediate to high signal on T2-weighted images

Commonly solid, although may exhibit cystic change

Avid arterial enhancement on postcontrast imaging

Variable enhancement pattern, including heterogenous or ringlike enhancement

Pancreatic ductal obstruction uncommon

Vascular invasion uncommon

Liver and peripancreatic lymph nodes are common locations for metastases

---

T2-weighted images, these tumors generally demonstrate relative hyperintensity to the background pancreas; however, uncommonly, they can be T2 hypointense, with larger lesions exhibiting cystic or necrotic changes. On dynamic gadolinium-enhanced images, the masses characteristically demonstrate avid arterial enhancement. The enhancement pattern is varied and can be homogenous, heterogenous, or ringlike.[9,14] Gastrinomas, in particular, commonly demonstrate ringlike enhancement.[13] On the portal venous and equilibrium phases, enhancement is variable, and these tumors can be hypointense, isointense, or hyperintense to the surrounding pancreatic tissue. PNETs typically demonstrate restricted diffusion on DWI, although this may be variable based on tumor grade and amount of fibrosis, as is discussed later. In general, however, they will not demonstrate diffusion restriction greater than the spleen.

Because PNETs do not arise from ductal epithelium, pancreatic ductal obstruction is uncommon, except in cases where the tumor is large and obstructs the duct by mass effect. A second uncommon cause of ductal obstruction can be seen in small serotonin-secreting tumors, because fibrotic stricturing may occur secondary to serotonin secretion.[42] Vascular invasion is also uncommon, although intravascular venous extension can be seen, which can be a clue to the diagnosis.

Several studies have used MR to identify imaging markers to recognize aggressiveness of PNET. Higher-grade tumors tend to have size greater than 2 cm, ill-defined margins, and atypical vascular appearance, including heterogeneous enhancement or nonenhancement on the arterial phase.[35–37,43] In addition, DWI with ADC quantification may be helpful in predicting higher grade tumors, with an inverse relationship between ADC values and tumor grade.[35–37,43,44] De Robertis and colleagues[35] suggest an ADC value cutoff of 1.21×10^{-3} mm^2/s for the identification of grades 2 and 3 tumors, with a sensitivity and specificity of 70.8% and 80.7%, respectively. Jang and colleagues[36] also used ADC ratios, calculated by ADC values of the tumor to background pancreas, with higher ADC ratios identified with grade 1 PNETs than with grade 2 or 3 PNETs, and an ADC cutoff ratio less than 1.03 associated with grade 2 or 3 PNETs, with a specificity of 100%.

Common sites of metastases include the liver and peripancreatic lymph nodes. In the liver, metastatic lesions are usually hypointense on T1-weighted images and hyperintense on T2-weighted images. Similar to lesions found in the pancreas, both hepatic and lymph node metastases often show early, avid arterial enhancement, and therefore, these metastases are more conspicuous on arterial phase imaging, with variable degrees of washout on later phases.[45] Some lesions are exclusively seen on the arterial phase, highlighting the importance of optimal timing of imaging. In addition, hepatic metastases may demonstrate early ringlike enhancement of liver lesions, which may be helpful in differentiating it from other hepatic neoplasms.[14,24] On delayed postcontrast imaging, however, there may be peripheral rim that is hypointense relative to the center of the lesion, creating a target appearance that has been reported to be highly specific for hypervascular metastases, especially neuroendocrine metastases.[45–47] The use of a hepatocyte-specific agent, such as gadoxetate disodium, has been shown to improve the detection of hepatic metastases, although not many studies have been performed specifically investigating its utility with neuroendocrine metastases. A recent study has suggested that hepatobiliary phase imaging may be helpful, with high levels of interobserver agreement; this contrast agent is most helpful in lesion detection when deciding whether cytoreductive surgery is an option rather than for lesion characterization.[48–50]

In additional to postcontrast arterial phase imaging, fat-suppressed T2-weighted images and DWI can be helpful for the detection of hepatic metastatic lesions.[9,39] Several studies have found that DWI improves detection of liver metastases from various primary malignancies, with superior detection of hepatic metastases also observed in patients with PNET on DWI over both T2-weighted images and dynamic gadolinium-enhanced imaging, with one study demonstrating sensitivities of up to 71%.[38,40,41] In fact, a study has proposed that DWI alone may be acceptable for visualization and measurement of PNET hepatic metastases.[39]

MONITORING RESPONSE TO THERAPY

Imaging plays a crucial role in tumor staging, allowing determination of lesion size, presence of local invasion, and presence of nodal and distant metastatic disease, particularly in the liver. PNET staging suggested by imaging along with tumor grade confirmed via tissue sampling helps determine therapy for patients with PNET.

Although several treatment options are available, the only potential curative option for PNET is surgery. In general, if the lesion is localized, most patients undergo pancreatectomy with lymphadenectomy, although if the tumor is low grade, small, and distant from the main pancreatic duct, enucleation may also be a viable option.[8,10] In patients with advanced locoregional, recurrent, or metastatic disease, cytoreductive surgery is a key treatment strategy, although other locoregional therapies (such as transarterial chemoembolization [TACE], radiofrequency ablation, internal radiotherapy, or infusional chemotherapy) and systemic therapies (such as somatostatin analogues like octreotide; cytotoxic chemotherapy; or targeted agents like sunitinib, everolimus, and bevacizumab) can be considered.[8,10] Occasionally, in patients with hepatic metastases and without extrahepatic disease, liver transplantation can be considered.[8] In nonoperative candidates, locoregional or systemic therapies are usually used to prolong survival and improve quality of life.

In patients undergoing locoregional or systemic therapy, MR imaging can be helpful in assessing treatment response, although the data in this realm are limited. Li and colleagues[51] have proposed that an increase in mean ADC, decrease in mean arterial enhancement, and increase in venous enhancement between baseline imaging before therapy and 1-month post-TACE imaging can help predict whether these patients would respond to therapy at the 6-month follow-up.

DIFFERENTIAL DIAGNOSIS OF SOLID NEUROENDOCRINE TUMORS

The differential diagnosis of solid pancreatic tumors is broad, including both benign and malignant processes (Table 1). In general, differentiating PNET from other solid pancreatic tumors

Table 1
Differential diagnosis of solid pancreatic tumors or masslike lesions

Common	PDAC
Uncommon	PNET
	Metastases to the pancreas
	Mass-forming pancreatitis
	IPAS
Rare	Pancreatoblastoma
	Pancreatic lymphoma
	Pancreatic sarcoidosis
	Castleman disease of the pancreas

can be based on the characteristic hypervascular nature of PNETs, although several notable diagnostic challenges include pancreatic ductal adenocarcinoma (PDAC), intrapancreatic accessory spleen (IPAS), and hypervascular metastases to the pancreas.

With PDAC accounting for 85% to 95% of all solid pancreatic tumors, PNETs are relatively rare in comparison, although accurate diagnosis is crucial, because prognosis and treatment differ greatly.[1] Several imaging features may be helpful in differentiating the two solid tumors. PNETs will generally demonstrate avid arterial enhancement, which is uncommon with PDAC, a typically hypovascular tumor. In addition, presence of a ringlike enhancement pattern can often suggest PNET over PDAC.[14] However, differentiating hypovascular PNETs from PDAC remains a challenge.

Additional imaging features, such as the presence of vascular invasion and pancreatic ductal dilatation, will help to favor PDAC as the leading diagnosis. Alternatively, cystic degeneration and calcifications will help favor PNETs. Ultimately, tissue sampling is often needed to confirm the diagnosis.

Differentiating PNETs from IPAS can also be difficult. IPAS will demonstrate low signal on T1-weighted images, high signal on T2-weighted images, and avid enhancement on postcontrast sequences, all imaging features similar to PNETs (**Fig. 3**). However, IPAS will follow the same signal characteristics and contrast enhancement pattern as the spleen. Unlike PNETs, IPAS will demonstrate the arciform splenic enhancement pattern that the spleen demonstrates during the arterial phase, which is due to the perfusion differences between red and white pulp, because IPAS are supplied by the splenic artery and drained by the splenic vein.[1] Furthermore, IPAS should be located within the pancreas no further than 3 cm from the pancreatic tail; a lesion in the head or body is unlikely to be an IPAS[42] (**Table 2**). In addition, on DWI, PNETs are similar in appearance to IPAS, although IPAS will demonstrate lower mean ADC values compared with PNET.[52] In many cases, the arciform arterial enhancement pattern itself can be sufficient for diagnosis in large IPAS. In small IPAS, where it may be difficult to distinguish the enhancement pattern, confirmation can be made with a Technetium 99m (^{99m}Tc) sulfur colloid scintigraphy or ^{99m}Tc head-damaged red blood cell scintigraphy. In addition, a superparamagnetic iron oxide MR

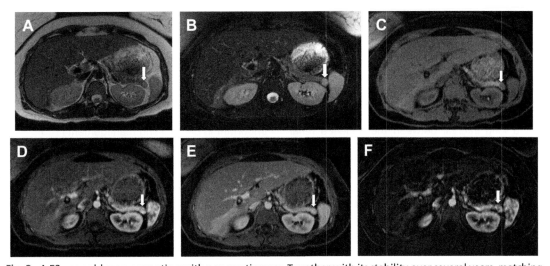

Fig. 3. A 52-year-old man presenting with pancreatic mass. Together with its stability over several years, matching of signal intensity between the lesion (*arrow*) and the spleen on T2-weighted imaging (*A*), fat-saturated T2-weighted imaging (*B*), T1-weighted imaging (*C*), arterial phase imaging (*D*), and portal venous phase imaging (*E*) favored intrahepatic accessory spleen. Subtracted postcontrast T1-weighted imaging (*F*) best demonstrates the typical arciform enhancement pattern in both the spleen and the IPAS.

Table 2
Comparison of imaging characteristics between pancreatic neuroendocrine tumor and intrapancreatic accessory spleen

	PNET	IPAS
T1 signal	Hypointense	Hypointense
T2 signal	Hyperintense	Hyperintense
Arterial enhancement	Commonly solid arterial enhancement, although can have heterogeneous or ringlike pattern	Arciform arterial enhancement, following the spleen
Venous enhancement	Variable	Follows the spleen
DWI and ADC	Often restricts diffusion, will not be as low as spleen on ADC	Restricts diffusion following the spleen, low on ADC
Location	Even distribution throughout the pancreas	Pancreatic tail

Table 3
Comparison of imaging characteristics between pancreatic neuroendocrine tumor and hypervascular metastases to the pancreas

	PNET	Hypervascular Metastases to the Pancreas
T1 signal	Hypointense	Hypointense
T2 signal	Hyperintense	Hyperintense
Arterial enhancement	Avid enhancement	Avid enhancement
Venous enhancement	Variable	Variable
DWI	Often restricts diffusion	Restricts diffusion
Ductal dilatation	Present if lesion is large or by the duct, resulting in mass effect	Present if lesion is large or by the duct, resulting in mass effect
Cystic change	Can be present	Can be present, particularly with renal cell metastases
Clinical history	Favored if hormone-secreting syndrome or presence of inherited disease	Favored if history of hypervascular primary tumor elsewhere, even if history is distant

contrast agent, ferumoxide, which is taken up by reticuloendothelial cells in the liver and spleen, may also help recognize IPAS.[53]

Finally, differentiating PNETs from hypervascular metastases can prove difficult. Renal cell carcinomas account for the most common hypervascular tumor to metastasize to the pancreas, although other primary hypervascular tumors, including hepatocellular carcinoma and thyroid cancer, can also spread to the pancreas[54] (Table 3). In these situations, a history of primary malignancy elsewhere can be strongly suggestive of the diagnosis, although tissue sampling is often necessary for confirmation.[42] It should be noted that renal cell carcinoma metastases to the pancreas can occur late, even 10 years after the initial diagnosis, and thus a long interval between the patient's renal cell carcinoma diagnosis and the presence of a new pancreatic lesion is not a sufficient reason to favor a new diagnosis or to exclude a metastatic lesion.[55] Hypervascular metastases can be solitary or multiple in number, similar to PNETs. Renal cell carcinoma, in particular, can also demonstrate cystic changes as seen in PNETs, and contrast enhancement can be solid in small tumors or ring-like in larger masses, also similar to PNETs[1] (Fig. 4). Renal cell metastases can be suggested if there is ductal dilatation, although as mentioned before, PNETs can also cause ductal dilatation on occasion if they are large enough.[56]

DIFFERENTIAL DIAGNOSIS OF CYSTIC NEUROENDOCRINE TUMORS

Cystic pancreatic lesions are considered uncommon, although technological advancement and expanded utilization of cross-sectional imaging, especially MR imaging, has increased detection of these lesions, many small in size and affecting up to 10% to 15% of patients undergoing imaging.[57] The differential diagnosis for cystic pancreatic tumors is also broad, ranging from benign to malignant, making accurate diagnosis extremely important in determining management (Table 4).

The most common cystic neoplasms represent greater than 90% of all cystic pancreatic tumors and include serous cyst adenomas (SCA), primary mucinous cystic neoplasms, and intraductal papillary mucinous neoplasms.[58] Less common cystic neoplasms include PNET, solid pseudopapillary neoplasm of the pancreas, and cystic degeneration of other solid neoplasms.

Although PNETs are predominantly solid, approximately 10% to 20% of PNETs demonstrate cystic change, commonly presenting with both cystic and solid components.[59,60] Controversy exists over whether this is truly cystic degeneration

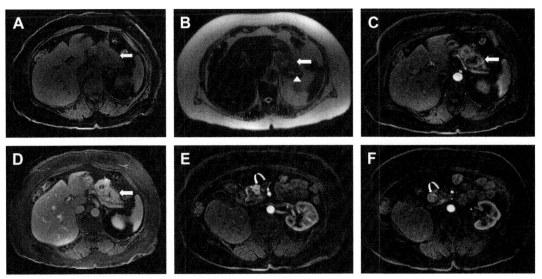

Fig. 4. A 61-year-old woman with history of right-sided clear cell renal cell carcinoma, status post right nephrectomy, presenting with several pancreatic masses. The dominant mass (*arrow*) in the pancreatic tail was hypointense on T1-weighted imaging (*A*), heterogeneous on T2-weighted imaging (*B*) with distal pancreatic ductal dilatation (*arrowhead*). On postcontrast imaging, the mass (*arrow*) demonstrated peripheral ringlike enhancement on the arterial phase (*C*), with persistent enhancement on the portal venous phase (*D*). Several smaller lesions (*curved arrows*) were seen on the arterial phase (*E, F*) with more solid enhancement. These masses were renal cell metastases.

of a solid PNET versus a de novo cyst formation or another distinct disease entity separate from PNET, because there is a lack of necrotic material in most resected specimens and a higher association with MEN-1.[57,61] Most cystic PNETs present larger in size than solid PNETs and commonly are nonfunctioning, unlike solid PNETs, which are more evenly split between functioning and nonfunctioning tumors.[61] Imaging of cystic PNETs often demonstrate a thick-walled, unilocular cystic

Table 4 Differential diagnosis of cystic pancreatic tumors	
Common	Serous cystadenoma Primary mucinous cystic neoplasm Intraductal papillary mucinous neoplasm
Uncommon	Solid psuedopapillary neoplasm Cystic neuroendocrine tumor Cystic degeneration of solid neoplasm
Rare	Acinar cell neoplasm Intraductal tubular neoplasm Angiomatous neoplasm Lymphoepithelial cysts Mesenchymal tumor

lesion, often with a solid component or septation, which cannot be always readily differentiated from other cystic pancreatic masses. A diagnosis of pancreatic PNETs can be suggested in the presence of a thick-enhancing wall, although other clues may be helpful, including the presence of an arterially enhancing septation or nodule, presence of concurrent hypervascular liver metastases, supportive findings on octreotide scan, or, less commonly, clinical symptoms associated with functioning PNETs.[62,63] Further characterization is often required with EUS and FNA to confirm the diagnosis and guide management.[58]

Classically, SCAs are hypointense on T1-weighted images and hyperintense on T2-weighted imaging, demonstrating a conglomerate of small cysts with thin septa that radiate from a central scar that may enhance on delayed phase imaging. However, a small subset of patients with SCAs may be somewhat solid appearing, making differentiation from PNET particularly important, because management is markedly different for these two entities. In these patients, the diagnosis of SCA can be suggested when the lesion is extremely T2 hyperintense versus moderately high in signal intensity seen in PNET. In addition, SCAs do not demonstrate restricted diffusion on subjective and objective evaluation with ADC maps, which can also set these lesions apart from PNETs.[64] These findings are summarized in **Table 5**.

Table 5
Comparison of imaging characteristics between pancreatic neuroendocrine tumor and serous cystadenoma

	PNET	Serous Cystadenoma
T1 signal	Hypointense	Hypointense
T2 signal	Moderately hyperintense	Markedly hyperintense, can demonstrate conglomerate of small cysts with central scar
Morphology	Variable, although often unilocular with or without internal septations; may be solid appearing or cystic appearing	Conglomerate of small cysts with thin septa and central scar; may be solid appearing or cystic appearing
Enhancement pattern	May have arterially enhancing thick walls, septations, or nodules	May have delayed enhancement of central scar
Cystic component	Variable, but will be moderately T2 hyperintense	Variable, but will be markedly T2 hyperintense
DWI	Often restricts diffusion	No restricted diffusion
Metastatic disease	May be present	Absent
Clinical symptoms	May be present	Absent

IMAGING SCREENING AND SURVEILLANCE
Multiple Endocrine Neoplasia Type 1

MEN-1 is one of the most common familial cancer syndromes and causes tumors in the parathyroid gland as well as neuroendocrine tumors in the pancreas, gastrointestinal tract, the anterior pituitary, thymus, lung and bronchus, and the adrenal cortex.[65] The incidence of PNETs in patients with MEN-1 varies from 30% to 80% in different studies, although malignant PNETs are reported to be the most common cause of death in patients with MEN-1.[5,65–67] Worse prognosis is seen with nonfunctioning tumors when compared with functioning tumors.[65] As such, early and frequent imaging screening for PNETs in patients with MEN-1 is suggested to begin by age 10 using CT, MR imaging, or EUS and to occur annually.[65,68]

von Hippel-Lindau Syndrome

VHL syndrome predisposes patients to benign and malignant tumors as well as cyst development, in several organs and systems, including the central nervous system, kidneys, pancreas, adrenal glands, and reproductive organs. The incidence of PNETs in patients with VHL syndrome ranges from 10% to 17%, with greater than 98% of PNETs found to be nonfunctioning.[5] Compared with MEN-1, PNETs seen in VHL are often solitary rather than multiple and are malignant in 8% to 50% of patients, although most deaths in VHL patients are secondary to metastatic renal cell carcinoma or complications of cerebellar hemangioblastomas.[5] Treatment is often based on presence of symptoms, which is rare in VHL patients, and risk of malignancy, including size of the tumor and presence of metastatic disease. Imaging screening for PNETs in patients with VHL is suggested to begin by age 8 with abdominal ultrasound with supplemental MR imaging as indicated, with either CT or MR imaging beginning at least by age 18.[69] Surveillance has been recommended at yearly intervals for tumors less than 1 cm; tumors greater than 1 cm are managed based on location, often surgically.[5,69]

Neurofibromatosis Type 1

NF-1, also known as von Recklinghausen disease, causes benign and malignant tumors of the skin, central and peripheral nervous system, as well as neurodegenerative and musculoskeletal abnormalities. PNETs can occur in NF-1 patients though are relatively uncommon, occurring in 0% to 10% of patients.[5] Given its rarity in this patient population, no dedicated screening recommendations have been established.

Tuberous Sclerosis Complex

TSC is a highly variable disease that causes tumors of several organs and organ groups, including the skin, brain, kidneys, lung, heart, and gastrointestinal system. Specific to the pancreas, PNETs are relatively uncommon, with approximately 2% to 9% of TSC patients found to have PNETs, which is only slightly increased incidence compared with the general population.[5,70,71] Routine dedicated pancreatic imaging surveillance is not uniformly recommended, although these patients receive routine renal MR imaging for angiomyolipomas. Either expansion of the renal mass protocol to a more complete abdominal protocol is recommended for adequate surveillance of the pancreas or, at minimum, attention to the pancreatic parenchyma on renal mass protocol MR imaging is advised.[71]

SUMMARY

PNETs are uncommon pancreatic tumors that can be classified as functioning or nonfunctioning tumors based on the presence or absence of associated clinical symptoms. All PNETs are potentially malignant neoplasms, and a WHO classification system based on the proliferative rate has been developed to help predict tumor aggressiveness. Tumor detection, localization, and staging with diagnostic imaging are crucial to determine treatment strategy. With superior soft tissue contrast and contrast resolution, MR imaging offers improved detection of small tumors (<2 cm) and hepatic metastatic lesion detection over CT, particularly with the use of fat-saturated T2-weighted, diffusion-weighted, and arterial phase postcontrast imaging. In addition, in patients who will undergo repeated examinations for surveillance or screening, which often begins at a young age for those with inherited familial syndromes, MR imaging allows patients to avoid radiation exposure. With ongoing improvements to MR technology and scan time, as well as increasing accessibility to MR scanners, MR imaging will continue to expand its role as an important tool in diagnostic imaging of PNETs.

REFERENCES

1. Low G, Panu A, Millo N, et al. Multimodality imaging of neoplastic and nonneoplastic solid lesions of the pancreas. Radiographics 2011;31(4):993–1015.
2. Oberg K, Eriksson B. Endocrine tumours of the pancreas. Best Pract Res Clin Gastroenterol 2005;19(5):753–81.
3. Kloppel G, Anlauf M. Pancreatic endocrine tumors. Pathol Case Rev 2006;11(6):256–67.
4. O'Grady HL, Conlon KC. Pancreatic neuroendocrine tumours. Eur J Surg Oncol 2008;34(3):324–32.
5. Jensen RT, Berna MJ, Bingham DB, et al. Inherited pancreatic endocrine tumor syndromes: advances in molecular pathogenesis, diagnosis, management, and controversies. Cancer 2008;113(7 suppl):1807–43.
6. Tamm EP, Bhosale P, Lee JH, et al. State-of-the-art imaging of pancreatic neuroendocrine tumors. Surg Oncol Clin N Am 2016;25(2):375–400.
7. Kim JY, Hong SM. Recent updates on neuroendocrine tumors from the gastrointestinal and pancreatobiliary tracts. Arch Pathol Lab Med 2016;140(5):437–48.
8. Burns WR, Edil BH. Neuroendocrine pancreatic tumors: guidelines for management and update. Curr Treat Options Oncol 2012;13(1):24–34.
9. Lewis RB, Lattin GE Jr, Paal E. Pancreatic endocrine tumors: radiologic-clinicopathologic correlation. Radiographics 2010;30(6):1445–64.
10. Milan SA, Yeo CJ. Neuroendocrine tumors of the pancreas. Curr Opin Oncol 2012;24(1):46–55.
11. Service FJ, McMahon MM, O'Brien PC, et al. Functioning insulinoma–incidence, recurrence, and long-term survival of patients: a 60-year study. Mayo Clin Proc 1991;66(7):711–9.
12. Mansour JC, Chen H. Pancreatic endocrine tumors. J Surg Res 2004;120(1):139–61.
13. Semelka RC, Custodio CM, Cem Balci N, et al. Neuroendocrine tumors of the pancreas: spectrum of appearances on MRI. J Magn Reson Imaging 2000;11(2):141–8.
14. Semelka RC, Cumming MJ, Shoenut JP, et al. Islet cell tumors: comparison of dynamic contrast-enhanced CT and MR imaging with dynamic gadolinium enhancement and fat suppression. Radiology 1993;186(3):799–802.
15. Yang RH, Chu YK. Zollinger-Ellison syndrome: revelation of the gastrinoma triangle. Radiol Case Rep 2015;10(1):827.
16. Klimstra DS, Modlin IR, Coppola D, et al. The pathologic classification of neuroendocrine tumors: a review of nomenclature, grading, and staging systems. Pancreas 2010;39(6):707–12.
17. Strosberg JR, Cheema A, Weber J, et al. Prognostic validity of a novel American Joint Committee on Cancer staging classification for pancreatic neuroendocrine tumors. J Clin Oncol 2011;29(22):3044–9.
18. Strosberg JR, Cheema A, Weber JM, et al. Relapse-free survival in patients with nonmetastatic, surgically resected pancreatic neuroendocrine tumors: an analysis of the AJCC and ENETS staging classifications. Ann Surg 2012;256(2):321–5.
19. Cho JH, Ryu JK, Song SY, et al. Prognostic validity of the American Joint Committee on Cancer and the European Neuroendocrine Tumors Staging classifications for pancreatic neuroendocrine tumors: a retrospective nationwide multicenter study in South Korea. Pancreas 2016;45(7):941–6.
20. Luo G, Javed A, Strosberg JR, et al. Modified staging classification for pancreatic neuroendocrine tumors on the basis of the American Joint Committee on Cancer and European Neuroendocrine Tumor Society Systems. J Clin Oncol 2017;35(3):274–80.
21. McAuley G, Delaney H, Colville J, et al. Multimodality preoperative imaging of pancreatic insulinomas. Clin Radiol 2005;60(10):1039–50.
22. Reznek RH. CT/MRI of neuroendocrine tumours. Canc Imag 2006;6:S163–77.

23. Stark DD, Moss AA, Goldberg HI, et al. CT of pancreatic islet cell tumors. Radiology 1984; 150(2):491–4.

24. Herwick S, Miller FH, Keppke AL. MRI of islet cell tumors of the pancreas. AJR Am J Roentgenol 2006; 187(5):W472–80.

25. Ichikawa T, Peterson MS, Federle MP, et al. Islet cell tumor of the pancreas: biphasic CT versus MR imaging in tumor detection. Radiology 2000;216(1): 163–71.

26. Thoeni RF, Mueller-Lisse UG, Chan R, et al. Detection of small, functional islet cell tumors in the pancreas: selection of MR imaging sequences for optimal sensitivity. Radiology 2000;214(2):483–90.

27. Rosch T, Lightdale CJ, Botet JF, et al. Localization of pancreatic endocrine tumors by endoscopic ultrasonography. N Engl J Med 1992;326(26):1721–6.

28. Pitre J, Soubrane O, Palazzo L, et al. Endoscopic ultrasonography for the preoperative localization of insulinomas. Pancreas 1996;13(1):55–60.

29. Sotoudehmanesh R, Hedayat A, Shirazian N, et al. Endoscopic ultrasonography (EUS) in the localization of insulinoma. Endocrine 2007;31(3):238–41.

30. Kim YH, Saini S, Sahani D, et al. Imaging diagnosis of cystic pancreatic lesions: pseudocyst versus nonpseudocyst. Radiographics 2005;25(3):671–85.

31. Sandrasegaran K, Lin C, Akisik FM, et al. State-of-the-art pancreatic MRI. AJR Am J Roentgenol 2010;195(1):42–53.

32. Coppens E, Metens T, Winant C, et al. Pineapple juice labeled with gadolinium: a convenient oral contrast for magnetic resonance cholangiopancreatography. Eur Radiol 2005;15(10):2122–9.

33. Papanikolaou N, Karantanas A, Maris T, et al. MR cholangiopancreatography before and after oral blueberry juice administration. J Comput Assist Tomogr 2000;24(2):229–34.

34. Riordan RD, Khonsari M, Jeffries J, et al. Pineapple juice as a negative oral contrast agent in magnetic resonance cholangiopancreatography: a preliminary evaluation. Br J Radiol 2004;77(924):991–9.

35. De Robertis R, Cingarlini S, Tinazzi Martini P, et al. Pancreatic neuroendocrine neoplasms: magnetic resonance imaging features according to grade and stage. World J Gastroenterol 2017;23(2): 275–85.

36. Jang KM, Kim SH, Lee SJ, et al. The value of gadoxetic acid-enhanced and diffusion-weighted MRI for prediction of grading of pancreatic neuroendocrine tumors. Acta Radiol 2014;55(2):140–8.

37. Lotfalizadeh E, Ronot M, Wagner M, et al. Prediction of pancreatic neuroendocrine tumour grade with MR imaging features: added value of diffusion-weighted imaging. Eur Radiol 2017;27(4):1748–59.

38. d'Assignies G, Fina P, Bruno O, et al. High sensitivity of diffusion-weighted MR imaging for the detection of liver metastases from neuroendocrine tumors: comparison with T2-weighted and dynamic gadolinium-enhanced MR imaging. Radiology 2013;268(2):390–9.

39. Lavelle LP, O'Neill AC, McMahon CJ, et al. Is diffusion-weighted MRI sufficient for follow-up of neuroendocrine tumour liver metastases? Clin Radiol 2016;71(9):863–8.

40. Low RN, Gurney J. Diffusion-weighted MRI (DWI) in the oncology patient: value of breathhold DWI compared to unenhanced and gadolinium-enhanced MRI. J Magn Reson Imaging 2007;25(4): 848–58.

41. Soyer P, Boudiaf M, Place V, et al. Preoperative detection of hepatic metastases: comparison of diffusion-weighted, T2-weighted fast spin echo and gadolinium-enhanced MR imaging using surgical and histopathologic findings as standard of reference. Eur J Radiol 2011;80(2):245–52.

42. Raman SP, Hruban RH, Cameron JL, et al. Pancreatic imaging mimics: part 2, pancreatic neuroendocrine tumors and their mimics. AJR Am J Roentgenol 2012;199(2):309–18.

43. Canellas R, Lo G, Bhowmik S, et al. Pancreatic neuroendocrine tumor: correlations between MRI features, tumor biology, and clinical outcome after surgery. J Magn Reson Imaging 2018;47(2):425–32.

44. Kim M, Kang TW, Kim YK, et al. Pancreatic neuroendocrine tumour: correlation of apparent diffusion coefficient or WHO classification with recurrence-free survival. Eur J Radiol 2016;85(3):680–7.

45. Kamaya A, Maturen KE, Tye GA, et al. Hypervascular liver lesions. Semin Ultrasound CT MR 2009; 30(5):387–407.

46. Danet IM, Semelka RC, Leonardou P, et al. Spectrum of MRI appearances of untreated metastases of the liver. AJR Am J Roentgenol 2003;181(3): 809–17.

47. Mahfouz AE, Hamm B, Wolf KJ. Peripheral washout: a sign of malignancy on dynamic gadolinium-enhanced MR images of focal liver lesions. Radiology 1994;190(1):49–52.

48. Jeong HT, Kim MJ, Park MS, et al. Detection of liver metastases using gadoxetic-enhanced dynamic and 10- and 20-minute delayed phase MR imaging. J Magn Reson Imaging 2012;35(3):635–43.

49. Scharitzer M, Ba-Ssalamah A, Ringl H, et al. Preoperative evaluation of colorectal liver metastases: comparison between gadoxetic acid-enhanced 3.0-T MRI and contrast-enhanced MDCT with histopathological correlation. Eur Radiol 2013;23(8): 2187–96.

50. Morse B, Jeong D, Thomas K, et al. Magnetic resonance imaging of neuroendocrine tumor hepatic metastases: does hepatobiliary phase imaging improve lesion conspicuity and interobserver agreement of lesion measurements? Pancreas 2017; 46(9):1219–24.

51. Li Z, Bonekamp S, Halappa VG, et al. Islet cell liver metastases: assessment of volumetric early response with functional MR imaging after transarterial chemoembolization. Radiology 2012;264(1):97–109.

52. Kang BK, Kim JH, Byun JH, et al. Diffusion-weighted MRI: usefulness for differentiating intrapancreatic accessory spleen and small hypervascular neuroendocrine tumor of the pancreas. Acta Radiol 2014; 55(10):1157–65.

53. Wang YX. Superparamagnetic iron oxide based MRI contrast agents: current status of clinical application. Quant Imaging Med Surg 2011;1(1):35–40.

54. Triantopoulou C, Kolliakou E, Karoumpalis I, et al. Metastatic disease to the pancreas: an imaging challenge. Insights Imaging 2012;3(2):165–72.

55. De Riese W, Goldenberg K, Allhoff E, et al. Spontaneous regression of metastatic renal carcinoma with long-term survival. Br J Urol 1991;68(1):98–100.

56. Vincenzi M, Pasquotti G, Polverosi R, et al. Imaging of pancreatic metastases from renal cell carcinoma. Canc Imag 2014;14:5.

57. Kim TS, Fernandez-del Castillo C. Diagnosis and management of pancreatic cystic neoplasms. Hematol Oncol Clin North Am 2015;29(4):655–74.

58. Sakorafas GH, Smyrniotis V, Reid-Lombardo KM, et al. Primary pancreatic cystic neoplasms of the pancreas revisited. Part IV: rare cystic neoplasms. Surg Oncol 2012;21(3):153–63.

59. Kawamoto S, Johnson PT, Shi C, et al. Pancreatic neuroendocrine tumor with cystlike changes: evaluation with MDCT. AJR Am J Roentgenol 2013;200(3):W283–90.

60. Singhi AD, Chu LC, Tatsas AD, et al. Cystic pancreatic neuroendocrine tumors: a clinicopathologic study. Am J Surg Pathol 2012;36(11):1666–73.

61. Bordeianou L, Vagefi PA, Sahani D, et al. Cystic pancreatic endocrine neoplasms: a distinct tumor type? J Am Coll Surg 2008;206(6):1154–8.

62. Graziani R, Mautone S, Vigo M, et al. Spectrum of magnetic resonance imaging findings in pancreatic and other abdominal manifestations of Von Hippel-Lindau disease in a series of 23 patients: a pictorial review. JOP 2014;15(1):1–18.

63. Barral M, Soyer P, Dohan A, et al. Magnetic resonance imaging of cystic pancreatic lesions in adults: an update in current diagnostic features and management. Abdom Imaging 2014;39(1):48–65.

64. Park HS, Kim SY, Hong SM, et al. Hypervascular solid-appearing serous cystic neoplasms of the pancreas: differential diagnosis with neuroendocrine tumours. Eur Radiol 2016;26(5):1348–58.

65. Sadowski SM, Triponez F. Management of pancreatic neuroendocrine tumors in patients with MEN 1. Gland Surg 2015;4(1):63–8.

66. Brandi ML, Gagel RF, Angeli A, et al. Guidelines for diagnosis and therapy of MEN type 1 and type 2. J Clin Endocrinol Metab 2001;86(12):5658–71.

67. Dralle H, Krohn SL, Karges W, et al. Surgery of resectable nonfunctioning neuroendocrine pancreatic tumors. World J Surg 2004;28(12):1248–60.

68. Thakker RV, Newey PJ, Walls GV, et al. Clinical practice guidelines for multiple endocrine neoplasia type 1 (MEN1). J Clin Endocrinol Metab 2012;97(9):2990–3011.

69. Libutti SK, Choyke PL, Bartlett DL, et al. Pancreatic neuroendocrine tumors associated with von Hippel Lindau disease: diagnostic and management recommendations. Surgery 1998;124(6):1153–9.

70. Koc G, Sugimoto S, Kuperman R, et al. Pancreatic tumors in children and young adults with tuberous sclerosis complex. Pediatr Radiol 2017;47(1):39–45.

71. Larson AM, Hedgire SS, Deshpande V, et al. Pancreatic neuroendocrine tumors in patients with tuberous sclerosis complex. Clin Genet 2012;82(6):558–63.

Cystic Pancreatic Tumors

Kristine S. Burk, MD*, David Knipp, MD, Dushyant V. Sahani, MD

KEYWORDS

- Cystic pancreatic neoplasm • Intraductal papillary mucinous neoplasm • Serous cystadenoma
- Mucinous cystadenoma and cystadenocarcinoma • Solid pseudopapillary tumor

KEY POINTS

- Cystic pancreatic lesions are common and often incidentally detected. Correct identification of lesions by clinical history and imaging, and differentiation of benign from malignant neoplasms are critical.
- With its superior soft tissue contrast and multi-parametric nature, MR imaging/magnetic resonance cholangiopancreatography is an ideal single imaging modality for complete characterization of cystic pancreatic lesions. Other imaging modalities can offer additional, specific information, including multi-detector computed tomography for detection of calcification, PET for metabolic assessment, and endoscopic ultrasound for fluid and tissue sampling.
- Main-duct intraductal papillary mucinous neoplasms, mucinous cystic neoplasms, and solid pseudopapillary tumors all carry significant risk for malignant degeneration and, in amenable patients, are typically immediately resected.
- The appropriate follow-up/screening algorithm for cystic pancreatic lesions has undergone multiple revisions in the last few years. The most up-to-date recommendations incorporate lesion size, communication with the main pancreatic duct, and age of patients at the initial presentation.

INTRODUCTION

Cystic pancreatic lesions are common, present in 2.5% of the population[1] and incidentally detected on 2.2% of computed tomography (CT) examinations of the abdomen and pelvis and up to 19.6% of MR imaging examinations of the abdomen.[2] Most lesions, on the order of 70%, are asymptomatic, and most are benign. However, some of these benign lesions have malignant potential as high as 68%[3]; therefore, correct identification, complete characterization, and adequate follow-up/management of these lesions are paramount.

This review addresses the most common imaging modalities used for the evaluation of cystic pancreatic lesions, with a focus on MR imaging. Following this is a discussion of the epidemiology, pathology, and imaging characteristics of the most common cystic pancreatic neoplasms, including intraductal papillary mucinous neoplasm (IPMN), serous cystic neoplasm (SCN), mucinous cystic neoplasm (MCN),

and solid pseudopapillary tumor (SPT), and a brief discussion of other causes of cystic pancreatic lesions, including cystic degeneration of solid malignant masses, pancreatitis-related pseudocysts, and pancreatic cysts associated with systemic disease. Finally, the authors conclude with a discussion about how to follow cystic pancreatic lesions, incorporating the most up-to-date guideline recommendations.

IMAGING MODALITIES USED TO EVALUATE CYSTIC PANCREATIC LESIONS

Because most pancreatic cystic lesions are asymptomatic, they are most often found incidentally on cross-sectional CT or MR imaging studies. Occasionally a cystic lesion may be found by transabdominal ultrasound in the pancreatic head or neck, though evaluation of the body and tail is often limited by overlying bowel gas. This limitation also decreases the utility of transabdominal ultrasound for lesion characterization and

Disclosure Statement: The authors have nothing to disclose.
Department of Radiology, Massachusetts General Hospital, 55 Fruit Street, Boston, MA 02114, USA
* Corresponding author.
E-mail address: ksburk@partners.org

Magn Reson Imaging Clin N Am 26 (2018) 405–420
https://doi.org/10.1016/j.mric.2018.03.006

follow-up.[4] The major modalities used for cystic pancreatic lesion characterization are multi-detector CT (MDCT), MR imaging/magnetic resonance cholangiopancreatography (MRCP), and endoscopic ultrasound (EUS) with or without cyst fluid sampling, with PET/CT being reserved for select cases. For pancreatic cyst follow-up, in which a less invasive examination is preferred, MDCT and MR imaging/MRCP are most commonly used. Technical considerations, strengths, and weakness of each modality are presented here.

MR Imaging/Magnetic Resonance Cholangiopancreatography

The multi-parametric nature of MR imaging/MRCP examinations allows for complete characterization of cystic pancreatic lesions. The pancreas MR imaging protocol used for lesion characterization at the authors' institution includes in- and out-of-phase gradient echo sequences, postcontrast images in multiple phases of contrast enhancement, and thick slab and 3-dimensional (3D) MRCP sequences, as shown on the left in **Table 1**.[5] Once the cystic lesion is fully characterized, an abbreviated protocol can be considered for subsequent follow-up examinations, as shown on the right in **Table 1**.[6] Advanced MRCP techniques may incorporate negative oral contrast and/or secretin stimulation of the exocrine cells to further aid with more nuanced characterization of particular cystic pancreatic pathologies, such as IPMN and pseudocyst,[7,8] though these are often not necessary for initial lesion characterization.

MR imaging/MRCP offers a few general advantages over MDCT evaluation, including a lack of ionizing radiation exposure; superior evaluation of the pancreatic ductal system allowing characterization of complex fistulous connections between cystic lesions and surrounding structures, as seen in **Fig. 1**; and superior characterization of cyst morphology, including detection of septa and solid nodular components, as described in **Table 2**. General disadvantages of MR imaging/MRCP include the high cost of the examination, poorer temporal resolution, patient cooperation, and limited evaluation of calcification.[5]

Other Imaging Modalities

A multi-phase pancreatic protocol including arterial (30 seconds), pancreatic parenchymal (45 seconds), and portal venous (70 seconds) phases of contrast enhancement can be used to characterize cystic pancreatic lesions. Dose reduction techniques to consider include limiting the field of view to the abdomen and use of a dual-energy CT scanner with creation of virtual noncontrast, monochromatic low-kilovolt multiparametric and virtual iodine map reconstructions.[9–13] With this protocol, MDCT has a few advantages over MR imaging/MRCP, namely, temporal resolution, lower cost, greater availability, and a better ability to see calcifications.[5] However, the radiation involved and renal and allergic risks associated with iodinated contrast have led to MR imaging/MRCP being the more frequently used examination.[14]

EUS can also be used for characterization of cystic pancreatic lesions. Although it performs similarly to MR imaging/MRCP for detection of septa, solid nodules, and main pancreatic ductal dilatation, it is relatively limited in its assessment of main pancreatic ductal communication and

---

Table 1
Complete and abbreviated MR imaging/magnetic resonance cholangiopancreatography protocols

Complete MR Imaging/MRCP Protocol	Abbreviated MR Imaging/MRCP Protocol
Axial T2 FSE ± fat suppression	Axial T2 FSE ± fat suppression
Coronal T2 FSE ± fat suppression	Coronal T2 FSE ± fat suppression
Axial T1 in-phase and opposed-phase GRE	Axial 3D T1 fat-suppressed spoiled GRE
Axial diffusion-weighted imaging	Axial diffusion-weighted imaging
Axial 3D T1 fat-suppressed spoiled GRE	Coronal thick slab T2-weighted MRCP
Axial T1 post–pancreatic phase	Coronal 3D T2-weighted MRCP
Axial T1 post–portal venous phase	
Axial T1 post–equilibrium/delayed phase	
Coronal thick slab T2-weighted MRCP	
Coronal 3D T2-weighted MRCP	

Abbreviations: FSE, fast spin echo; GRE, gradient echo.

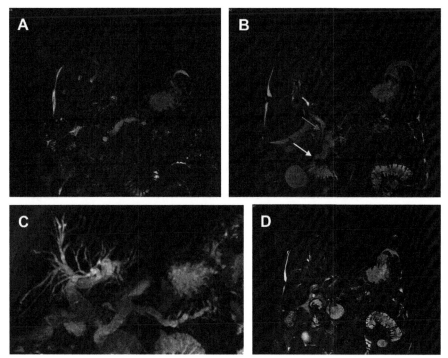

Fig. 1. MR imaging and MRCP of a complex, combined-type IPMN. Single slice from a coronal 3D MRCP demonstrates diffuse enlargement of the main pancreatic duct with multiple dilated side branches (*A*). A different single slice from this 3D MRCP shows a fistulous connection between a dilated side branch in the pancreatic head and the proximal common bile duct (*red arrow*), with a normal joining of the distal common bile duct and pancreatic duct just proximal to the ampulla (*yellow arrow*) (*B*). Thick slab MRCP of the same lesion (*C*). Coronal T2-weighted image shows multiple solid nodular components (*blue arrows*) are seen within the dilated main pancreatic duct and side-branch ducts (*D*).

Table 2
Performance of common imaging modalities in the identification and characterization of cystic pancreatic lesions

	Lesion Identification	Lesion Characterization
MDCT	100% Specificity differentiating SCN from MCN[58] 90% Specificity differentiating SCN from IPMN[59] 70%–81% Specificity for SB-IPMN demonstrating communication with the main pancreatic duct[60] 86% Specificity identifying IPMN[61]	Sensitivity for detection of septa 74% and main duct communication 86%[62] 74%–78% Accuracy differentiating malignant from benign IPMN[63] 83% Specificity differentiating malignant from benign MCN[25]
MR imaging/ MRCP	91% Specificity identifying IPMN[61]	Sensitivity for detection of septa 91% and main duct communication 100%[62] 74%–75% Accuracy differentiating malignant from benign IPMN[63]
EUS	76% Accuracy identifying SCN[64] 84%–96% Accuracy identifying MCN[64]	68% Accuracy differentiating malignant from benign IPMN[63]
PET	—	94% Accuracy differentiating malignant from benign cystic lesions[65,66] 97% Sensitivity and 91% specificity differentiating malignant from benign IPMN[67]

Abbreviations: MCN, mucinous cystic neoplasm; SB-IPMN, side-branch IPMN.

Table 3
Summary of characteristics of cystic pancreatic neoplasms

	IPMN	SCN	MCN	SPT
Sex	M > F	F > M	F	F
Age	Sixth–seventh decades	Sixth–seventh decades	Fourth–fifth decades	Second–third decades
Location	SB: head/uncinate MD: Head > body > diffuse > tail	Head > body	Tail/body	Tail/body
Morphology	SB: cystic oval or lobulated MD: cystic tubular	Honeycomb Cystic Lobulated	Cystic Oval	Cystic and solid Oval Large
Cyst size	Macro ± solid nodularity	Micro > macro	Macro	Micro or macro
Walls/loculations	Variable	>6	<6 Uniformly thick	Thick capsule
Solid components	When malignant	Central scar	When malignant	Present
Calcifications	+/− Within the duct	Within central scar in 30%	Peripheral/septal	Peripheral
MR imaging signal intensity	T1 hypo/hyper T2 hyper	T1 hypo T2 hyper	T1 hypo/hyper T2 hyper	T1 hyper T2 hyper
Enhancement	Walls, nodules if malignant	Central scar, septa	Variable enhancement of walls/septa	Heterogeneously enhancing solid components
Main pancreatic duct communication	SB: present MD: dilated ± tapering	Absent	Absent	Absent
Cyst fluid	Highly viscous fluid with elevated amylase; high cyst fluid CEA or CA-125 suggests malignancy	Low amylase, CEA, and CA 19-9 levels	Highly viscous fluid with low amylase; high cyst fluid CEA suggests malignancy	—

Abbreviations: CA, cancer antigen; CEA, carcinoembryonic antigen; MD, main duct; SB, side branch; SPT, solid pseudopapillary tumor.

evaluation of microcystic lesions, which may appear solid.[15,16] A major drawback is the invasive nature of EUS, which requires conscious sedation, though this also allows for cyst fluid sampling or biopsy, when appropriate.

PET with F^{18}-fludeoxyglucose is not used routinely for lesion characterization in part because of radiation, availability, and cost; however, the information added by this functional examination can significantly impact clinical decisions, especially in cases where surgeons are debating whether to take patients for resection or not. In the future, PET/MR imaging may play a significant role in lesion characterization as this combines the benefits of both modalities. Early studies have shown PET/MR imaging can be used to identify malignant degeneration within IPMN.[17] A summary of MDCT, EUS, and PET performance in the identification and

characterization of cystic pancreatic lesions can be found in **Table 2**.

INTRADUCTAL PAPILLARY MUCINOUS NEOPLASMS
Epidemiology

IPMNs account for 21% to 33% of all cystic pancreatic lesions.[4] There is a slight male to female predominance, with 60% of these lesions occurring in men. They typically occur in the sixth to seventh decades, resulting in their nickname as the *grandfather* lesion of the pancreas.[3] There are 2 major types of IPMNs, which differ slightly in morphology and aggressiveness: side-branch IPMNs (SB-IPMN), which involve *only* the side-branch pancreatic ducts and are typically asymptomatic, and main-duct IPMNs (MD-IPMN), which involve the main pancreatic duct and may cause low-grade obstruction and symptoms of pancreatitis. Combined-type IPMNs, which involve both the main and side-branch ducts, are considered a subtype of MD-IPMNs.[3]

Pathology

Histologically, IPMNs are composed of papillary growths of mucin-producing neoplastic cells with varying degrees of atypia within the pancreatic ducts.[16] The degree of cellular atypia determines the aggressiveness of the lesion, with low-grade atypia correlating with clinical benignity and high-grade atypia correlating with the eventual development of an invasive malignant component.[18] MD-IPMNs are most often segmental affecting only the pancreatic head (58% of cases), followed by segmental involving only the pancreatic body (23% of cases), diffusely involving the gland all

the way to the ampulla as seen in **Fig. 2** (12% of cases), and least commonly segmental affecting only the pancreatic tail (7% of cases). Similarly, SB-IPMNs most commonly occur in the head or uncinate process of the pancreas, seen in 60% of cases.[4,19–23] Fluid analysis will show a viscous mucinous fluid with elevated amylase levels; if the carcinoembryonic antigen (CEA), cancer antigen (CA) 19-9, or CA 72.4 levels are elevated, this is suggestive of a malignant component.[24]

Imaging Characteristics

As their name implies, SB-IPMNs involve only the side branch ducts. They are macrocystic, sometimes lobulated lesions that may or may not contain internal septations, as seen in **Fig. 3**. They are distinguished from the other macrocystic lesions in the pancreas by their characteristic connection

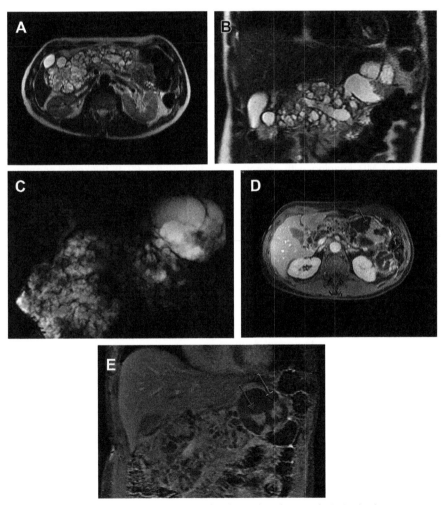

Fig. 2. Diffuse IPMN involving the entire pancreatic gland. Axial and coronal T2 single-shot sequences (*A*, *B*) and 3D coronal MRCP (*C*) show dilatation of both the main pancreatic duct and innumerable side branches. Axial T1 postcontrast images in the axial (*D*) and coronal (*E*) planes show enhancement of a solid nodular component in the pancreatic tail (*blue arrows*), which was a pathologically invasive malignant component.

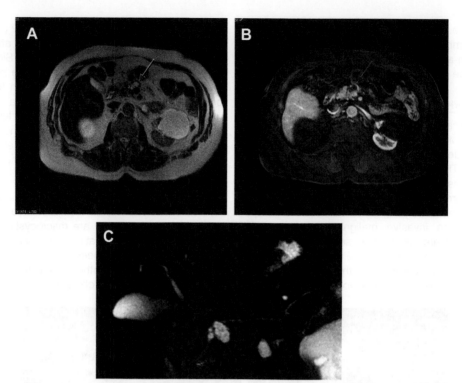

Fig. 3. MR imaging of an side-branch IPMN showing cyst lobulations and septations (*blue arrow*) on axial T2 single-shot fast spin echo (*A*), wall enhancement (*blue arrow*) on postcontrast axial T1 FS postcontrast images in the pancreatic phase (*B*), and MRCP showing a connection to a normal caliber main pancreatic duct (*C*).

to the main pancreatic duct, which may or may not be easily visualized.[8] MR imaging with secretin stimulation may better delineate the connection to the main pancreatic duct, though this is often not necessary to make the diagnosis of SB-IPMN.[7]

MD-IPMNs involve the main pancreatic duct either focally or diffusely, and as a result look quite different. When they involve the pancreatic head, they often extend all the way to the ampulla causing it to bulge into the duodenal lumen giving it a characteristic appearance on endoscopy.[25] Ductal dilatation relating to an MD-IPMNs can be distinguished from dilatation due to chronic pancreatitis by the transition point to normal duct caliber: In an MD-IPMN it will taper without focal transition point, whereas in chronic pancreatitis there will be a focal stricture present. In both, gland atrophy around and distal to the dilated ductal segment is seen and is secondary to low-grade obstruction.[4] Combined-type IPMNs have imaging features of both MD-IPMNs and SB-IPMNs, as depicted in **Fig. 1**.

For both MD-IPMN and SB-IPMN, features associated with a high risk of malignant degeneration and a moderate risk of malignant degeneration have been described. High-risk features include an enhancing mural nodule and main ductal dilatation greater than 10 mm.[26] Moderate-risk features

include an SB-IPMN size greater than 3 cm (odds ratio [OR] 2.3–62.4), thickened or enhancing septa (OR 2.3), a nonenhancing mural nodule (OR 6.0–9.3), or main duct dilatation greater than 7 mm (OR 3.4–7.6).[26–29]

Management

The different subtypes of IPMNs are managed differently, because the risk of malignant transformation is much higher for an MD-IPMN or combined-type IPMN than for an SB-IPMN: 38% to 68% versus 12% to 47% within 5 years.[2] So long as patients are healthy enough to undergo surgery, MD-IPMNs and combined-type IPMNs typically get immediately resected.[26] In contrast, SB-IPMNs are often followed with imaging to asses for the development of worrisome features over time, as discussed later in this article. In addition to reassessment of the IPMN, screening the remainder of the pancreatic parenchyma is paramount, as these patients are at increased risk for the development of pancreatic ductal adenocarcinomas in other parts of the gland.[5]

SEROUS CYSTIC NEOPLASMS
Epidemiology

SCNs account for approximately 1% to 2% of all pancreatic neoplasms and up to one-third of all pancreatic cysts.[30] There is a strong female to male predominance, with 80% of these lesions occurring in women.[16] The mean age of occurrence in the sixth to seventh decades, giving rise to their nickname as the *grandmother* lesion. Although most patients are asymptomatic (80%), symptoms arising from mass effect on adjacent organs may be present.[31–34]

Pathology

Most SCNs are asymptomatic and incidentally found. They are most often located in the head of the pancreas (40%), followed by the body (34%), and occur least commonly in the tail (26%). Diffuse pancreatic involvement is even more rare (3%).[31,34] Classically, SCNs are composed of multiple microcysts of a few millimeters in size with a polycystic (70%) or honeycomb (20%) appearance.[35] Larger cysts may be seen at the periphery, measuring up to 2 cm in size and accounting for the classic lobulated contour and cluster of grapes appearance.[16] In less than 10% of cases, SCNs may have an oligocystic appearance; these lesions can be mistaken for a mucinous cystic neoplasm.[35] On histopathologic evaluation, these cysts are lined by cuboidal or flat epithelial cells, which, in 20% to 50% of cases, stain positive for periodic acid-Schiff because of glycogen-rich components.[36] A link between biallelic inactivation of the von Hippel-Lindau (VHL) gene has been found in both VHL-associated and sporadic forms of SCNs.[19,32–34] If performed, cyst fluid analysis shows low amylase, CEA, and CA 19.9 levels.[37]

Imaging Appearance

Classically, SCNs appear as a well-circumscribed, lobulated, microcystic mass with a characteristic honeycomb appearance and greater than 6 loculations, as seen in **Fig. 4**. Less commonly, they can present as a macrocyctic or even an oligocystic mass; this variant appearance is more often found in a younger population.[34] The cystic components are typically T2 hyperintense and can vary in T1 intensity based on the amount of hemorrhage within the fluid. In up to 20% of cases, the microcysts are so small that SCNs appear as soft tissue–density or mixed-density masses that enhance uniformly after the administration of iodinated contrast or gadolinium.[38] In these cases, MR imaging may be particularly helpful in revealing the multiple underlying cysts.[32,33,39] The presence of true solid components suggests other causes.

A central T1 and T2 hypointense, stellate, fibrous scar is thought to be a specific feature of SCNs but is only seen in about 33% of cases, as shown in **Fig. 4**. When present, the central scar and septa should show enhancement in the portal venous phase and persistence of enhancement in the more delayed phases of intravenous contrast.[16] There may be calcifications associated

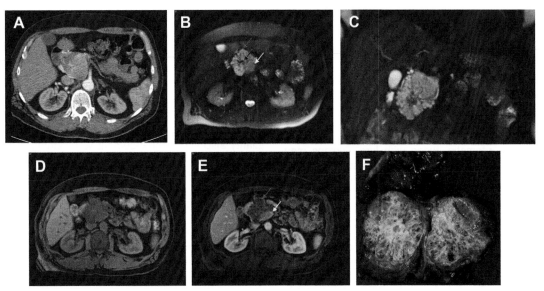

Fig. 4. Mixed polycystic and honeycomb SCN in the pancreatic neck shown on CT (*A*). T2-weighted and fat-saturated fast spin echo MR imaging in the axial (*B*) and coronal (*C*) planes demonstrate a characteristic central scar (*blue arrow*) and that the polycystic component (*red arrow*) is slightly more T2 hyperintense than the honeycomb component (*yellow arrow*). T1 fat-saturated precontrast (*D*) and postcontrast images (*E*) show enhancement of the septa in the polycystic component (*red arrow*) and denser enhancement of the honeycomb component, which almost appears solid (*yellow arrow*). Correlative gross pathologic specimen seen in (*F*).

with the scar; if present, these are typically better visualized on CT than on MR imaging. Lack of communication with the pancreatic duct is another important differentiating feature to distinguish SCN from IPMN, although compression of the duct may occur in larger masses.[19,33,39]

Management

SCNs are considered benign lesions, although rare cases of malignant transformation have been reported (<1%).[34] Surgery is indicated for appropriate candidates presenting with lesions greater than 4 cm in size or lesions with a macrocystic appearance, as these are more likely to be symptomatic and demonstrate faster growth rates.[40,41] Recurrence after resection of an SCN is rare.[31] For indeterminate lesions on cross-sectional imaging, endoscopic or percutaneous sampling may be obtained. Neither amylase nor CEA levels should be elevated.[42] For nonsurgical candidates or for patients with lesions with low-risk features, the follow-up interval of imaging surveillance remains debated.

MUCINOUS CYSTIC NEOPLASMS
Epidemiology

MCNs are a group of tumors, including benign cystadenomas (72% of MCNs), borderline mucinous cystic tumors (10.5% of MCNs), mucinous cystic tumor with carcinoma in situ (5.5% of MCNs), and mucinous cystadenocarcinomas (12% of MCNs).[16,25] Together, these make up 10% to 45% of all cystic pancreatic masses and 2.5% of all exocrine pancreatic neoplasms.[4,43] They are almost exclusively found in women, with the mean age of occurrence in the fourth to fifth decades and, therefore, are termed the *mother* lesion.[23] Only a handful of cases have been reported in men, in which they occur in older age range, approximately the 70s.[43] Although most patients are asymptomatic, those with large lesions may develop symptoms related to mass effect and those with malignant MCN types may present with abdominal pain and weight loss.[19,33,39,44]

Pathology

MCNs are typically large on initial presentation, with mean diameters reported in the literature ranging from 6 to 11 cm.[45] They are most commonly found in the pancreatic tail (72%), followed by the pancreatic body (13%) and least often the head (6%); in 9% of cases they can involve the gland diffusely.[43,44,46] They classically are round or oval macrocystic masses, which may be multi-locular with a few septations or unilocular. They also have a thick, fibrous pseudo-capsule around their periphery, which may or may not contain calcifications.[25] Although benign MCNs have smooth borders, malignant subtypes demonstrate solid components, mural nodules, and papillary projections.[39,44,47]

On histopathology, the walls are uniquely lined by ovarianlike stroma. It is hypothesized that proximity of the left primordial gonad to the dorsal pancreatic bud is what accounts for this phenomenon.[19,44,46,47] The remainder of the mucin-producing, columnar epithelial lining may show various degrees of dysplasia, resulting in the benign and malignant subtypes described earlier. Furthermore, both benign and malignant dysplastic regions can reside in a single tumor.[19,44,47] If performed, fluid analysis demonstrates viscous fluid with a high level of extracellular mucin but low amylase content given the lack of communication with the main pancreatic duct. CEA and CA 19-9 levels are variable but when elevated suggest a malignant component to the lesion.[48]

Imaging Characteristics

MCNs most commonly manifest as macrocystic masses, either unilocular (80% of cases) or with fewer than 6 loculations (20% of cases), each measuring greater than 2 cm in size.[8] When present, the septa are typically less organized than in SCAs and are typically more peripherally located in the tumor.[49] The cyst fluid appears T1 hypointense and T2 hyperintense on MR imaging. However, hemorrhagic components may be present and may increase the cyst T1 hyperintensity.[19,33,39,47] The thick, fibrous tumor capsule is hypointense on T2-weighted images, retains gadolinium on delayed phases of contrast, and may be the only characteristic present to differentiate an MCN from benign lymphoepithelial or functional cyst. When present, septa and areas of mural nodularity also show enhancement with retention on the delayed phases postcontrast.[16] An example of a septated MCN is seen in **Fig. 5**, and unilocular MCN in **Fig. 6**. Peripheral calcifications are present within the capsule in 15% of cases and appear dark on both T1- and T2-weighed sequences.[25] MRCP may also be helpful to rule out communication with the main pancreatic duct and differentiate a unilocular MCN from SB-IPMN.[8] If incidentally discovered on transabdominal ultrasound, MCNs appear as well-defined, round/oval, multilocular masses with associated cyst hypoechogenicity and increased posterior acoustic transmission.

Although most MCNs are benign, malignant transformation is suspected with the presence of wall thickening/irregularity, solid enhancing

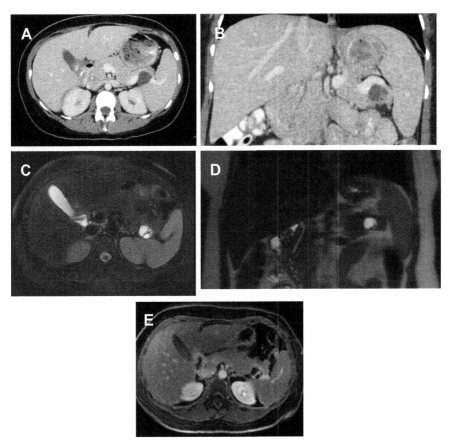

Fig. 5. MCN in the pancreatic tail. CT images (*A, B*) show a cystic lesion in the pancreatic tail with a few septations and possible solid nodular component. T2-weighted MR imaging in the axial plane with fat saturation (*C*) and in the coronal plane without fat saturation (*D*) better show the T2 bright cyst with slightly thickened T2 hypointense septations and nodular component. T1 fat-saturated postcontrast images in the delayed phase show persistent enhancement of the cyst pseudocapsule and septa (*E*).

components, mural nodularity, papillary projections, size greater than 4 cm, patients aged greater than 55 years, or peripheral eggshell calcifications.[46,47,50]

These features can distinguish malignant from benign MCNs with 81% sensitivity and 83% specificity, with the presence of a thick surrounding

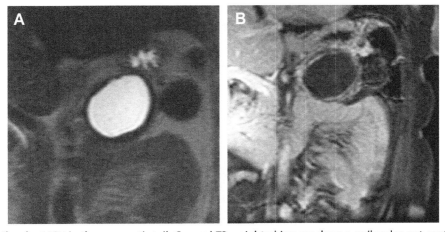

Fig. 6. Unilocular MCN in the pancreatic tail. Coronal T2-weighted images show a unilocular cyst containing T2 hyperintense fluid and a T2 hypointense thick capsule (*A*). Postcontrast T1-weighted images show enhancement of the tumor capsule (*B*).

wall, internal septations, and calcifications of the wall or septa associated with a 95% chance of malignancy and the presence of 2 of these 3 characteristics corresponding to a 56% to 74% chance of malignancy.[25]

Management

All MCNs have the potential to transform into an invasive carcinoma; therefore, surgical resection is typically pursued for both diagnostic and therapeutic purposes.[43] Prognosis in noninvasive cases is excellent, and recurrence is rare.[19,39] For those patients who are not surgical candidates, follow-up periodicity and duration are debated.[8]

SOLID PSEUDOPAPILLARY TUMOR
Epidemiology

SPTs, formerly known as solid and papillary epithelial neoplasm, is a rare tumor accounting for approximately 9% of all cystic pancreatic neoplasms.[2] They most commonly occur in young women with a peak incidence in the third decade, leading to their nickname the *daughter* lesion of the pancreas, though have been seen in women in the seventh decade.[16] Most SPTs are benign, with low-grade carcinoma seen in only 10% to 15% of cases.[51,52] They are most often asymptomatic and incidentally found. However, larger tumors may cause symptoms, such as pain and mechanical obstruction, because of their size.[51,52]

Pathology

SPTs are classically well circumscribed and large at the time of diagnosis, on the order of 5 to 10 cm.[53] They are typically heterogeneous in appearance with both solid and cystic components, with areas of internal hemorrhage, central necrosis, and calcifications seen in 30%.[16] Histologically they are characterized by their pseudopapillary architecture and lack of endocrine or exocrine components. This observation has led to the belief that these tumors arise directly from primordial pancreatic stem cells rather than from more differentiated components of the gland.[16] Progesterone receptors are seen in 81% of tumors, as are a specific subset of estrogen receptors, possibly accounting for the sex and age predilection of these tumors.[51]

Imaging Characteristics

The heterogeneous histology of SPTs is reflected in its imaging appearance, as seen in **Fig. 7**. On MR imaging, T1 and T2 signal hyperintensity is variable and depends on the amount of hemorrhage and cystic degeneration within the lesion.[54] The solid components of the tumor tend to be peripheral in location and typically demonstrate arterial followed by progressive enhancement on MR imaging.[53] Calcifications, though present in one-third of tumors histologically, are not always seen on imaging. A characteristic and more reliable imaging finding in SPTs is the fibrous capsule around the tumor, which accounts for its well-demarcated appearance. The capsule is intrinsically T1 and T2 hypointense and demonstrates intense arterial enhancement and progressive enhancement on postcontrast MR imaging.[54] A summary of the imaging appearances and salient clinical features of IPMN, SCN, MCN, and SPT can be found in **Table 3**.

Management

On account of the high rate of benignity and the young population of patients affected, the 5-year survival rate of SPTs is quite favorable. Even in setting of malignant carcinoma, the 5-year survival rate is 96%.[53] Surgical resection is generally the

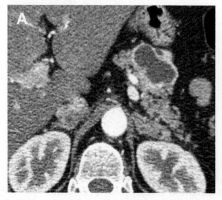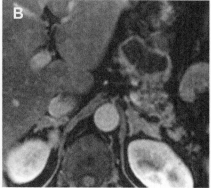

Fig. 7. Cystic SPT on CT (*A*) and T1-weighted postcontrast MR imaging (*B*) demonstrating a cystic lesion in the pancreatic tail with a thick, enhancing wall and enhancing septations.

recommended course of treatment, even in the uncommon setting of metastatic disease.

OTHER COMMON CYSTIC PANCREATIC LESIONS
Cystic Presentations of Solid Masses

Pancreatic neuroendocrine tumors (PNETs) present as cystic rather than solid masses in 10% of cases.[49] Compared with their solid-appearing counterparts, cystic PNETs tend to be larger, averaging 8.4 cm in size, and are nonfunctioning in 64% of cases.[55] The cyst walls are made of viable tumor and maintain the signal characteristics of solid PNETs, specifically hyperenhancement related to the pancreatic parenchyma in the arterial phase, intrinsic T2 hyperintense signal, and intrinsic T1 hypointensity relative to the background pancreatic parenchyma,[16] as seen in **Fig. 8**. Pancreatic ductal adenocarcinoma presents as a cystic rather than a solid mass in 8% of cases.[49] A macrocystic appearance is more common than a microcystic appearance, as seen in **Fig. 9**. The cystic component is variable in cause, at times representing tumor necrosis, a retention cyst related to obstructed adjacent pancreatic parenchyma, or a true neoplastic component.[49]

Pseudocysts

Pancreatitis-related pseudocysts are the most common cystic lesions in the pancreas across the population, accounting for 34% of all pancreatic cystic lesions.[8] They may or may not communicate with the pancreatic ductal system.[7] They are typically distinguished from other cystic lesions of the pancreas by the history of recent pancreatitis. For further discussion of the imaging appearance of pancreatitis and pseudocysts, please see the dedicated article in this issue.

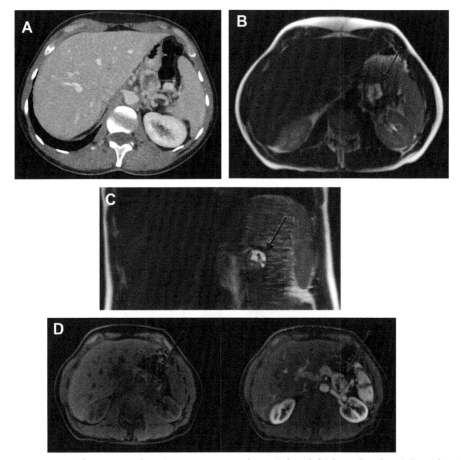

Fig. 8. Cystic PNET on CT has a central cystic component and a peripheral thickened and nodular enhancing solid component (A). On T2-weighted MR imaging sequences the cystic components are T2 hyperintense (*blue arrows*) (B, C), and on postcontrast T1 fat-saturated images the solid components are hyperenhancing relative to the pancreatic parenchyma in the arterial phase (*blue arrows*) (D).

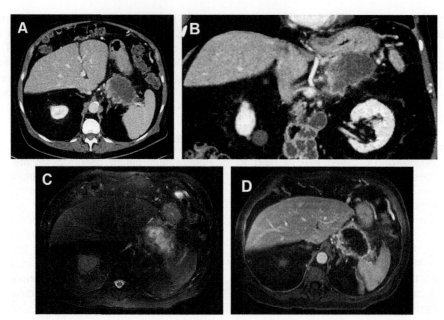

Fig. 9. Cystic pancreatic ductal adenocarcinoma in the pancreatic tail appears as a lobulated, heterogeneous, predominantly cystic lesion on CT (*A*, *B*). The cyst fluid was sampled and positive for malignant cells. On MR imaging the fluid components are heterogeneously T2 hyperintense (*C*), and the periphery of the tumor demonstrates irregular enhancement postcontrast (*D*).

Epithelial Cysts

Benign epithelial cysts are simple cysts of the pancreatic parenchyma that develop as a result of endocrine or exocrine gland dysfunction. They are T2 hyperintense and T1 hypointense on MR imaging unless they hemorrhage, in which case they may have some T1 intrinsic signal hyperintensity. They are nonenhancing and have no communication to the pancreatic ductal system. These cysts can be difficult to distinguish from small SB-IPMNs, though clinical history may be helpful. They are seen in 71% of patients with VHL syndrome, as seen in **Fig. 10**, and are also frequently seen in patients with polycystic kidney disease, cystic fibrosis, and other syndromes.[8,16]

IMAGING FOLLOW-UP OF CYSTIC PANCREATIC LESIONS

The appropriate screening algorithm for cystic lesions of the pancreas has undergone multiple revisions since the publication of the Fukuoka guidelines in 2006.[26,56] The most recently released screening algorithm recommendations, published by the American College of Radiology Incidental Findings Committee in *Journal of the American College of Radiology* in 2017, is summarized in **Fig. 11**.[5,57] These guidelines distinguish lesions by size (less than 1.5 cm, 1.5 to 2.5 cm, and greater than 2.5 cm), confident characterization as an SB-IPMN via the presence of a clear connection to the main pancreatic duct, and by age of patients at the initial presentation (less than 65 years of age, 65 to 79 years of age, and greater than 80 years of age).

In general, the larger the lesion and the younger the patient, the more frequently the cyst should be reimaged. Any interval growth or development of concerning features should trigger consideration of an EUS with fine-needle aspiration and cyst aspiration. Lesions should be followed for 9 to

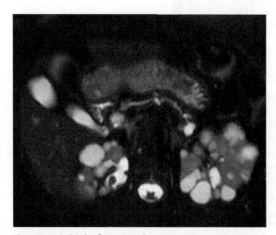

Fig. 10. Multiple functional pancreatic cysts seen on T2-weighted MR imaging in a patient with VHL. Multiple bilateral renal cysts help make the diagnosis of the syndrome in this patient.

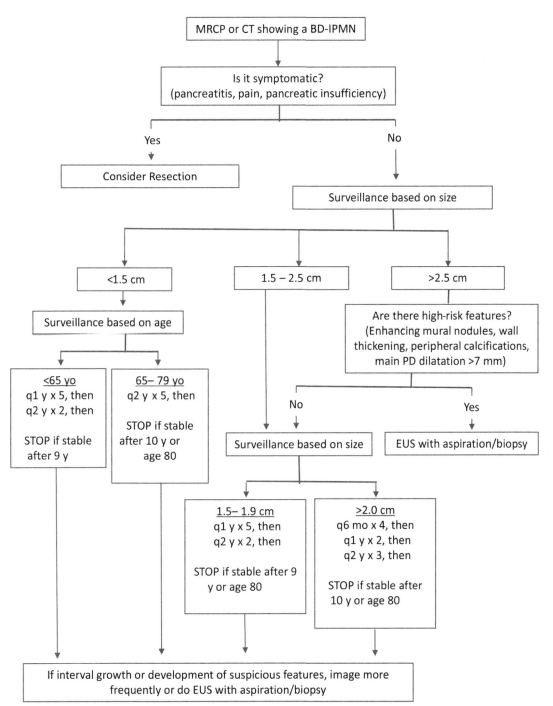

Fig. 11. Algorithm for follow-up of incidental cystic pancreatic lesions, which can be applied to SB-IPMNs. yo, years old. (*From* Burk KS, Lo GC, Gee MS, et al. Imaging and screening of pancreatic cancer. Radiol Clin North Am 2017;55(6):1227; with permission.)

10 years or until patients are 80 years old, whichever comes first. If the cyst is symptomatic or if it contains or develops characteristic features distinguishing it as an SCN, MCN, or SPT, and so forth, the algorithm no longer applies.[57]

SUMMARY

Cystic pancreatic lesions are common and often incidentally detected on cross-sectional imaging. It is important to fully characterize cystic lesions of the pancreas, using MR imaging/MRCP, MDCT, and EUS/ERCP when necessary, as a subset of cystic lesions carry significant malignant potential. Understanding the strengths and limitations of the different imaging modalities and having a firm knowledge of the clinical implications of our interpretations, namely, management and follow-up recommendations, enables the radiologist to contribute significantly to patient care.

REFERENCES

1. Gardner TB, Glass LM, Smith KD, et al. Pancreatic cyst prevalence and the risk of mucin-producing adenocarcinoma in US adults. Am J Gastroenterol 2013;108(10):1546–50.
2. Stark A, Donahue TR, Reber HA, et al. Pancreatic cyst disease: a review. JAMA 2016;315(17):1882–93.
3. Sahani DV, Kambadakone A, Macari M, et al. Diagnosis and management of cystic pancreatic lesions. AJR Am J Roentgenol 2013;200(2):343–54.
4. Catalano O, Price M, Sahani DV. Cystic lesions of the pancreas. In: Sahani DV, Samir A, editors. Abdominal imaging. 2nd edition. Philadelphia: Elsevier; 2017. p. 489–508.
5. Burk KS, Lo GC, Gee MS, et al. Imaging and screening of pancreatic cancer. Radiol Clin North Am 2017;55(6):1223–34.
6. Pozzi-Mucelli RM, Rinta-Kiikka I, Wunsche K, et al. Pancreatic MRI for the surveillance of cystic neoplasms: comparison of a short with a comprehensive imaging protocol. Eur Radiol 2017;27(1):41–50.
7. Tirkes T, Sandrasegaran K, Sanyal R, et al. Secretin-enhanced MR cholangiopancreatography: spectrum of findings. Radiographics 2013;33(7):1889–906.
8. Barral M, Soyer P, Dohan A, et al. Magnetic resonance imaging of cystic pancreatic lesions in adults: an update in current diagnostic features and management. Abdom Imaging 2014;39(1):48–65.
9. Macari M, Spieler B, Kim D, et al. Dual-source dual-energy MDCT of pancreatic adenocarcinoma: initial observations with data generated at 80 kVp and at simulated weighted-average 120 kVp. AJR Am J Roentgenol 2010;194(1):W27–32.
10. Marin D, Nelson RC, Barnhart H, et al. Detection of pancreatic tumors, image quality, and radiation dose during the pancreatic parenchymal phase: effect of a low-tube-voltage, high-tube-current CT technique–preliminary results. Radiology 2010; 256(2):450–9.
11. Klauss M, Stiller W, Pahn G, et al. Dual-energy perfusion-CT of pancreatic adenocarcinoma. Eur J Radiol 2013;82(2):208–14.
12. Frellesen C, Fessler F, Hardie AD, et al. Dual-energy CT of the pancreas: improved carcinoma-to-pancreas contrast with a noise-optimized monoenergetic reconstruction algorithm. Eur J Radiol 2015;84(11):2052–8.
13. Matsumoto K, Jinzaki M, Tanami Y, et al. Virtual monochromatic spectral imaging with fast kilovoltage switching: improved image quality as compared with that obtained with conventional 120-kVp CT. Radiology 2011;259(1):257–62.
14. Canto MI, Harinck F, Hruban RH, et al. International Cancer of the Pancreas Screening (CAPS) consortium summit on the management of patients with increased risk for familial pancreatic cancer. Gut 2013;62(3):339–47.
15. Kim YC, Choi JY, Chung YE, et al. Comparison of MRI and endoscopic ultrasound in the characterization of pancreatic cystic lesions. AJR Am J Roentgenol 2010;195(4):947–52.
16. Dewhurst CE, Mortele KJ. Cystic tumors of the pancreas: imaging and management. Radiol Clin North Am 2012;50(3):467–86.
17. Huo L, Feng F, Liao Q, et al. Intraductal papillary mucinous neoplasm of the pancreas with high malignant potential on FDG PET/MRI. Clin Nucl Med 2016;41(12):989–90.
18. Adsay NV. Cystic neoplasia of the pancreas: pathology and biology. J Gastrointest Surg 2008;12(3): 401–4.
19. Brugge WR, Lauwers GY, Sahani D, et al. Cystic neoplasms of the pancreas. N Engl J Med 2004; 351(12):1218–26.
20. Suzuki Y, Atomi Y, Sugiyama M, et al. Cystic neoplasm of the pancreas: a Japanese multi-institutional study of intraductal papillary mucinous tumor and mucinous cystic tumor. Pancreas 2004; 28(3):241–6.
21. Tanaka M, Sawai H, Okada Y, et al. Clinicopathologic study of intraductal papillary-mucinous tumors and mucinous cystic tumors of the pancreas. Hepatogastroenterology 2006;53(71):783–7.
22. Tanno S, Nakano Y, Nishikawa T, et al. Natural history of branch duct intraductal papillary-mucinous neoplasms of the pancreas without mural nodules: long-term follow-up results. Gut 2008;57(3):339–43.
23. Hruban RH, Pitman MB, Klimstra DS. Atlas of tumor pathology. Washington, DC: Armed forces institute of pathology; 2007.
24. Maire F, Voitot H, Aubert A, et al. Intraductal papillary mucinous neoplasms of the pancreas: performance of pancreatic fluid analysis for positive diagnosis and the prediction of malignancy. Am J Gastroenterol 2008;103(11):2871–7.
25. Procacci C, Carbognin G, Accordini S, et al. CT features of malignant mucinous cystic tumors of the pancreas. Eur Radiol 2001;11(9):1626–30.
26. Tanaka M, Fernandez-del Castillo C, Adsay V, et al. International consensus guidelines 2012 for the management of IPMN and MCN of the pancreas. Pancreatology 2012;12(3):183–97.
27. Kang MJ, Jang JY, Lee S, et al. Clinicopathological meaning of size of main-duct dilatation in intraductal

papillary mucinous neoplasm of pancreas: proposal of a simplified morphological classification based on the investigation on the size of main pancreatic duct. World J Surg 2015;39(8):2006–13.

28. Anand N, Sampath K, Wu BU. Cyst features and risk of malignancy in intraductal papillary mucinous neoplasms of the pancreas: a meta-analysis. Clin Gastroenterol Hepatol 2013;11(8):913–21 [quiz: e59–60].

29. Kim KW, Park SH, Pyo J, et al. Imaging features to distinguish malignant and benign branch-duct type intraductal papillary mucinous neoplasms of the pancreas: a meta-analysis. Ann Surg 2014;259(1):72–81.

30. Solicia E, Capella C, Kloppel G. Atlas of tumor pathology. Washington, DC: Armed forces institute of pathology; 1997.

31. Tseng JF, Warshaw AL, Sahani DV, et al. Serous cystadenoma of the pancreas: tumor growth rates and recommendations for treatment. Ann Surg 2005;242(3):413–9 [discussion: 9–21].

32. Sakorafas GH, Smyrniotis V, Reid-Lombardo KM, et al. Primary pancreatic cystic neoplasms revisited. Part I: serous cystic neoplasms. Surg Oncol 2011;20(2):e84–92.

33. Demos TC, Posniak HV, Harmath C, et al. Cystic lesions of the pancreas. AJR Am J Roentgenol 2002;179(6):1375–88.

34. Jais B, Rebours V, Malleo G, et al. Serous cystic neoplasm of the pancreas: a multinational study of 2622 patients under the auspices of the International Association of Pancreatology and European Pancreatic Club (European Study Group on Cystic Tumors of the Pancreas). Gut 2016;65(2):305–12.

35. Choi JY, Kim MJ, Lee JY, et al. Typical and atypical manifestations of serous cystadenoma of the pancreas: imaging findings with pathologic correlation. AJR Am J Roentgenol 2009;193(1):136–42.

36. Belsley NA, Pitman MB, Lauwers GY, et al. Serous cystadenoma of the pancreas: limitations and pitfalls of endoscopic ultrasound-guided fine-needle aspiration biopsy. Cancer 2008;114(2):102–10.

37. Bhosale P, Balachandran A, Tamm E. Imaging of benign and malignant cystic pancreatic lesions and a strategy for follow up. World J Radiol 2010;2(9):345–53.

38. Takeshita K, Kutomi K, Takada K, et al. Unusual imaging appearances of pancreatic serous cystadenoma: correlation with surgery and pathologic analysis. Abdom Imaging 2005;30(5):610–5.

39. Sahani DV, Kadavigere R, Saokar A, et al. Cystic pancreatic lesions: a simple imaging-based classification system for guiding management. Radiographics 2005;25(6):1471–84.

40. Farrell JJ, Fernandez-del Castillo C. Pancreatic cystic neoplasms: management and unanswered questions. Gastroenterology 2013;144(6):1303–15.

41. Malleo G, Bassi C, Rossini R, et al. Growth pattern of serous cystic neoplasms of the pancreas: observational study with long-term magnetic resonance surveillance and recommendations for treatment. Gut 2012;61(5):746–51.

42. Khashab MA, Kim K, Lennon AM, et al. Should we do EUS/FNA on patients with pancreatic cysts? The incremental diagnostic yield of EUS over CT/MRI for prediction of cystic neoplasms. Pancreas 2013;42(4):717–21.

43. Scott J, Martin I, Redhead D, et al. Mucinous cystic neoplasms of the pancreas: imaging features and diagnostic difficulties. Clin Radiol 2000;55(3):187–92.

44. Zamboni G, Scarpa A, Bogina G, et al. Mucinous cystic tumors of the pancreas: clinicopathological features, prognosis, and relationship to other mucinous cystic tumors. Am J Surg Pathol 1999;23(4):410–22.

45. Buetow PC, Rao P, Thompson LD. From the archives of the AFIP. Mucinous cystic neoplasms of the pancreas: radiologic-pathologic correlation. Radiographics 1998;18(2):433–49.

46. Goh BK, Tan YM, Chung YF, et al. A review of mucinous cystic neoplasms of the pancreas defined by ovarian-type stroma: clinicopathological features of 344 patients. World J Surg 2006;30(12):2236–45.

47. Manfredi R, Ventriglia A, Mantovani W, et al. Mucinous cystic neoplasms and serous cystadenomas arising in the body-tail of the pancreas: MR imaging characterization. Eur Radiol 2015;25(4):940–9.

48. Bhutani MS, Gupta V, Guha S, et al. Pancreatic cyst fluid analysis–a review. J Gastrointestin Liver Dis 2011;20(2):175–80.

49. D'Onofrio M, De Robertis R, Capelli P, et al. Uncommon presentations of common pancreatic neoplasms: a pictorial essay. Abdom Imaging 2015;40(6):1629–44.

50. Sarr MG, Carpenter HA, Prabhakar LP, et al. Clinical and pathologic correlation of 84 mucinous cystic neoplasms of the pancreas: can one reliably differentiate benign from malignant (or premalignant) neoplasms? Ann Surg 2000;231(2):205–12.

51. Geers C, Moulin P, Gigot JF, et al. Solid and pseudopapillary tumor of the pancreas–review and new insights into pathogenesis. Am J Surg Pathol 2006;30(10):1243–9.

52. Hernandez JM, Centeno BA, Kelley ST. Solid pseudopapillary tumors of the pancreas: case presentation and review of the literature. Am Surg 2007;73(3):290–3.

53. Balthazar EJ, Subramanyam BR, Lefleur RS, et al. Solid and papillary epithelial neoplasm of the pancreas. Radiographic, CT, sonographic, and angiographic features. Radiology 1984;150(1):39–40.

54. Cantisani V, Mortele KJ, Levy A, et al. MR imaging features of solid pseudopapillary tumor of the

pancreas in adult and pediatric patients. AJR Am J Roentgenol 2003;181(2):395–401.

55. Horton KM, Hruban RH, Yeo C, et al. Multi-detector row CT of pancreatic islet cell tumors. Radiographics 2006;26(2):453–64.

56. Tanaka M, Chari S, Adsay V, et al. International consensus guidelines for management of intraductal papillary mucinous neoplasms and mucinous cystic neoplasms of the pancreas. Pancreatology 2006; 6(1–2):17–32.

57. Megibow AJ, Baker ME, Morgan DE, et al. Management of incidental pancreatic cysts: a white paper of the ACR incidental findings committee. J Am Coll Radiol 2017;14(7):911–23.

58. Cohen-Scali F, Vilgrain V, Brancatelli G, et al. Discrimination of unilocular macrocystic serous cystadenoma from pancreatic pseudocyst and mucinous cystadenoma with CT: initial observations. Radiology 2003;228(3):727–33.

59. Kim SY, Lee JM, Kim SH, et al. Macrocystic neoplasms of the pancreas: CT differentiation of serous oligocystic adenoma from mucinous cystadenoma and intraductal papillary mucinous tumor. AJR Am J Roentgenol 2006;187(5):1192–8.

60. Waters JA, Schmidt CM, Pinchot JW, et al. CT vs MRCP: optimal classification of IPMN type and extent. J Gastrointest Surg 2008;12(1):101–9.

61. Song SJ, Lee JM, Kim YJ, et al. Differentiation of intraductal papillary mucinous neoplasms from other pancreatic cystic masses: comparison of multirow-detector CT and MR imaging using ROC analysis. J Magn Reson Imaging 2007;26(1):86–93.

62. Sainani NI, Saokar A, Deshpande V, et al. Comparative performance of MDCT and MRI with MR cholangiopancreatography in characterizing small pancreatic cysts. AJR Am J Roentgenol 2009; 193(3):722–31.

63. Choi SY, Kim JH, Yu MH, et al. Diagnostic performance and imaging features for predicting the malignant potential of intraductal papillary mucinous neoplasm of the pancreas: a comparison of EUS, contrast-enhanced CT and MRI. Abdom Radiol (NY) 2017;42(5):1449–58.

64. Brugge WR. Evaluation of pancreatic cystic lesions with EUS. Gastrointest Endosc 2004;59(6):698–707.

65. Kauhanen S, Rinta-Kiikka I, Kemppainen J, et al. Accuracy of 18F-FDG PET/CT, Multidetector CT, and MR imaging in the diagnosis of pancreatic cysts: a prospective single-center study. J Nucl Med 2015; 56(8):1163–8.

66. Sperti C, Pasquali C, Decet G, et al. F-18-fluorodeoxyglucose positron emission tomography in differentiating malignant from benign pancreatic cysts: a prospective study. J Gastrointest Surg 2005;9(1):22–8 [discussion: 8–9].

67. Sultana A, Jackson R, Tim G, et al. What is the best way to identify malignant transformation within pancreatic IPMN: a systematic review and meta-analyses. Clin Transl Gastroenterol 2015;6:e130.

Rare Pancreatic Tumors

Anup S. Shetty, MD[a],*, Christine O. Menias, MD[b]

KEYWORDS

- Pancreatic cancer • Rare pancreatic tumors • Rare pancreatic lesions • MR imaging
- Computed tomography

KEY POINTS

- Pancreatic ductal adenocarcinoma is the most common pancreatic malignancy and represents greater than 90% of all pancreatic neoplasms.
- Magnetic resonance (MR) and computed tomography (CT) imaging provide complementary high contrast, spatial, and temporal resolution for imaging and characterization of pancreatic tumors.
- The absence of classic imaging features of pancreatic ductal adenocarcinoma, such as hypoenhancement, ductal dilation, and distal pancreatic atrophy, should raise consideration for a nonductal tumor.
- Tissue sampling is often required to make a definitive diagnosis, but MR and CT imaging can potentially narrow the differential diagnosis and guide management.

INTRODUCTION

Pancreatic ductal adenocarcinoma (PDAC) (90%) and neuroendocrine tumors (5%) comprise most malignant pancreatic neoplasms.[1] A variety of cystic neoplasms of the pancreas, ranging from intraductal papillary mucinous neoplasms to serous and mucinous cystadenomas to solid pseudopapillary neoplasms, are also well known to most radiologists. However, a variety of rare benign and malignant pancreatic tumors may be encountered that radiologists are unfamiliar with. An important consideration in evaluating solid pancreatic lesions is an appearance atypical of PDAC, such as the lack of pancreatic ductal dilation or distal atrophy, that might lead the radiologist to consider a rare tumor. Pancreatic neoplasms may be of exocrine, endocrine, mesenchymal, or extrapancreatic origin; imaging features of the rare pancreatic tumors are often nonspecific. Knowledge of the patients' history for clues to guide the radiologist is key,

such as a history of neurofibromatosis type I or a primary renal cell carcinoma (RCC) or melanoma; but in many cases tissue sampling will be required to confirm the diagnosis. An MR imaging protocol for comprehensive evaluation of the pancreas is described in **Table 1**. This article reviews a variety of rare pancreatic tumors (**Table 2**) with magnetic resonance (MR) and computed tomography (CT) case examples.

ACINAR CELL CARCINOMA

The exocrine pancreas is composed primarily of ductal cells, the precursors for PDAC, and acinar cells, which secrete enzymes such as amylase and lipase.[2] Carcinomas arising from acinar cells, also known as acinic cell carcinomas (ACCs), represent less than 1% of adult pancreatic neoplasms but 15% of pediatric pancreatic exocrine neoplasms.[3] These tumors have a male predominance in the sixth and seventh decades of life.[4]

Disclosure Statement: The authors have nothing to disclose.

[a] Mallinckrodt of Institute Radiology, Washington University School of Medicine, Campus Box 8131, 510 South Kingshighway Boulevard, St Louis, MO 63110, USA; [b] Department of Radiology, Mayo Clinic in Arizona, 1300 East Shea Boulevard, Scottsdale, AZ 85259, USA
* Corresponding author.
E-mail address: anup.shetty@wustl.edu

Magn Reson Imaging Clin N Am 26 (2018) 421–437
https://doi.org/10.1016/j.mric.2018.03.007

Table 1
Magnetic resonance protocol

Sequence	TR (ms)	Base TE (ms)	FOV (mm)	Matrix	Slice Thickness (mm)
T2W coronal SSTSE	1300	90	400 × 400	640 × 640	6 mm
T2W coronal SSTSE FS (thin slice)	1000	84	320 × 350	320 × 300	4 mm
T2W axial SSTSE (thin slice)	1000	84	320 × 260	260 × 320	4 mm
T2W sagittal SSTSE (thin slice)	1000	84	284 × 350	320 × 260	4 mm
T2W coronal/oblique thick slab MRCP × 3	4500	750	300 × 300	384 × 348	70 mm
T1W axial GRE in and out of phase	112	2.38	320 × 260	520 × 640	7 mm
EPI axial DWI (b = 50, 400, 800)	5800	65	380 × 285	144 × 192	6 mm
PD axial GRE multi-echo Dixon	122	2.38	320 × 320	192 × 192	10 mm
T1W 3D FS spoiled GRE axial	4.62	2.3	340 × 255	480 × 640	3.2 mm
Administer 0.1 mmol/kg intravenous gadolinium contrast agent at 2 mL/s, with bolus tracking on the abdominal aorta					
T1W 3D FS spoiled GRE axial × 3	4.62	2.3	340 × 255	480 × 640	3.2 mm
T1W 3D FS spoiled GRE coronal	4.62	2.3	330 × 380	320 × 280	3 mm
T1W 3D FS spoiled GRE axial 5 min	4.62	2.3	340 × 255	480 × 640	3.2 mm
T2W 3D TSE free breathing MRCP	4084	703	380 × 380	384 × 384	1 mm

Abbreviations: 3D, 3 dimensional; DWI, diffusion-weighted imaging; EPI, echo planar imaging; FOV, field of view; FS, fat suppressed; GRE, gradient echo; MRCP, magnetic resonance cholangiopancreatography; PD, proton density; SSTSE, single-shot turbo spin echo; TE, echo time; T1W, T1 weighted; TR, repetition time; T2W, T2 weighted.

Table 2
Rare pancreatic tumors

Pancreatic Tumor	Key Features
Acinar cell carcinoma	Exocrine malignancy arising from acinar cells; usually well-circumscribed, large, hypoenhancing on early postcontrast phases, less likely to see ductal dilation than with ductal adenocarcinoma
Hepatoid carcinoma	Extrahepatic malignancy resembling hepatocellular carcinoma with arterial phase hyperenhancement and delayed washout
Nerve sheath tumors	Schwannomas may be cellular and solidly enhancing or hyaline/myxoid with a cystic appearance; neurofibromas have characteristic T2 target appearance and if plexiform may resemble a bag of worms
Plasma cell tumors	Multiple myeloma or solitary plasmacytoma may be infiltrative or masslike and may be T1 hyperintense from proteinaceous content
Leiomyoma	Benign smooth muscle tumor, well circumscribed with intermediate T2 hypointensity and delayed enhancement
Lipoma	Benign fatty tumor following fat intensity on all sequences
Metastatic disease	Renal cell and melanoma notoriously metastasize to the pancreas but also from common cancers (lung, breast, colon)
Lymphangioma	Benign lymphatic tumor, circumscribed cystic mass with thin septations; may not be distinguishable from more common cystic lesions by imaging
Dermoid	Mature cystic teratoma; imaging appearance varies depending on composition between fat, calcification, and soft tissue
Lymphoma	Usually secondary, may present as diffuse or segmental masslike enlargement, frequently without pancreatic ductal dilation or atrophy
Sarcoma	Variable imaging appearance depending on histology, frequently locally aggressive and prone to metastasize to liver and lymph nodes
Pancreatoblastoma	Most common malignant pancreatic tumor in young children; circumscribed, lobulated heterogeneous mass with peripheral calcification, central hemorrhage/necrosis, and mild enhancement

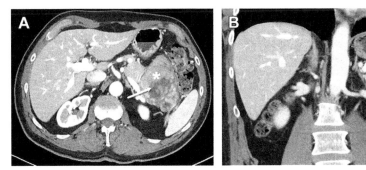

Fig. 1. Acinar cell carcinoma. Arterial phase (*A*) and portal venous phase (*B*) CT images demonstrate a bulky enhancing pancreatic tail mass (*asterisks*) with central necrosis (*arrows*).

ACCs can present in up to 15% of cases with an unusual paraneoplastic syndrome of lipase hypersecretion to levels greater than 10,000 U/dL, resulting in multifocal regions of subcutaneous fat necrosis, bony fat necrosis resulting in polyarthralgias, and eosinophilia.[3,5] However, clinical manifestations are typically more nonspecific and include weight loss, abdominal pain, nausea, and vomiting.

ACCs are usually well circumscribed and large at presentation (**Figs. 1** and **2**), averaging greater than 6 cm in size.[6,7] MR-specific features are T1 hypointensity and T2 hyperintensity relative to the normal pancreas.[8] Tumors are isodense on noncontrast imaging and hypoenhancing to normal pancreas on arterial and portal venous phase imaging, with peak enhancement earlier than ductal adenocarcinomas (arterial or portal venous vs delayed phase for ductal adenocarcinomas).[5,9] Internal necrosis and cystic change can be seen, but pancreatic and biliary ductal dilation are less common with proximal tumors compared with ductal adenocarcinomas, because of the less infiltrative nature of ACC compared with PDAC.[5] Metastatic disease is unfortunately present in 50% to 60% of cases,[1] most frequently to the liver[5]; ACC is an aggressive tumor with a prognosis slightly better than that of PDAC and a median survival for resectable nonmetastatic cancer of 47 months with surgery and adjuvant therapy.[2]

HEPATOID CARCINOMA

Hepatoid carcinomas are extrahepatic neoplasms with morphologic and immunohistochemical features of hepatocellular carcinoma.[10] Cases have

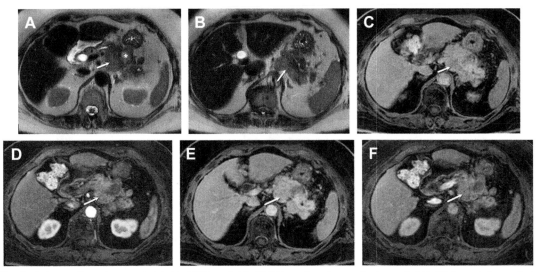

Fig. 2. Acinar cell carcinoma. Axial, (*A, B*) T2-weighted MR imaging demonstrates a slightly T2 hyperintense, heterogeneous pancreatic tail mass (*arrows*) with internal cystic necrosis (*asterisk*). T1-weighted images demonstrate precontrast hypointensity (*C*) and hypoenhancement on arterial (*D*), portal venous (*E*), and delayed phase (*F*) images.

been described initially in the stomach and subsequently in other sites, including the colon, lung, kidney, and genitourinary tract.[11] Pancreatic hepatoid carcinoma is rare, described in case series in approximately 25 patients in the medical literature.[10–13] The clinical signs are nonspecific, including epigastric pain, nausea, and vomiting[11]; serum alpha-fetoprotein may be elevated.[14] Hepatoid carcinoma is thought to arise in ectopic liver tissue and in the pancreas is often admixed with a primary pancreatic component of ductal, acinar, or endocrine subtype.[14]

Pancreatic hepatoid carcinomas are typically large at the time of diagnosis (**Figs. 3** and **4**), with a mean size of 6 cm, with a slight male predilection.[11] They occur slightly more frequently in the pancreatic body and tail than the head. Imaging features overlap with those of primary hepatocellular carcinomas, including arterial phase hyperenhancement, delayed washout, and the potential presence of intravoxel lipid, but are not well defined in the literature[11,15] and may be variable because of an admixed pancreatic cell type. Gastrointestinal hepatoid carcinomas are aggressive but may have a better prognosis than orthotopic hepatocellular carcinoma.[14]

NERVE SHEATH TUMORS

Schwannomas are benign nerve sheath tumors, typically slow growing, with Schwann cell differentiation.[16] Although they may occur virtually anywhere in the body, visceral schwannomas are rare. Several nerve plexuses in the peripancreatic region, including the pancreatic head, superior mesenteric, celiac, and splenic plexuses, serve as a potential nidus for development of a schwannoma.[17] A true pancreatic schwannoma is even rarer, and is thought to arise from branches of the vagus nerve.[18] Patients are usually asymptomatic or experience vague abdominal pain.[19] No sex predilection has been described with pancreatic schwannomas.

Schwannomas (**Fig. 5**) are characterized by 2 distinct growth patterns: cellular Antoni A, which are typically more vascular and solidly enhancing, and Antoni B, which are loosely distributed cells with hyaline or myxoid degeneration and are more frequently cystic or multiseptated.[16] The imaging features of pancreatic schwannomas overlap with other cystic pancreatic neoplasms and include cystic degeneration, necrosis, and calcification.[16,18] If patients do not have a predisposing risk factor, such as neurofibromatosis, accurate preoperative diagnosis is challenging and tissue sampling via

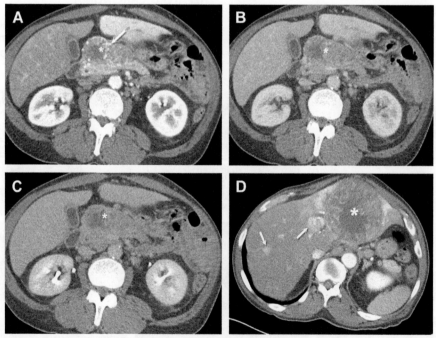

Fig. 3. Hepatoid carcinoma of the pancreas. Axial arterial (*A*), portal venous (*B*), and 4-minute delay (*C*) CT images demonstrate a centrally necrotic, peripherally enhancing pancreatic head mass (*asterisks*) with foci of internal hypervascularity (*arrows*). A more superior image through the liver (*D*) demonstrates a segment 2 liver mass with similar imaging characteristics (*asterisk*) and smaller arterially enhancing liver masses (*arrows*) consistent with liver metastases. Alpha fetoprotein was elevated at 3449.3 ng/mL.

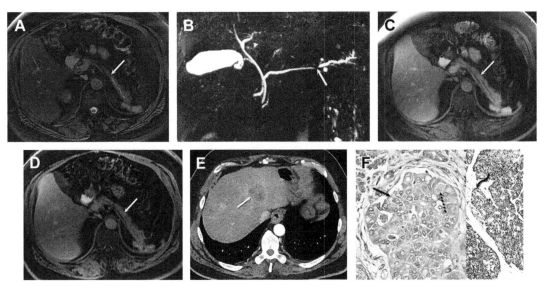

Fig. 4. Hepatoid carcinoma of the pancreas. Axial fat-suppressed balanced steady-state free precession MR (A) demonstrates a pancreatic body mass (arrow) obstructing the distal pancreatic duct. Coronal 3-dimensional MR cholangiopancreatography (B) demonstrates focal pancreatic duct cutoff in the body (arrow) with distal dilation. Axial T1-weighted fat-suppressed MR imaging (C, D) demonstrates enhancement of the pancreatic body mass (arrows). Axial CT 6 months after resection (E) reveals hepatic metastatic disease (arrow). Histologic sections (F) demonstrate large epithelioid cells with abundant cytoplasm and frequent mitotic activity arranged in sheets and focally rosettes (solid black arrow) (hematoxylin-eosin, original magnification ×100). Bile production is noted by tumor cells (dashed black arrow). Immunohistochemical staining with a hepatocyte-specific antigen is strongly and diffusely positive (curved black arrow), supporting hepatoid differentiation (immunohistochemical stain, original magnification ×10).

endoscopic ultrasound (US) is key.[19] Simple enucleation can be performed if anatomically feasible.

Neurofibromas (**Fig. 6**) are also benign nerve sheath tumors but include all components of the peripheral nerve and are the characteristic lesion of patients with neurofibromatosis type I.[20] In the abdomen, neurofibromas are typically paraspinal or sacral in location.[21] Neurofibromas may be

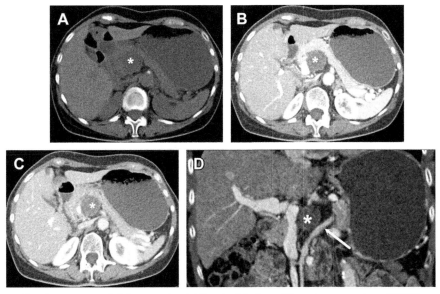

Fig. 5. Pancreatic schwannoma. Axial noncontrast (A), arterial phase (B), and venous phase (C) CT images demonstrate a low-attenuation mass posterior to the pancreatic body (asterisk) with modest enhancement and no invasive features. Coronal arterial phase CT (D) demonstrates proximity of this mass (asterisk) to the superior mesenteric artery (arrow), as it likely arises from the superior mesenteric plexus.

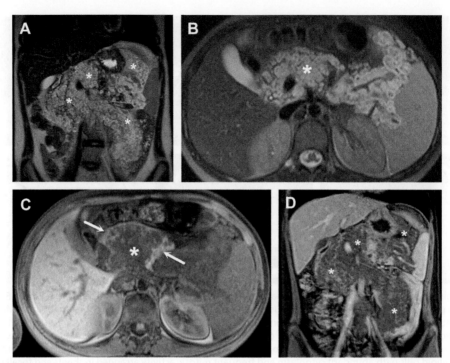

Fig. 6. Plexiform abdominal neurofibroma. Coronal T2-weighted single-shot fast spin echo MR imaging (*A*) demonstrates an extensive bag-of-worms appearance of a plexiform neurofibroma occupying much of the abdomen (*asterisks*), without readily discernible pancreatic tissue. Axial fat-suppressed T2-weighted MR imaging (*B*) through the level of the pancreas demonstrates a similar appearance in the expected region of the pancreas (*asterisk*). Axial fat-suppressed T1-weighted precontrast MR imaging (*C*) demonstrates T1 hyperintense normal pancreatic tissue (*arrows*) surrounded by the T1 hypointense plexiform neurofibroma (*asterisk*). Coronal fat-suppressed T1-weighed postcontrast MR imaging (*D*) redemonstrates the extent of the abdominal plexiform neurofibroma (*asterisks*).

localized, plexiform, or diffuse and rarely involve the pancreas.[20] The characteristic imaging features depend on composition; but most neurofibromas are T1 hypointense and heterogeneously T2 hyperintense, with a target appearance of central T2 hypointensity and a whorled appearance of curvilinear T2 hypointensity. Cystic changes, hemorrhage, calcification, and myxoid degeneration may also be present.[20] Plexiform neurofibromas may resemble a bag of worms and serpiginously interdigitate along the course of nerves.[21]

PLASMA CELL TUMORS

Multiple myeloma is the second most common hematologic malignancy[22] and is characterized by unordered clonal proliferation of plasma cells.[23] Extramedullary disease is uncommon at the time of initial diagnosis, occurring in only 10% to 15% of patients,[24] but occurs with greater frequency in patients with multiple myeloma who relapse.[22] Pancreatic involvement is rare, with a prevalence rate at autopsy of 2.3% of patients with multiple myeloma.[25] In a

systematic literature review of case reports, no sex predilection was present, jaundice was present twice as frequently as pain at the time of diagnosis (70% vs 36%), and most cases involved the pancreatic head.[24]

The imaging features of pancreatic myeloma (**Fig. 7**) have been gleaned from case reports and institutional experience. Pancreatic involvement may be infiltrative or masslike.[26] Early enhancement is similar to the normal pancreas like lymphoma but, in contrast to primary pancreatic adenocarcinoma, are typically isodense on CT. On MR imaging, lesions are T1 hyperintense, thought to be due to the light chain proteinaceous content, and T2 hyperintense. Biliary obstruction will result from mass effect on the pancreatic head. Lesions enhance homogeneously with intravenous contrast.[27]

Solitary plasmacytomas, representing extramedullary proliferation of plasma cells without the presence of systemic myeloma, may also develop in the pancreas and confer a better prognosis than systemic myeloma.[27] Biopsy is often required in either case to confirm the diagnosis, as the imaging features are nonspecific.

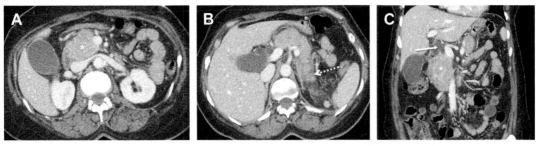

Fig. 7. Pancreatic plasmacytoma. Axial CT images (*A, B*) demonstrate enlargement of the pancreatic head (*asterisk*) and likely infiltrative involvement of the pancreatic body and tail (*dashed arrow*). Coronal CT image (*C*) redemonstrates the pancreatic head mass (*asterisk*) causing biliary ductal obstruction (*solid arrow*).

LEIOMYOMA

Leiomyomas are benign tumors of smooth muscle origin, arising in the gastrointestinal tract from the esophagus and small bowel or from the uterus. Primary pancreatic leiomyoma (**Fig. 8**) is exceedingly rare, described in only a handful of case reports.[28] As the pancreas itself does not contain smooth muscle, these tumors are thought to arise from blood vessels within the pancreas.[20] Like leiomyomas elsewhere in the body, pancreatic leiomyomas are well circumscribed.[20] Other

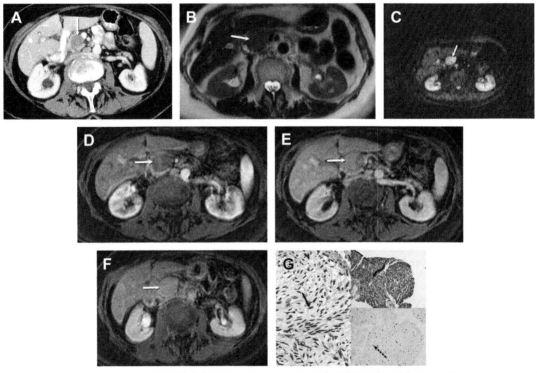

Fig. 8. Pancreatic leiomyoma. Axial CT (*A*) demonstrates a pancreatic head mass (*arrow*). Hypoenhancing to normal adjacent pancreas. Axial T2-weighted MR imaging (*B*) demonstrates intermediate T2 signal of the pancreatic head mass (*arrow*). Axial diffusion-weighted MR imaging (*C*) with b-value of 500 demonstrates marked diffusion restriction of the mass (*arrow*). Axial T1-weighted fat-suppressed postcontrast MR imaging in the arterial, venous, and delayed phases (*D–F*) demonstrates arterial phase hypoenhancement with delayed enhancement of the pancreatic head mass (*arrows*). Histopathology images (*G*) demonstrate interlacing bundles of uniform spindle cells with long oval nuclei and no significant hypercellularity, mitoses or necrosis (*solid black arrow*) (hematoxylin-eosin, original magnification ×100), corresponding to a spindle smooth muscle neoplasm. Subsequent immunoperoxidase stains show the neoplastic cells to be positive for muscle-specific actin, vimentin, and desmin (*curved black arrow*) (original magnification ×10). The Ki-67 proliferation rate is 5% to 10% (*dashed black arrow*) (original magnification ×40), and stains for cytokeratin, S-100, CD-34, and CD117 were negative.

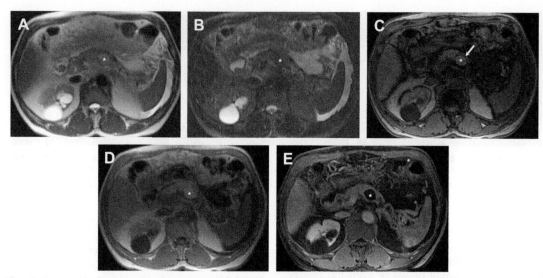

Fig. 9. Pancreatic lipoma. T2-weighted single shot fast spin echo MR imaging (*A*) demonstrates a well-circumscribed, T2 hyperintense lesion posterior to the pancreatic body (*asterisk*) which loses signal on fat-suppressed T2-weighted MR imaging achieved with short tau inversion recovery (*B*). T1-weighted opposed-phase (*C*) and in-phase (*D*) MR imaging demonstrates T1 hyperintensity (*asterisk*) and an India-ink artifact (*arrow*) around the periphery of the lesion at fat-water interfaces. Postcontrast fat-suppressed T1-weighted MR imaging (*E*) demonstrates no enhancement within the lesion (*asterisk*).

imaging features are not well defined; but in the authors' example, the pancreatic leiomyoma restricts diffusion similar to uterine leiomyomas due to the smooth muscle content, is of intermediate T2 hypointensity, and enhances in a delayed fashion.

LIPOMA

Mesenchymal tumors of the pancreas are thought to be rare, reported to constitute only 1% to 2% of pancreatic neoplasms,[29] but are likely underreported[30] due to their incidental nature.[27] Lipomas can be readily diagnosed on CT as well-circumscribed lesions, owing to their thin collagenous capsule,[31] with homogenous CT attenuation values of −80 to −120 confirming the presence of fat.[30] MR imaging demonstrates a T1 and T2 hyperintense, well-circumscribed lesion with loss of signal on fat-suppressed imaging and peripheral India ink artifact at the interface between the lipoma and adjacent pancreas.[20] On US, pancreatic lipomas appear similar to elsewhere in the body, ranging from hypoechoic to hyperechoic depending on the composition and amount of fat, with thin linear striations.[32]

Lipomas (**Figs. 9** and **10**) can usually be differentiated from pancreatic lipomatosis that

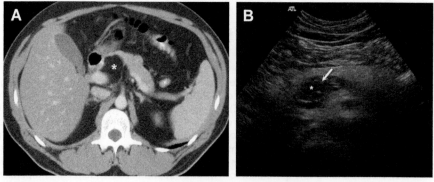

Fig. 10. Pancreatic lipoma. Axial CT (*A*) demonstrates a well-circumscribed fat attenuation mass (*asterisk*) posterior to the pancreatic neck. US of the same lesion (*B*) demonstrates a hypoechoic mass (*asterisk*) with thin internal striations (*arrow*).

occurs in the setting of aging, cystic fibrosis, Shwachman-Diamond syndrome or chronic pancreatitis by its well defined margins.[20] Liposarcomas of the pancreas can overlap in appearance with simple lipomas but are distinguished by their large size (>5 cm), irregular borders, infiltrative nature, and soft tissue or enhancing components and are exceedingly rare.[30,33] In a longitudinal single-institution evaluation of pancreatic lipomas, most patients were asymptomatic and no patients either underwent a change in diagnosis or required intervention over a median follow-up of 31 months.[33]

METASTATIC DISEASE

Metastatic disease to the pancreas is rare, accounting for only 2% to 4% of pancreatic masses[6]; even in patients with widespread metastatic disease, pancreatic metastases are only seen in 3% to 12% of patients in autopsy studies and 2% to 5% in imaging studies.[34] Primary malignancies that frequently metastasize to the pancreas include lung, breast, kidney, gastrointestinal tract, thyroid, and melanoma. Imaging features are frequently not sufficiently specific to distinguish metastases from primary pancreatic neoplasms,

with knowledge of a preexisting primary malignancy and multiplicity of lesions lending support to the diagnosis of metastatic disease.[6,34] Metastases are frequently asymptomatic unless obstructive symptoms develop.[35] Patterns of disease include solitary masses, diffuse pancreatic involvement or enlargement, or multiple discrete lesions[35] (**Fig. 11**).

RCC metastases (**Figs. 12 and 13**) to the pancreas are among the most common[35] and are unique in that there is occasionally a lead time of 10 to 20 years between initial diagnosis of RCC and development of pancreatic metastases.[6] As the clear cell subtype is the most common variant of RCC, metastases will resemble the primary tumor as hypervascular lesions with early enhancement, T1 hypointensity, and T2 hyperintensity.[35] Distinguishing typical RCC metastases to the pancreas from neuroendocrine tumors by imaging is challenging, requiring knowledge of prior RCC or risk factors for pancreatic neuroendocrine tumors, such as von Hippel Lindau syndrome. If the primary tumor contains intravoxel lipid, clear cell metastases can also be diagnosed using chemical shift imaging. RCC metastases from other subtypes, such as papillary RCC, may be hypoenhancing relative to the

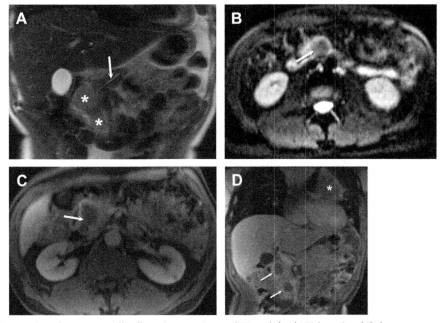

Fig. 11. Metastatic pulmonary small cell carcinoma. Coronal T2-weighed MR imaging (*A*) demonstrates 2 intermediate T2 intensity pancreatic head and uncinated process masses (*asterisks*) with normal caliber pancreatic duct (*arrow*). Axial apparent diffusion coefficient map from diffusion-weighted MR imaging (*B*) demonstrates diffusion restriction of the pancreatic head mass (*arrow*). Axial T1-weighted fat-suppressed postcontrast MR imaging (*C*) demonstrates peripheral enhancement and central necrosis of the pancreatic head mass (*arrow*). Coronal T1-weighted fat-suppressed postcontrast MR imaging (*D*) demonstrates the 2 peripherally enhancing, centrally necrotic pancreatic masses (*arrows*) and necrotic mediastinal lymphadenopathy in the chest (*asterisk*).

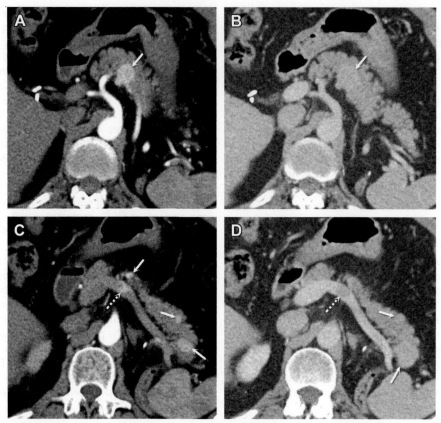

Fig. 12. Metastatic RCC. Arterial phase CT images (*A, B*) demonstrate multiple avidly enhancing pancreatic masses (*solid arrows*), the largest of which invades the splenic vein (*dashed arrow*). Venous phase CT images (*C, D*) are included to demonstrate how subtle the masses are on the more delayed phase of imaging.

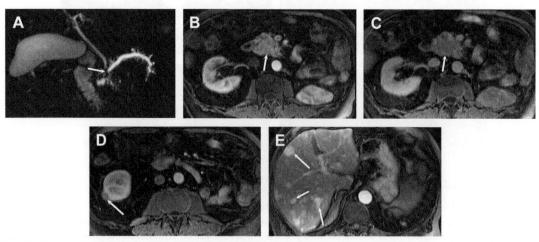

Fig. 13. Metastatic RCC. Coronal 3D MR cholangiopancreatography (*A*) demonstrates pancreatic duct obstruction (*arrow*) with distal dilation. Axial T1-weighted fat-suppressed arterial and delayed-phase MR imaging (*B, C*) demonstrate an arterially enhancing pancreatic head mass (*arrow*) with delayed-phase hypoenhancement, along with an absent left kidney. Axial T1-weighed fat-suppressed MR imaging (*D, arrow*) demonstrates a right renal metastasis along with numerous liver metastases (*E, arrows*).

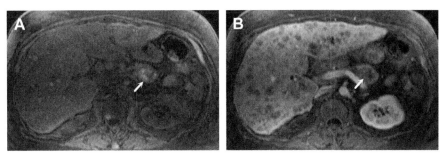

Fig. 14. Metastatic melanoma. Precontrast T1-weighted MR imaging (*A*) demonstrates a T1 hyperintense mass in the distal pancreatic body (*arrow*) along with innumerable T1 hyperintense hepatic lesions. Postcontrast portal venous T1-weighted MR imaging (*B*) demonstrates hypoenhancement of the pancreatic lesion (*arrow*) and innumerable hepatic metastases.

normal background pancreas rather than hypervascular. PET-CT with gallium-68 dota-tate, a somatostatin analogue, can be useful in differentiating metastatic clear cell RCC from neuroendocrine tumors.[36]

Metastatic melanoma to the pancreas (**Fig. 14**) can often be more specifically suggested from T1 hyperintensity due to the paramagnetic properties of melanin.[34] However, this may not always be present, especially in the amelanotic variant of melanoma, and should not be discounted as a diagnostic possibility if absent.

LYMPHANGIOMA

Lymphangiomas are benign congenital lymphatic malformations that obstruct lymphatic channels leading to lymphangiectasia.[37,38] More common sites include the neck and axilla, with less than 1% presenting in the abdomen.[39] The mesentery and retroperitoneum are typical sites of lymphangiomas in the abdomen, with primary pancreatic lymphangiomas being extremely rare. Symptoms range from abdominal pain to nausea, vomiting, early satiety and a palpable mass.[37,40] There is a female predilection, and the tail of the pancreas is more commonly involved.[41] Tumors can be quite large at the time of presentation, up to 25 cm.[38]

By imaging, pancreatic lymphangiomas (**Fig. 15**) are typically well-circumscribed, lobulated, cystic masses with thin walls and septations, either arising from or insinuating around the pancreas and adjacent structures.[39,40] The

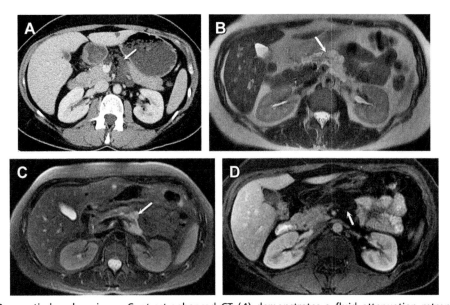

Fig. 15. Pancreatic lymphangioma. Contrast-enhanced CT (*A*) demonstrates a fluid attenuation retroperitoneal lesion (*arrow*) insinuating adjacent to the pancreatic tail. T2-weighted MR imaging (*B*) demonstrates a T2 hyperintense lesion (*arrow*) with thin internal septations in the lesser sac (this image is slightly below the plane of the CT to illustrate the full extent). T2-weighted fat-suppressed MR imaging (*C*) also confirms the fluid nature of the lesion (*arrow*). T1-weighted fat-suppressed postcontrast MR imaging (*D*) demonstrates no enhancement within the lesion.

cystic components are usually simple fluid but may contain T1 hyperintense material representing hemorrhage or proteinaceous content on MR.[39] Calcification is not typical but can occur.[42] Enhancement of the wall and septa are variable.[39,40] The imaging appearance overlaps considerably with primary pancreatic cystadenomas, pseudocysts, or intraductal papillary mucinous neoplasms of the pancreas; surgical excision is often required rather than cyst aspiration to definitively make the diagnosis histologically by endothelial cell factor VIII/R antigen reactivity, CD31 positivity, and CD34 negativity.[37,38,41] Total excision is curative, either by enucleation if anatomically feasible or more extensive resection if needed.[38,41]

DERMOID

Mature cystic teratomas, also known as dermoid cysts, are benign congenital germ cell neoplasms containing all 3 germ layers, with most ectodermal components, hence, their cystic nature.[43,44] Most commonly found in the ovaries and testes, they can occur anywhere along the germ cell migration pathway along the midline, with pancreatic origin being the least common.[20] Dermoids are one of 3 squamous-lined cysts of the pancreas, which also include lymphoepithelial cysts and epidermoid

cysts.[45] Pancreatic dermoid cysts are diagnosed at a relatively young age (mean 36 years), without a sex predilection; symptoms are nonspecific[45] but frequently present.[44]

The imaging appearance of a pancreatic dermoid (Fig. 16) depends greatly on internal composition, which typically will include fluid with or without fat, calcification, and soft tissue. Mature cystic teratomas are rounded, well-circumscribed, thin-walled lesions, either unilocular or with septations. Fat is readily detectable on CT with attenuation of less than −50 Hounsfield units, or on MR with signal loss on fat-suppressed T1- and T2-weighted imaging.[20,45] Fat, although pathognomonic for diagnosing a pancreatic teratoma, is frequently not present.[43] In the absence of fat, other cystic pancreatic neoplasms have to be considered in the differential diagnosis. Treatment with simple enucleation if a preoperative diagnosis can be made or more radical resection are curative.[46,47]

LYMPHOMA

Secondary involvement of the pancreas by lymphoma can be seen in autopsy of up to 30% of patients with non-Hodgkin lymphoma; but primary pancreatic lymphoma is rare and defined by a lack of mediastinal or superficial lymphadenopathy,

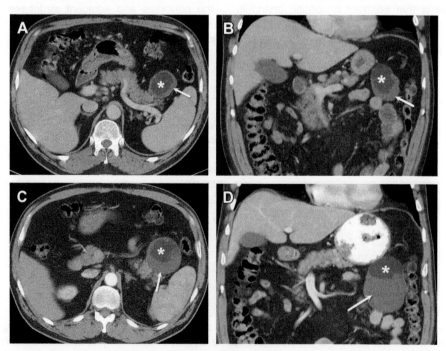

Fig. 16. Pancreatic dermoid. Axial and coronal CT (A, B) demonstrate a well-circumscribed mass adjacent to the pancreatic tail with cystic (asterisk) and soft tissue (arrow) components. Follow-up axial and coronal CT (C, D) 18 months later demonstrates interval growth of the mass.

no leukocytosis or evidence of bone marrow involvement, and absence of hepatosplenomegaly.[26] The pancreatic head contains the most abundant lymphoid tissue in the pancreas and is the most common site of segmental pancreatic involvement.[48] B-cell phenotypes of non-Hodgkin lymphoma are the most common subtype of primary pancreatic lymphoma, particularly diffuse large B-cell lymphoma.[26] Abdominal pain is the most common presenting symptoms, followed by B symptoms, jaundice, and gastrointestinal obstruction.[48]

Pancreatic lymphoma (**Fig. 17**) typically manifests as either diffuse homogeneous enlargement or segmental masslike enlargement of the pancreas.[26] Enhancement is uniform and typically less than that of uninvolved pancreas. Marked hypointensity on apparent diffusion coefficient maps with diffusion-weighted MR imaging would be expected because of the lymphoid tissue. T2-weighted signal intensity is intermediate and typical of lymphoma anywhere in the body. Biliary ductal obstruction can be seen with pancreatic lymphoma. The imaging appearance may overlap somewhat with PDAC; but distinguishing features can include a lack of pancreatic ductal dilation or occlusion/invasion of adjacent vascular structures, lack of distal atrophy, infrarenal lymphadenopathy, and loss of the margins of the pancreas from local lymphadenopathy.[26,48] Tumor markers can also be helpful in differentiation as an elevated serum lactate dehydrogenase and beta-2 microglobulin with normal carbohydrate antigen 19 to 9 and carcinoembryonic antigen level favor the diagnosis of lymphoma over ductal adenocarcinoma.[48] Autoimmune pancreatitis (immunoglobulin G4 [IgG4] related) is another consideration, and PET/CT may be helpful as lymphoma is much more fludeoxyglucose avid than autoimmune pancreatitis[26]; serum IgG4 elevation, delayed pancreatic enhancement, distal bile duct enhancement, and a capsulelike rim would be expected in autoimmune pancreatitis but not lymphoma.[26,48]

SARCOMA

Primary pancreatic sarcomas are exceedingly rare, described in the literature primarily as case reports. Histologic varieties include leiomyosarcoma, liposarcoma, clear cell sarcoma, carcinosarcoma, and spindle cell sarcoma, with leiomyosarcoma the most frequent.[49] Clinical features are nonspecific, depending on location and local involvement; incidence is equal between the head and body/tail.[50] The sex

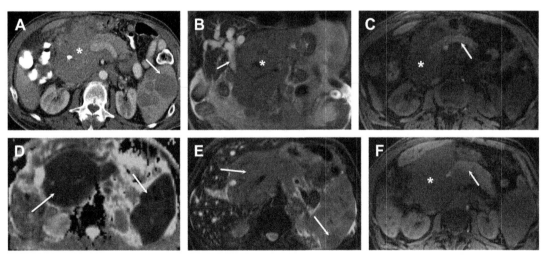

Fig. 17. Pancreatic lymphoma. Axial CT (*A*) demonstrates a large homogeneous mass in the region of the pancreatic head (*asterisk*), without distal pancreatic atrophy or ductal dilation, and multiple splenic masses (*arrow*). Coronal T2-weighted MR imaging (*B*) demonstrates an intermediate T2 intensity mass (*asterisk*) causing biliary ductal obstruction (*arrow*). Axial T1-weighted fat-suppressed precontrast MR imaging (*C*) demonstrates normal T1 hyperintense signal within the distal pancreas (*arrow*), distinguishing it from the T1 hypointense pancreatic head mass (*asterisk*). Apparent diffusion coefficient map from diffusion-weighted MR imaging (*D*) demonstrates marked hypointensity in the pancreatic head mass and spleen from lymphomatous involvement (*arrows*). Axial T2-weighted short tau inversion recovery MR imaging (*E*) demonstrates intermediate T2 signal of the pancreatic mass and splenic masses (*arrows*). Axial T1-weighted fat-suppressed postcontrast MR imaging (*F*) demonstrates hypoenhancement of the pancreatic mass (*asterisk*) compared with normal pancreas (*arrow*).

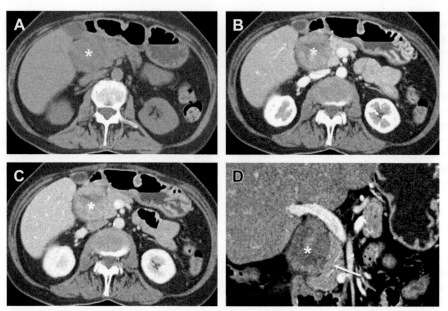

Fig. 18. Pancreatic dedifferentiated liposarcoma. Axial precontrast (A), arterial phase (B), and portal venous phase (C) CT demonstrate a heterogeneously enhancing mass (asterisks) in the pancreaticoduodenal groove. Coronal arterial phase CT (D) demonstrates the relationship of the mass (asterisk) to the pancreatic head (arrow).

distribution is fairly equal with a wide age spectrum.[51] Depending on the histology and grade of tumor, sarcomas can be locally aggressive and metastasize to the liver and lymph nodes.[51,52]

Imaging features of pancreatic sarcoma (Figs. 18 and 19) are also generally nonspecific. Pancreatic sarcomas have been described as well-defined masses[34] with variable size.[50,51,53]

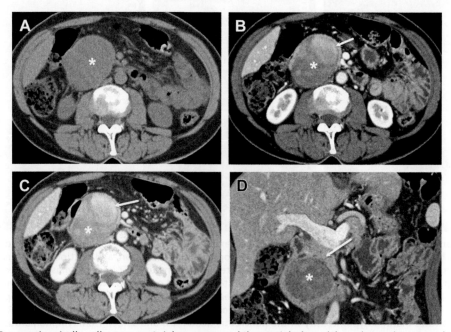

Fig. 19. Pancreatic spindle cell sarcoma. Axial precontrast (A), arterial phase (B), and portal venous phase (C) CT demonstrate a pancreaticoduodenal groove mass (asterisks) with heterogeneous enhancement, including a markedly enhancing component medially (arrows). Coronal arterial phase CT (D) demonstrates the relationship of the mass (asterisk) to the pancreatic head (arrow).

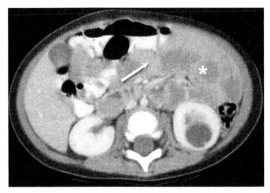

Fig. 20. Pancreatoblastoma. Axial CT demonstrates a large enhancing mixed solid and cystic mass (*asterisk*) in the region of the pancreatic tail distal to normal pancreatic body (*arrow*).

Some lesions enhance avidly, such as leiomyosarcomas,[54] and may resemble neuroendocrine tumors; others, such as clear cell sarcomas, may be hypoenhancing[53]; and others may be centrally necrotic or contain fat if a well-differentiated liposarcoma component is present.[52] Surgical resection is considered the only curative therapy.[49,52]

PANCREATOBLASTOMA

Pancreatic malignancy is fortunately rare in children, but pancreatoblastoma is the most common malignant pancreatic tumor in young children typically presenting in the first decade of life.[55] Even more rarely, pancreatoblastoma can occur in the adult population.[56,57] Thought to arise from pancreatic acinar cells,

pancreatoblastoma occurs most frequently in the pancreatic head.[57] Pancreatoblastoma is differentiated histologically from acinar cell carcinoma by the presence of squamoid corpuscles or nests.[58] Cases may either be sporadic or associated with Beckwith-Wiedemann syndrome.[59] A 2:1 male predilection has been described,[55,60] along with preponderance in those of Asian descent. Similar to hepatoblastoma, serum alpha fetoprotein may be elevated in up to a third of cases.[55] Clinically presenting symptoms are often the result of mass effect, as these slow-growing tumors can be quite large at the time of diagnosis[56,59]; but jaundice is unusual in pediatric patients. Tumors invade adjacent organs and vascular structures and metastasize to the liver and lungs.

On imaging, pancreatoblastoma (**Figs. 20 and 21**) is a circumscribed, often lobulated mass with heterogeneous mixed solid and cystic internal contents.[59] Calcification is often observed peripherally, with central hemorrhage and necrosis. Enhancement is typically mild.[60] Surgical resection is the goal of treatment, and various chemotherapeutic regimens have been used to treat unresectable, metastatic or recurrent disease.[55,57] Radiation is also potentially beneficial for palliation for patients with metastatic disease.[57]

SUMMARY

Although PDAC and neuroendocrine tumors comprise most malignant pancreatic neoplasms, a variety of rare benign and malignant pancreatic neoplasms can occur. Given their rarity, radiologists may be unfamiliar with the clinical

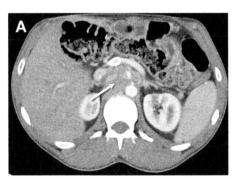
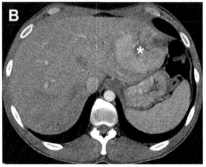

Fig. 21. Recurrent, metastatic pancreatoblastoma in an adult. Axial CT (*A*) demonstrates recurrent pancreatoblastoma (*arrow*) in a retropancreatic location after Whipple procedure, abutting the inferior vena cava and superior mesenteric artery. Axial CT (*B*) demonstrates a hyperenhancing segment 2 liver metastasis (*asterisk*).

characteristics and imaging appearance of these lesions. The imaging appearance of these tumors may overlap with more common pancreatic neoplasms, but awareness of their unique characteristics can aid in recognizing and diagnosing these lesions to guide appropriate management.

REFERENCES

1. Hackeng WM, Hruban RH, Offerhaus JA, et al. Surgical and molecular pathology of pancreatic neoplasms. Diagn Pathol 2016;11:47–63.
2. Glazer ES, Neill KG, Frakes JM, et al. Systemic review and case series report of acinar cell carcinoma of the pancreas. Cancer Control 2016;23:446–54.
3. Chaudhary P. Acinar cell carcinoma of the pancreas: a literature review and update. Indian J Surg 2015; 77:226–31.
4. Wang Y, Wang S, Zhou X, et al. Acinar cell carcinoma: a report of 19 cases with a brief review of the literature. World J Surg Oncol 2016;14:172–9.
5. Bhosale P, Balachandran A, Wang H, et al. CT imaging features of acinar cell carcinoma and its hepatic metastases. Abdom Imaging 2013;38:1383–90.
6. Raman SP, Hruban RH, Cameron JL, et al. Pancreatic imaging mimics: part 2, pancreatic neuroendocrine tumors and their mimics. Am J Roentgenol 2012;199:309–18.
7. Raman SP, Hruban RH, Cameron JL, et al. Acinar cell carcinoma of the pancreas: computed tomography features-a study of 15 patients. Abdom Imaging 2013;38:137–43.
8. Tian L, Lv XF, Dong J, et al. Clinical features and CT/MRI findings of pancreatic acinar cell carcinoma. Int J Clin Exp Med 2015;8:14846–54.
9. Sumiyoshi T, Shima Y, Okabayashi T, et al. Comparison of pancreatic acinar cell carcinoma and adenocarcinoma using multidetector-row computed tomography. World J Gastroenterol 2013;19:5713–9.
10. Marchegiani G, Gareer H, Parisi A, et al. Pancreatic hepatoid carcinoma: a review of the literature. Dig Surg 2013;30:425–33.
11. Kuo PC, Chen SC, Shyr YM, et al. Hepatoid carcinoma of the pancreas. World J Surg Oncol 2015; 13:185–92.
12. Majumder S, Dasanu CA. Hepatoid variant of pancreatic cancer: insights from a case and literature review. JOP 2013;14:442–5.
13. Chang JM, Katariya NN, Lam-Himlin DM, et al. Hepatoid carcinoma of the pancreas: case report, next-generation tumor profiling, and literature review. Case Rep Gastroenterol 2016;10:605–12.
14. Kelly PJ, Spence R, Dasari BV, et al. Primary hepatocellular carcinoma of the pancreas: a case report and review of the heterogeneous group of

15. Chang MY, Kim JH, Park SH, et al. CT features of hepatic metastases from hepatoid adenocarcinoma. Abdom Radiol (NY) 2017. https://doi.org/10.1007/s00261-017-1150-3.
16. Lee NJ, Hruban R, Fishman EK. Abdominal schwannomas: review of imaging findings and pathology. Abdom Radiol (NY) 2017;42:1864–70.
17. Kuo TC, Yang CY, Wu JM, et al. Peripancreatic schwannoma. Surgery 2012;153:542–8.
18. Duma N, Ramirez DC, Young G, et al. Enlarging pancreatic schwannoma: a case report and review of the literature. Clin Pract 2015;5:124–7.
19. Gupta A, Subhas G, Mittal VK, et al. Pancreatic schwannoma: literature review. J Surg Educ 2009; 66:168–73.
20. Manning MA, Srivastava A, Paal EE, et al. Nonepithelial neoplasms of the pancreas: radiologic-pathologic correlation, part 1-benign tumors. Radiographics 2016;36:123–41.
21. Levy AD, Patel N, Dow N, et al. Abdominal neoplasms in patients with neurofibromatosis type 1: radiologic-pathologic correlation. Radiographics 2005;25:455–80.
22. Sher T, Bhat S, Jitawatanarat P, et al. Multiple myeloma mimicking metastatic pancreatic cancer. J Clin Oncol 2013;31:e297–9.
23. Coss A, Zhou C, Byrne MF, et al. Relapse of multiple myeloma presenting with biliary obstruction. Can J Gastroenterol 2010;24:237–8.
24. Williet N, Kassir R, Cuilleron M, et al. Difficult endoscopic diagnosis of a pancreatic plasmacytoma: case report and review of the literature. World J Clin Oncol 2017;8:91–5.
25. Pallavi R, Ravella PM, Popescu-Martinez A. An unusual pancreatic mass: a case report and literature review. Transl Gastrointest Cancer 2014;3:106–10.
26. Sandrasegaran K, Tomasian A, Elsayes KM, et al. Hematologic malignancies of the pancreas. Abdom Imaging 2015;40:411–23.
27. Hammond NA, Miller FH, Day K, et al. Imaging features of the less common pancreatic masses. Abdom Imaging 2013;38:561–72.
28. Sato T, Kato S, Watanabe S, et al. Primary leiomyoma of the pancreas diagnosed by endoscopic ultrasound-guided fine-needle aspiration. Dig Endosc 2012;24:380.
29. Stadnik A, Cieszanowski A, Bakon L, et al. Pancreatic lipoma: an incydentaloma which can resemble cancer – analysis of 13 cases studied with CT and MRI. Pol J Radiol 2012;77:9–13.
30. Shaaban AM, Rezvani M, Tubay M, et al. Fat-containing retroperitoneal lesions: imaging characteristics, localization, and differential diagnosis. Radiographics 2016;36:710–34.

31. Xhan HX, Zhang TP, Liu BN, et al. A systematic review of pancreatic lipoma: how come there are so few cases? Pancreas 2010;39:257–9.

32. Sitharama SA, Bashini M, Gunasekaran K, et al. Pancreatic lipoma: a pancreatic incidentaloma; diagnosis with ultrasound, computed tomography and magnetic resonance imaging. BJR Case Rep 2016;2:20150507.

33. Butler JR, Fohtung TM, Sandrasegaran K, et al. The natural history of pancreatic lipoma: does it need observation? Pancreatology 2016;16:95–8.

34. Franz D, Esposito I, Kapp AC, et al. Magnetic resonance imaging of less common pancreatic malignancies and pancreatic tumors with malignant potential. Eur J Radiol Open 2014;1: 49–59.

35. Sikka A, Adam SZ, Wood C, et al. Magnetic resonance imaging of pancreatic metastases from renal cell carcinoma. Clin Imaging 2015;39:945–53.

36. Mojtahedi A, Thamake S, Tworowska I, et al. The value (68)Ga-DOTATATE PET/CT in diagnosis and management of neuroendocrine tumors compared to current FDA approved imaging modalities: a review of the literature. Am J Nucl Med Mol Imaging 2014;4:426–34.

37. Nodit L, Johnson M, Gray KD, et al. Pancreatic lymphangioma: a diagnostic and treatment dilemma. Am Surg 2017;7:e255–7.

38. Sakorafas GH, Smyrniotis V, Reid-Lombardo KM, et al. Primary pancreatic cystic neoplasms of the pancreas revisited. Part IV: rare cystic neoplasms. Surg Oncol 2012;21:153–63.

39. Mortele KJ. Cystic pancreatic neoplasms: imaging features and management strategy. Semin Roentgenol 2013;48:253–63.

40. Koenig TR, Loyer EM, Whitman GJ, et al. Cystic lymphangioma of the pancreas. Am J Roentgenol 2001; 177:1090.

41. Colovic RB, Grubor NM, Micev MT, et al. Cystic lymphangioma of the pancreas. World J Gastroenterol 2008;14:6873–5.

42. Bihari C, Rastogi A, Rajesh S, et al. Cystic lymphangioma of pancreas. Indian J Surg Oncol 2016;7: 106–9.

43. Lane J, Vance A, Finelli D, et al. Dermoid cyst of the pancreas: a case report with literature review. J Radiol Case Rep 2012;6:17–25.

44. Scheele J, Barth TF, Wittau M, et al. Cystic teratoma of the pancreas. Anticancer Res 2012;32:1075–80.

45. Kubo T, Takeshita T, Shimono T, et al. Squamous-lined cyst of the pancreas: radiological-pathologic correlation. Clin Radiol 2014;69:880–6.

46. Chakaravarty KD, Venkata CD, Manicketh I, et al. Matura cystic teratoma of the pancreas. ACG Case Rep J 2016;3:80–1.

47. Degrate L, Misani M, Mauri G, et al. Mature cystic teratoma of the pancreas. Case report and review of the literature of a rare pancreatic cystic lesion. JOP 2012;13:66–72.

48. Anand D, Lall C, Bhosale P, et al. Current update on primary pancreatic lymphoma. Abdom Radiol (NY) 2016;41:347–55.

49. Ambe P, Kautz C, Shadouh S, et al. Primary sarcoma of the pancreas, a rare histopathological entity. A case report with review of the literature. World J Surg Oncol 2011;9:85–8.

50. Xu J, Zhang T, Wang T, et al. Clinical characteristics and prognosis of primary leiomyosarcoma of the pancreas: a systematic review. World J Surg Oncol 2011;11:290–3.

51. Jia Z, Zhang K, Huang R, et al. Pancreatic carcinosarcoma with rare long-term survival: case report and review of the literature. Medicine (Baltimore) 2017;96(4):e5966.

52. Cesar Machado MC, Fonseca GM, Rodrigues de Meirelles L, et al. Primary liposarcoma of the pancreas: a review illustrated by findings from a recent case. Pancreatology 2016;16:715–8.

53. Huang J, Luo RK, Min D, et al. Clear cell sarcoma of the pancreas: a case report and review of the literature. Int J Clin Exp Pathol 2015;8:2171–5.

54. Soreide JA, Undersrud ES, Al-Saiddi MS, et al. Primary leiomyosarcoma of the pancreas – a case report and a comprehensive review. J Gastrointest Cancer 2016;47:358–65.

55. Glick RD, Pashankar FD, Pappo A, et al. Management of pancreatoblastoma in children and young adults. J Pediatr Hematol Oncol 2012;34:s47–S50.

56. Omiyale AO. Clinicopathological review of pancreatoblastoma in adults. Gland Surg 2015;4:322–8.

57. Salman B, Brat G, Yoon YS, et al. The diagnosis and surgical treatment of pancreatoblastoma in adults: a case series and review of the literature. J Gastrointest Surg 2013;17:2153–61.

58. Cavallini A, Falconi M, Bortesi L, et al. Pancreatoblastoma in adults: a review of the literature. Pancreatology 2009;9:73–80.

59. Shet NS, Cole BL, Iyer RS. Imaging of pediatric pancreatic neoplasms with radiologic-histopathologic correlation. Am J Roentgenol 2014; 202:1337–48.

60. Papaioannou G, Sebire NJ, McHugh K. Imaging of the unusual pediatric 'blastomas'. Cancer Imaging 2009;9:1–11.

Acute Pancreatitis
How Can MR Imaging Help

Kristin K. Porter, MD, PhD*, Daniel E. Cason, MD, Desiree E. Morgan, MD

KEYWORDS

- Acute pancreatitis • Pancreas • MR imaging
- Magnetic resonance cholangiopancreatography (MRCP)

KEY POINTS

- Imaging is often needed to diagnose acute pancreatitis when the clinical situation is unclear, to determine the underlying cause of acute pancreatitis, to evaluate complications and disease severity, and to guide intervention.
- MR imaging allows for noninvasive evaluation of the pancreatic parenchyma, biliary and pancreatic ducts, exocrine function, peripancreatic soft tissues, and vascular structures in a single examination.
- MR imaging is at least comparable and arguably superior to CT for the diagnosis and assessment of acute pancreatitis.

INTRODUCTION

Acute pancreatitis is the most frequent gastrointestinal cause of hospital admissions in the United States, with approximately 275,000 admissions each year.[1] The incidence of acute pancreatitis is increasing and has been linked with the increasing incidence of obesity. Obesity is known to contribute to gallstone formation, and gallstones are the most common cause of acute pancreatitis in the United States.[1] The most common cause worldwide is alcohol consumption.[2] Acute pancreatitis affects men and women in similar proportion; however, the etiology is different. Alcohol-related pancreatitis is more common in men, whereas women are more likely to develop pancreatitis related to gallstones, autoimmune diseases, endoscopic retrograde cholangiopancreatography (ERCP), or an idiopathic origin.[1]

DIAGNOSING ACUTE PANCREATITIS

Patients with acute pancreatitis typically present with epigastric abdominal pain that may radiate to the back. The abdominal pain is often associated with nausea and vomiting and physical examination reveals severe upper abdominal tenderness, sometimes with guarding. Laboratory abnormalities indicating acute pancreatitis are elevated serum amylase and lipase and, if the origin is biliary, elevated alanine aminotransferase (ALT).

The clinical diagnosis of acute pancreatitis requires 2 of these 3 features: (1) abdominal pain consistent with acute pancreatitis (acute onset of persistent, severe, epigastric pain often radiating to the back); (2) serum lipase or amylase levels at least 3 times greater than the upper limits of normal; and (3) characteristic findings of acute pancreatitis on contrast-enhanced CT, MR imaging, or transabdominal ultrasonography (US).[3] As such, if the abdominal pain is characteristic of pancreatitis and the amylase and/or lipase levels are not elevated to at least 3 times above normal, imaging is required for diagnosis.

TYPES AND SEVERITY OF PANCREATITIS

Acute pancreatitis is divided into 2 types: interstitial edematous pancreatitis and necrotizing pancreatitis (**Table 1**). Interstitial edematous pancreatitis is characterized by diffuse (or sometimes localized)

Disclosure Statement: The authors have nothing to disclose.
Department of Radiology, University of Alabama at Birmingham, 619 19th Street South, JT N325, Birmingham, AL 35249, USA
* Corresponding author.
E-mail address: kkporter@uabmc.edu

Magn Reson Imaging Clin N Am 26 (2018) 439–450
https://doi.org/10.1016/j.mric.2018.03.011

Table 1
Classification terms

1992 Atlanta Classification	2013 Revised Atlanta Terms
Within 4 weeks onset of acute pancreatitis: Acute fluid collection Sterile pancreatic necrosis Infected pancreatic necrosis	**Within 4 weeks onset of acute pancreatitis:** Acute fluid collection Acute necrotic collection[a]: Sterile acute necrotic collection Infected acute necrotic collection
After 4 weeks onset of acute pancreatitis: Pancreatic pseudocyst Pancreatic abscess	**After 4 weeks onset of acute pancreatitis:** Sterile pseudocyst (arises from interstitial edematous pancreatitis) Infected pseudocyst (arises from interstitial edematous pancreatitis) Walled-off necrosis (arises from acute necrotic collection)
Notes: There was no terminology in the Atlanta classification for the evolving collections arising from necrotizing pancreatitis that are now known as walled-off necrosis.	**Notes:** On presentation for each patient, the diagnosis of either interstitial edematous pancreatitis OR acute necrotizing pancreatitis should be made. Walled-off necrosis arises from acute necrotizing pancreatitis and, therefore, should not be confused with a pancreatic pseudocyst, which arises from interstitial edematous pancreatitis (or later from disconnected duct syndrome).

[a] Sterile or infected acute necrotic collection may be pancreatic, extrapancreatic, or both (most common).

inflammatory enlargement of the pancreas, typically with inflammatory changes of the peripancreatic fat and usually some peripancreatic fluid (**Fig. 1**). Most patients hospitalized with acute pancreatitis (85%) have interstitial edematous pancreatitis[4] and the symptoms of interstitial edematous pancreatitis usually resolve within 1 week.[3] The other 5% to 15% of patients develop necrotizing pancreatitis (**Fig. 2**), which is further subdivided by whether the necrosis involves the

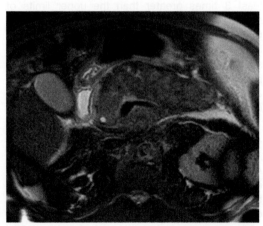

Fig. 1. A 37-year-old man with hypertriglyceridemia and history of recurrent acute pancreatitis presents with epigastric pain of 2 days' duration and elevated lipase. Axial T2-weighted fat-saturated MR image of the abdomen demonstrates inflammation within the pancreatic parenchyma and peripancreatic soft tissues, consistent with interstitial edematous pancreatitis.

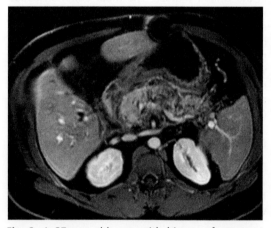

Fig. 2. A 37-year-old man with history of recurrent alcohol-induced acute pancreatitis presents with severe epigastric pain with associated nausea and vomiting of 3 days' duration and elevated lipase. Axial T1-weighted fat-saturated postcontrast MR image demonstrates hypoenhancement of the pancreatic body and tail, consistent with pancreatic necrosis. No acute necrotic collection was seen.

pancreatic parenchyma, the peripancreatic tissues, or both.[3] Necrosis involving both the pancreatic parenchyma and the peripancreatic tissues is most common, whereas necrosis only involving the pancreatic parenchyma is least common.[3] The overall mortality in pancreatitis is approximately 5%, with a mortality of 3% in interstitial pancreatitis and 17% in necrotizing pancreatitis.[5]

The severity of acute pancreatitis can be divided clinically into mild, moderately severe, and severe.[3] Mild acute pancreatitis is characterized by no organ failure or local or systemic complications. Moderately severe acute pancreatitis is characterized by transient (less than 48 hours) organ failure, local complications in the retroperitoneum, or exacerbation of comorbid diseases (eg, chronic lung disease). Severe acute pancreatitis is characterized by persistent organ failure (greater than 48 hours) that may involve 1 or more organ systems, most commonly renal, pulmonary or cardiovascular, and local and/or systemic complications.[3]

Mild pancreatitis is typically only seen with interstitial edematous pancreatitis, which is predominately nonsevere; interstitial edematous pancreatitis is severe in only 1% to 3% of cases, usually in patients with underlying comorbid conditions.[4] Mild pancreatitis is self-limited and requires only supportive care with low associated morbidity and mortality. Severe pancreatitis occurs in approximately 15% to 20% of patients with acute pancreatitis and is characterized by a protracted clinical course, multiorgan failure, and pancreatic necrosis.[6] Severe clinical pancreatitis is by and large seen only in necrotizing pancreatitis and can be life threatening, with morbidity and mortality as high as 36% to 50%.[3,7] Classifying the degree of severity of pancreatitis is an essential component of managing patients with acute pancreatitis, to identify the approximately 15% of patients who are likely to have a severe courses. Patients with severe acute pancreatitis need aggressive treatment, often including transfer to an ICU. Both clinical data and morphologic information provided by imaging are used in staging moderately severe and severe acute pancreatitis.[3,5,7]

THE CLINICAL COURSE OF ACUTE PANCREATITIS

The revised Atlanta classification divides the clinical course of pancreatitis into an early phase and late phase, and the timing of imaging is based on the clinical phase (see **Table 1**).[3] The onset of pancreatitis is defined by the onset of abdominal pain (not presentation or admission to the hospital).[3] The early phase of pancreatitis lasts approximately 1 week and the late phase starts after the first week and can last for weeks to months after the initial onset of abdominal pain. During the early phase, the severity of pancreatitis (mild, moderately severe, and severe) is based entirely on clinical criteria, care is supportive, and imaging findings have a lesser role, the exception being for diagnosis in cases without enzyme elevation. There is no direct correlation between the severity of organ failure in the early phase and the morphologic changes seen on imaging.[3,8]

The Early Phase

The early phase of acute pancreatitis is characterized by the systemic response to cytokine release from the initial pancreatic injury, or the systemic inflammatory response syndrome (SIRS).[3,8] SIRS is the main cause of early complications in acute pancreatitis, whereas superimposed infection and fluid collections are the cause of late complications. SIRS is present if 2 or more of these criteria are met: (1) heart rate greater than 90 beats/min; (2) core temperature less than 36°C or greater than 38°C; (3) white blood cell count less than 4000/mm^3 or greater than 12,000/mm^3; or (4) respirations greater than 20/min or P_{CO_2} 32 mm Hg.[3] If SIRS is present and persistent, organ failure is likely to develop. The presence, extent, and duration of organ failure determine the severity of pancreatitis in the early phase (first week), and clinical scoring methods are used to direct patient care independent of imaging.[3,7] Clinical scoring methods frequently used include the Acute Physiology and Chronic Health Evaluation (APACHE), Marshall, and the Bedside Index of Severity in Acute Pancreatitis (BISAP).[7]

The Late Phase

The late phase only occurs in patients with moderately severe or severe pancreatitis, because it occurs after the first week and is characterized by local complications and persistent systemic inflammatory response (SIRS).[3] Persistent organ failure continues to be the main determinant of severity in the late phase; however, local complications have important implications for management and their morphology is characterized by imaging.[3,7] Local complications evolve over time and may include sterile or infected peripancreatic collections, pseudoaneurysms, splenic or portal vein thrombosis, obstruction or ileus of the gastrointestinal tract, reactive colitis, bowel perforation, pancreatic or biliary duct strictures, ascites and pleural effusion; these complications are best characterized by imaging.[7,9]

A majority of patients with acute pancreatitis recover completely with appropriate therapy; however, approximately 25% to 30% of patients are diagnosed with recurrent acute pancreatitis.[10,11] Recurrent acute pancreatitis is characterized by at least 2 separate documented episodes of pancreatitis with interval resolution between them. Alcohol abuse is the most common cause of recurrent acute pancreatitis with additional, less frequent etiologies including gallstones, genetic predisposition, hypertriglyceridemia, autoimmune pancreatitis, among others.[11]

IMAGING IN ACUTE PANCREATITIS

Although the diagnosis of acute pancreatitis can be made based on nonimaging clinical criteria in most patients, atypical presentations of acute pancreatitis are frequent.[6,12,13] Serum amylase level is the most commonly used biochemical marker of acute pancreatitis and it may be within normal limits in 19% to 32% of patients at the time of hospital admission.[13] Levels of amylase less than 3 times normal can be related to delayed presentation because elevated amylase levels peak within the first 12 hours after the onset of symptoms, to elevated triglyceride levels interfering with the assay, or as a result of poor pancreatic exocrine function (eg, in chronic alcohol abuse).[13] As a result, early imaging is often needed to confirm or exclude the diagnosis of acute pancreatitis. In addition to diagnosing/confirming acute pancreatitis when the clinical situation is unclear, imaging in acute pancreatitis is also used to determine the underlying cause of acute pancreatitis, to evaluate complications and disease severity, and to follow-up complications and guide intervention.[7]

Imaging techniques commonly used in acute pancreatitis include transabdominal US, CT, and MR imaging. The morphologic findings of acute pancreatitis include changes in the pancreatic parenchyma (interstitial edema and necrosis), peripancreatic tissues (inflammatory retroperitoneal fat stranding and collections), and extrapancreatic complications (involvement of the biliary system, vascular structures, gastrointestinal tract, or other organs). The findings on imaging relate to these morphologic changes.

Sometimes the pancreas can be seen well enough on US to demonstrate features of acute pancreatitis, including diffuse glandular enlargement, hypoechoic echotexture of the pancreas consistent with edema, and ascites. US, however, is limited in the majority of patients with acute pancreatitis, often due to overlying bowel gas, particularly in the setting of associated focal adynamic ileus.[6,7] As such, US has limited effectiveness in the evaluation of pancreatic inflammation, peripancreatic inflammation and fluid, and pancreatic necrosis. The primary utility of US in patients with acute pancreatitis is to identify gallstones or biliary ductal dilatation/choledocholithiasis with a sensitivity for the detections of gallstones in patients with acute biliary pancreatitis of approximately 70%.[6] US has limited sensitivity (20%) for choledocholithiasis, however, compared with 40% for CT and 80% for magnetic resonance cholangiopancreatography (MRCP).[14]

CT with intravenous contrast is currently the modality of choice for evaluating patients with acute pancreatitis due to widespread availability and rapid acquisition. CT has shown consistent clinical value in predicting disease severity and outcome in acute pancreatitis. The CT severity index (CTSI) is an imaging prognosticator based on the combined assessment of peripancreatic fluid collections and the degree of pancreatic necrosis.[15] The CTSI, together with other clinical scoring systems, is used for guiding patient care decisions.[7] CT, however, has limitations. Contrast-enhanced CT has been shown to have false-negative results in 20% to 30% of early-stage or less severe cases of acute pancreatitis, because it has poor sensitivity for identifying ductal abnormalities and subtle pancreatic parenchymal changes.[7,16–19] Furthermore, CT is associated with ionizing radiation.[7] Qualified contraindications to contrast enhanced CT include patient allergy to iodinated contrast and acute or chronic renal impairment. Additional limitations of CT include moderate sensitivity for detecting gallstones and limited characterization of the internal contents of pancreatic and peripancreatic collections.[20]

MR IMAGING

Advances in MR imaging techniques, including high field-strength magnets, high-performance gradients, phased-array body coils, power injectors, dynamic contrast-enhanced breath-hold (and more recent motion-insensitive free-breathing) fat-suppressed sequences, and MRCP make MR imaging at least comparable and arguably superior to CT for the diagnosis and assessment of acute pancreatitis.[16,17,21–23] MR imaging is unique in that it allows for noninvasive evaluation of the pancreatic parenchyma, biliary and pancreatic ducts, exocrine function, adjacent soft tissues, and vascular structures in a single examination. MR imaging has the added advantages of not using ionizing radiation or sedation and its gadolinium contrast is not nephrotoxic, making it particularly well suited for pregnant women, patients with renal compromise, and younger patients with acute pancreatitis (**Box 1**).

Diagnosis

MR imaging (**Table 2**) provides excellent soft tissue contrast in the abdomen. The normal intrinsic T1 signal of the pancreas is slightly higher than the liver and the normal T2 signal is intermediate signal intensity, similar to the liver. An edematous pancreas demonstrates higher than normal parenchymal signal on T2-weighted images and mildly decreased parenchymal signal on T1-weighted images. MR imaging can detect trace amounts of peripancreatic fluid, which is high signal on T2-weighted images. The pancreas is very vascular and demonstrates intense, normally homogeneous enhancement during the arterial phase. Maximal enhancement of the pancreas occurs shortly after peak aortic enhancement (15–20 s) with enhancement persisting during the portal venous phase.[24]

Pancreatic necrosis is readily identified as low signal on T1-weighted unenhanced images and as focal regions of nonenhancement with

---

Box 1
Value of MR imaging in acute pancreatitis

Advantages

Noninvasive single examination evaluation of

- Pancreatic parenchyma
- Biliary and pancreatic ducts
- Exocrine function
- Adjacent soft tissues
- Vascular structures

No ionizing radiation or sedation

Gadolinium contrast not nephrotoxic

Diagnosis and etiology

More sensitive than CT or US for

- Detection of mild pancreatitis
- Detection of pancreatic necrosis and hemorrhage
- Identifying choledocholithiasis
- Identifying pancreatic ductal anomalies, stricture, or discontinuity

Assessment of complications

More accurate characterization of the contents of pancreatic and peripancreatic collections than CT or US

Better detection of ductal disconnection than CT, especially with secretin-enhanced MRCP

Table 2
Example of routine MR imaging for evaluating acute pancreatitis

Protocol Step	Sequence
Precontrast	Axial T2-weighted turbo spin-echo Axial T1-weighted in-phase and opposed-phase gradient echo Axial T1-weighted 3-D gradient echo with fat suppression DWI
Postcontrast	Dynamic axial T1-weighted gradient echo with fat suppression in the following phases: • 35-s pancreatic parenchymal • 70-s portal venous • 3-min delayed/equilibrium Coronal T1-weighted gradient echo with fat suppression in delayed/equilibrium phase
MRCP	Coronal 3-D heavily T2-weighted turbo spin echo Coronal and bilateral coronal oblique (15°) fat-saturated single-shot fast spin-echo radial slabs (20–60 mm in thickness)

---

intravenous gadolinium administration. On T2-weighted images, necrosis can be low signal intensity or hyperintense when liquefied. Necrosis may be more easily identified on MR imaging compared with CT.[24] Similarly, hemorrhagic pancreatitis or hemorrhagic fluid collections are more easily recognized on MR imaging than CT because of the presence of T1 hyperintense methemoglobin, low signal intensity hemosiderin rim on T2-weighted images, and signal abnormalities related to hemorrhage persisting longer on MR imaging than CT (**Fig. 3**).[24,25]

Nonenhanced MR imaging has been shown superior to both nonenhanced and contrast-enhanced CT for depicting an inflamed pancreas in mild acute pancreatitis and for depicting peripancreatic fat necrosis.[16] MR imaging is more sensitive than CT in the detection of early pancreatitis, in particular mild cases, and it shows the development of morphologic changes of acute pancreatitis earlier than CT.[16,17,21–23] When MR imaging includes heavily T2-weighted MRCP images, it obviates multimodality imaging, because MRCP images of the biliary system are more sensitive than US for the detection of choledocholithiasis.[14] A severity index based on MR imaging findings

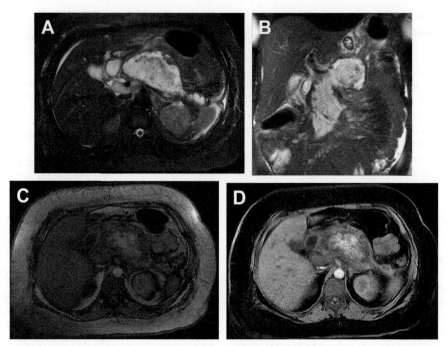

Fig. 3. A 37-year-old woman with alcohol-induced pancreatitis with symptom onset 2 weeks prior presents for further evaluation in the setting of persistent SIRS. (*A*) Axial T2-weighted fat saturated MR image demonstrates a T2-hyperintense acute necrotic collection involving the pancreas and peripancreatic soft tissues. (*B*) Coronal T2-weighted fat-saturated image better illustrates in the inflammatory stranding and involvement of the peripancreatic soft tissues. (*C*) Gradient-echo out-of-phase T1-weighted MR image demonstrates T1 hyperintensity within this collection, suggesting hemorrhage. (*D*) Axial T1-weighted fat-saturated MR image confirms hemorrhage in the acute necrotic collection.

(magnetic resonance severity index [MRSI]) significantly correlates with CTSI, the clinical variables associated with the severity of acute pancreatitis, and the clinical outcome.[17,26]

Identifying Etiology

Gallstones/choledocholithiasis and alcohol account for the majority of cases of acute pancreatitis (approximately 90% of cases) (**Fig. 4**).[27] Additional less frequent causes of acute pancreatitis include pancreatic cancer, blunt abdominal trauma (**Fig. 5**), and ductal anomalies, such as pancreas divisum and ansa pancreatica[28] (**Figs. 6 and 7**), among other causes. MR imaging with MRCP can facilitate the diagnosis of these entities and help guide therapeutic options.

For evaluation of the pancreatic duct and biliary tree, particularly when evaluating for choledocholithiasis or pancreatic ductal anomalies, MRCP

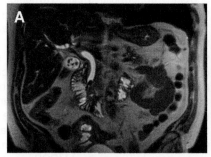
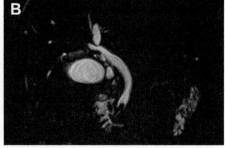

Fig. 4. A 74-year-old man presented to the emergency department with severe epigastric pain of 2 days' duration and elevated lipase, consistent with acute pancreatitis. (*A*) Coronal T2 nonfat saturation MR image demonstrates moderate intrahepatic and extrahepatic biliary ductal dilatation with choledocholithiasis and cholelithiasis. (*B*) Coronal MRCP image again demonstrates moderate extrahepatic biliary ductal dilatation and better depicts the stone within the distal common bile duct.

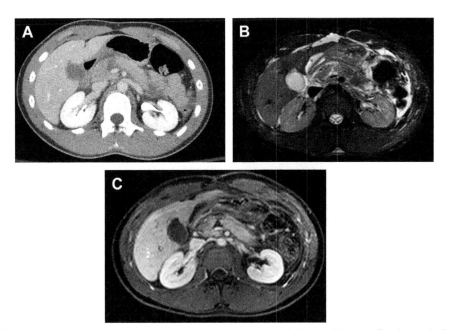

Fig. 5. A 21-year-old man presents with severe abdominal pain and elevated lipase after being kicked in the abdomen by a steer on the day of presentation. (*A*) Axial CT postcontrast image demonstrates peripancreatic fluid and linear hypoattenuation in the pancreatic neck, suspicious for focal inflammation or laceration. (*B*) Axial T2-weighted fat-saturated MR image demonstrates acute pancreatitis with hyperintense peripancreatic fluid and hyperintensity of the pancreatic parenchyma. There is a linear hyperintensity in the pancreatic neck, consistent with a pancreatic transection. (*C*) Postcontrast T1-weighted MR image confirms linear nonenhancement at the site of pancreatic transection in the pancreatic neck.

demonstrates high sensitivity and specificity and has the added benefit of potentially obviating the more invasive ERCP.[14,25,29,30] ERCP has a complication rate of approximately 5% to 10%, including post-ERCP pancreatitis, perforation, and hemorrhage.[31] Furthermore, ERCP may be technically challenging in the setting of acute pancreatitis when the duodenum and ampulla may be swollen. Also, in patients with ductal anomalies predisposing to them to acute pancreatitis or in patients with

traumatic injury to the pancreas, ERCP may be particularly challenging. As such, ERCP is almost exclusively reserved as a therapeutic modality, typically after MRCP, which is used for diagnosis.

Demonstrating Complications and Guiding Intervention

Local complications in acute pancreatitis include pancreatic and peripancreatic collections, which,

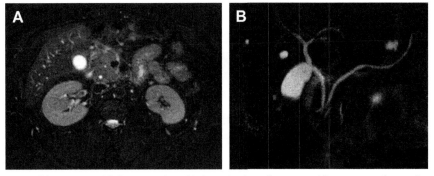

Fig. 6. A 48-year-old woman with history of multiple episodes of pancreatitis, presents for evaluation of the pancreatic duct. (*A*) Axial T2-weighted fat saturation MR image demonstrates enlargement of the pancreatic head with increased T2 signal within the pancreatic parenchyma and within the peripancreatic soft tissues, consistent with acute interstitial pancreatitis. (*B*) Coronal T2-weighted MRCP MIP image demonstrates pancreas divisum, an anatomic variant that predisposes patients to acute pancreatitis.

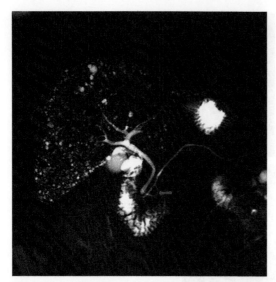

Fig. 7. A 57-year-old woman with recurrent acute pancreatitis presents for evaluation of the pancreatic duct. Heavily T2-weighted MRCP MIP image demonstrates a communication between the main pancreatic duct (of Wirsung) and the accessory pancreatic duct (of Santorini) (*red arrow*), consistent with ansa pancreatica. Ansa pancreatica is a predisposing anatomic variant for the onset of recurrent acute pancreatitis. Numerous biliary hamartomas are also incidentally seen in the liver.

depending on timing and the presence of necrosis, include acute peripancreatic fluid collection, pancreatic pseudocyst, acute necrotic collection, and walled-off necrosis. Acute peripancreatic fluid collections usually develop in the early phase of interstitial edematous pancreatitis. A pancreatic pseudocyst is a delayed (>4 weeks) complication of interstitial edematous pancreatitis, has a well-defined wall, and does not contain solid material. In necrotizing pancreatitis, a collection in the early phase is called an acute necrotic collection,

whereas walled-off necrosis, which is surrounded by a detectible capsule, usually does not develop until after 4 weeks.[3]

Differentiating collections that contain necrosis from those that do not has important implications for management, because residual necrotic debris after drainage may lead to secondary infection. The contents of pancreatic and peripancreatic collections can be more accurately assessed by MR imaging than by CT or US.[27,32] MR imaging is more sensitive for the detection of necrotic debris within pancreatic and peripancreatic collections and for predicting whether these collections can be drained by endoscopic, percutaneous, or surgical drainage procedures (**Figs. 8 and 9**).[32]

A pseudocyst may also be seen in necrotizing pancreatitis in the setting of "disconnected duct syndrome." A disconnected, or disrupted, pancreatic duct most commonly occurs as a complication of necrotizing pancreatitis. Focal necrosis of the pancreatic duct epithelium may lead to an isolated, functional, upstream pancreatic segment, which is not connected to the gastrointestinal system. This results in a persistent pancreatic fluid collection(s) or end pancreatic fistula.

Patients with a disconnected pancreatic duct typically present with an unresolving pseudocyst, a persistent pancreatic fistula, pancreatic ascites, a region of walled-off necrosis, or a combination of these findings. Although peripancreatic fluid collections may be treated conservatively or with drainage, these strategies most likely fail in the setting of a disconnected pancreatic duct or lead to persistent pancreatic fistula formation; therefore, early diagnosis of this condition leads to reduced morbidity and may avert unnecessary drainage procedures.[33] MRCP performed with secretin is emerging as the imaging study of choice for the diagnosis of a disconnected pancreatic duct, which

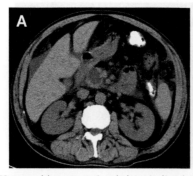
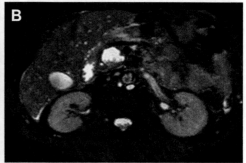

Fig. 8. A 62-year-old man previously hospitalized 6 months prior for acute pancreatitis presents for follow-up of a presumed acute peripancreatic collection. (*A*) Fluid collection in the pancreatic head appears simple on the CT examination, favoring pseudocyst. (*B*) Axial T2-weighted fat-saturated MR image demonstrates that the pancreatic head fluid collection contains layering dependent debris, which was not seen on the CT examination. This pancreatic fluid collection with debris is more consistent with walled-off necrosis.

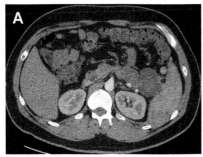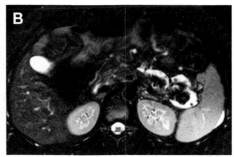

Fig. 9. A 31-year-old man with history of acute pancreatitis complicated by acute respiratory distress syndrome 10 months prior presents for evaluation of a pancreatic collection. (*A*) CT with contrast demonstrates a large hypoattenuating collection replacing the pancreatic tail, suspicious for walled-off necrosis. Subtle hyperattenuating areas are seen within the collection. (*B*) Axial T2-weighted fat-saturated MR image better demonstrates the extent of the necrotic material within the collection, consistent with walled-off necrosis.

demonstrates a cutoff of the downstream pancreatic duct with enhancing upstream pancreatic parenchyma.[34] Secretin stimulates pancreatic secretion and can improve detection of the site of pancreatic duct disruption or the continuity of the disrupted pancreatic duct with a fluid collection. MRCP has the advantage of being able to evaluate both the main pancreatic duct and the pancreatic parenchyma simultaneously compared with contrast-enhanced CT combined with ERCP.

Extravasation of pancreatic enzymes in acute pancreatitis can damage adjacent vascular structures resulting in vasculitis, pseudoaneurysm, or venous thrombosis. Magnetic resonance angiogram and/or magnetic resonance venogram and postcontrast images can be used to evaluate for these vascular abnormalities. Venous thrombosis is the most common vascular complication of pancreatitis and is well seen on contrast-enhanced MR images.[24] Venous thrombosis can also be evaluated on unenhanced balanced gradient-echo sequences (eg, BTFE [Balanced Turbo Field Echo], FIESTA [Fast Imaging Employing Steady State Acquisition, GE Healthcare, USA], and TrueFISP [True Fast Imaging with Steady Precession, Siemens, Germany]). Venous thrombosis typically affects the splenic vein and less frequently involves the portal and superior mesenteric veins. Pseudoaneurysms most frequently involve the splenic, gastroduodenal, and pancreaticoduodenal arteries and are best depicted on contrast-enhanced sequences when the enhancement is comparable to the arteries and the connection to the vessel can be seen.[24]

Follow-up

In the 10% to 30% of patients with acute pancreatitis who develop recurrent acute pancreatitis, identifying the underlying cause is particularly important to mitigate the progression to chronic pancreatitis.

Patients with recurrent acute pancreatitis benefit from secretin-enhanced MRCP, which facilitates detailed analysis of the pancreatic duct for anomalies, stricture/obstruction (**Fig. 10**), and discontinuity as well as for the assessment of decreased exocrine function of the pancreas.[10,17,34]

STANDARD MR IMAGING PROTOCOL

At the authors' institution, MR imaging of the pancreas is performed using a standardized protocol with a phased-array body surface coil. Acquired standard images include precontrast axial T2-weighted turbo spin-echo sequences through the liver and pancreas. Axial dual-echo sequences and precontrast T1-weighted 5-mm images are also acquired. Postcontrast axial T1-weighted images are acquired in the pancreatic parenchymal (35-s), portal venous (70-s), and delayed (3-min) phases. A delayed coronal postcontrast T1-weighted image extending from the diaphragm to the iliac crests is obtained as well as axial 5-mm diffusion-weighted images (DWIs). Gadoteridol is the typical contrast agent used; however, in select cases when improved delineation of the biliary tree is required or a ductal leak is suspected, the hepatobiliary agent, gadoxetate disodium, is used.

MRCP sequences are usually also included in the evaluation of the pancreas. Prior to MRCP, patients are held for 6 hours, nothing by mouth. High-resolution 3-D heavily T2-weighted images are acquired in the coronal plane using a 3-D turbo spin-echo technique. Additionally, fat-saturated single-shot fast spin-echo radial slabs (20–60 mm in thickness) are acquired in the straight coronal and bilateral coronal oblique positions (approximately 15° rotated in either direction). Maximum intensity projections (MIPs) are created from these slabs.

A synthetic analog of the hormone secretin is sometimes administered to augment the MRCP.

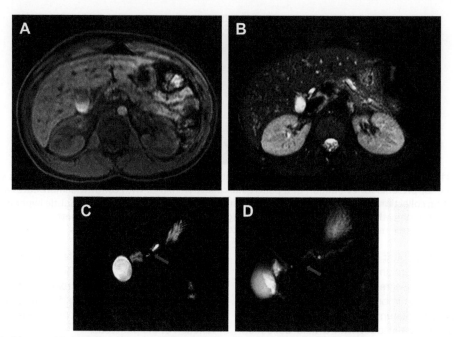

Fig. 10. A 24-year-old woman with worsening abdominal pain and nausea and vomiting. The patient has a history of recurrent acute pancreatitis, which began after a motor vehicle collision 2 years prior. (*A*) Axial T1-weighted fat-saturated MR image demonstrates hypointensity in the pancreatic neck and body, consistent with the patient's history of recurrent acute pancreatitis. (*B*) Axial T2-weighted fat-saturated MR image demonstrates increased signal in the pancreas consistent with acute pancreatitis. There is also dilation of the pancreatic duct in the body and tail. (*C*) Heavily T2-weighted MRCP image demonstrates a high-grade stricture of the pancreatic duct in the pancreatic neck (*red arrow*) with upstream dilation of the pancreatic duct. (*D*) Heavily T2-weighted MRCP MIP image confirms the stricture in the pancreatic neck (*red arrow*) with dilated upstream pancreatic duct and side branches in the body and tail.

Secretin stimulates water and bicarbonate secretions from the exocrine cells of the pancreas and transiently increases the tone of the sphincter of Oddi, leading to increased fluid signal in the pancreatic duct with subsequent fluid excretion into the duodenum.[34] Therefore, secretin-enhanced MRCP increases the conspicuity of the pancreatic duct and provides functional information regarding the pancreas. Secretin-enhanced MRCP is also used to evaluate for pancreatic ductal discontinuity, stricture, or pathologic communication with pancreatic or peripancreatic fluid collections. Coronal MRCP images are acquired prior to and after the slow intravenous injection of 0.2 μg/kg of secretin. Images are acquired every minute for 5 minutes after secretin injection.

FUTURE DIRECTIONS
Diffusion-Weighted Imaging

Standard MR imaging of the pancreas primarily emphasizes morphology. DWI focuses instead on pathologic changes within tissues that manifest as changes in the random molecular motion of water molecules, also known as brownian motion or diffusion. DWI is sensitive to changes in tissue composition that affect molecular motion, including edema and cellularity. The apparent diffusion coefficient (ADC) is the quantification of the magnitude of diffusion of water molecules within different tissues. DWI is commonly used in the evaluation of neoplastic processes, such as prostate cancer, and in inflammatory conditions, such as inflammatory bowel disease. Preliminary studies suggest that DWI may help in identifying mild acute pancreatitis with significantly reduced ADC values in patients with acute pancreatitis when compared with healthy controls.[35] Preliminary studies also suggest a prognostic role for ADC in patients with acute pancreatitis[36] and that normalized ADC values may help differentiate mass-forming pancreatitis from benign and malignant pancreatic neoplasms.[37] Diffusion tensor imaging, which is another MR imaging technique for measuring the restricted diffusion of water in tissue, has also preliminarily shown that ADC values of the pancreas have a negative correlation with the severity of acute pancreatitis.[38]

Magnetic Resonance Elastography

Magnetic resonance elastography (MRE) is an MR imaging technique that evaluates the stiffness of tissues in vivo. Continuous mechanical waves at a low frequency (40–60 Hz) are propagated from an acoustic driver to a passive driver on a patient's body, resulting in periodic tissue displacement.[39,40] The frequency and character of the propagated waves provide information about the target tissues stiffness. Recently, Shi and colleagues[39] demonstrated that patients with acute pancreatitis had significantly higher pancreatic stiffness values than healthy controls and that there was no overlap between the stiffness values between the 2 groups. Furthermore, MRE detected acute pancreatitis within 24 hours of admission better than contrast-enhanced CT and was comparable to clinical measures of disease severity (eg, CTSI, APACHE-II, and BISAP scores). The infiltration of inflammatory cells, interstitial edema, and increased perfusion are believed to contribute to increased pancreatic stiffness in acute pancreatitis. MRE may prove a useful, noninvasive method for diagnosing and assessing early severity in acute pancreatitis.

SUMMARY

Although CT is generally considered the workhorse for imaging of patients with known or suspected acute pancreatitis, MR imaging has several distinct advantages, including better sensitivity for detection of mild parenchymal and early inflammatory changes; complete evaluation of the pancreatic and biliary ductal systems and gall bladder; detection of pancreatic glandular necrosis on unenhanced examinations; improved identification of solid components in complex necrotizing collections before drainage; and lack of ionizing radiation. Physiologic evaluation with secretin stimulation and identification of ductal anatomy in disconnected duct syndrome, and the emerging value of MRE techniques as well as ADC assessment, further add to the high clinical impact of this modality.

REFERENCES

1. Yadav D, Lowenfels AB. The epidemiology of pancreatitis and pancreatic cancer. Gastroenterology 2013;144(6):1252–61.
2. Zyromski NJ. Etiology. Acute pancreatitis. Available at: https://online.epocrates.com/diseases/6624/Acute-pancreatitis/Etiology. Accessed September 26, 2017.
3. Banks PA, Bollen TL, Dervenis C, et al. Classification of acute pancreatitis–2012: revision of the Atlanta classification and definitions by international consensus. Gut 2013;62(1):102–11.
4. Singh VK, Bollen TL, Wu BU, et al. An assessment of the severity of interstitial pancreatitis. Clin Gastroenterol Hepatol 2011;9(12):1098–103.
5. Banks PA, Freeman ML, Practice Parameters Committee of the American College of Gastroenterology. Practice guidelines in acute pancreatitis. Am J Gastroenterol 2006;101(10):2379–400.
6. Forsmark CE, Baillie J, AGA Institute Clinical Practice and Economics Committee, AGA Institute Governing Board.. AGA institute technical review on acute pancreatitis. Gastroenterology 2007;132(5):2022–44.
7. Baker ME, Nelson RC, Rosen MP, et al. ACR appropriateness criteria® acute pancreatitis. Ultrasound Q 2014;30(4):267–73.
8. Thoeni RF. Imaging of acute pancreatitis. Radiol Clin North Am 2015;53(6):1189–208.
9. Thoeni RF. The revised Atlanta classification of acute pancreatitis: its importance for the radiologist and its effect on treatment. Radiology 2012;262(3):751–64.
10. Sandrasegaran K, Tahir B, Barad U, et al. The value of secretin-enhanced MRCP in patients with recurrent acute pancreatitis. AJR Am J Roentgenol 2017;208(2):315–21.
11. Machicado JD, Yadav D. Epidemiology of recurrent acute and chronic pancreatitis: similarities and differences. Dig Dis Sci 2017;62(7):1683–91.
12. Shinagare AB, Ip IK, Raja AS, et al. Use of CT and MRI in emergency department patients with acute pancreatitis. Abdom Imaging 2015;40(2):272–7.
13. Matull WR, Pereira SP, O'Donohue JW. Biochemical markers of acute pancreatitis. J Clin Pathol 2006;59(4):340–4.
14. Moon JH, Cho YD, Cha SW, et al. The detection of bile duct stones in suspected biliary pancreatitis: comparison of MRCP, ERCP, and intraductal US. Am J Gastroenterol 2005;100(5):1051–7.
15. Balthazar EJ, Robinson DL, Megibow AJ, et al. Acute pancreatitis: value of CT in establishing prognosis. Radiology 1990;174(2):331–6.
16. Amano Y, Oishi T, Takahashi M, et al. Nonenhanced magnetic resonance imaging of mild acute pancreatitis. Abdom Imaging 2001;26(1):59–63.
17. Arvanitakis M, Delhaye M, De Maertelaere V, et al. Computed tomography and magnetic resonance imaging in the assessment of acute pancreatitis. Gastroenterology 2004;126(3):715–23.
18. Staudacher C, Parolini D, Vanzulli A, et al. Computerized tomography versus nuclear magnetic resonance in acute pancreatitis. Chir Ital 1995;47(2):25–9 [in Italian].
19. Sica GT, Miller FH, Rodriguez G, et al. Magnetic resonance imaging in patients with pancreatitis: evaluation of signal intensity and enhancement changes. J Magn Reson Imaging 2002;15(3):275–84.

20. Bollen TL, van Santvoort HC, Besselink MG, et al. Update on acute pancreatitis: ultrasound, computed tomography, and magnetic resonance imaging features. Semin Ultrasound CT MR 2007;28(5):371–83.

21. Semelka RC, Ascher SM. MR imaging of the pancreas. Radiology 1993;188(3):593–602.

22. O'Neill E, Hammond N, Miller FH. MR imaging of the pancreas. Radiol Clin North Am 2014;52(4):757–77.

23. Morgan DE. Imaging of acute pancreatitis and its complications. Clin Gastroenterol Hepatol 2008; 6(10):1077–85.

24. Miller FH, Keppke AL, Dalal K, et al. MRI of pancreatitis and its complications: part 1, acute pancreatitis. AJR Am J Roentgenol 2004;183(6):1637–44.

25. Bates DD, LeBedis CA, Soto JA, et al. Use of magnetic resonance in pancreaticobiliary emergencies. Magn Reson Imaging Clin N Am 2016;24(2):433–48.

26. Lecesne R, Taourel P, Bret PM, et al. Acute pancreatitis: interobserver agreement and correlation of CT and MR cholangiopancreatography with outcome. Radiology 1999;211(3):727–35.

27. Balci NC, Bieneman BK, Bilgin M, et al. Magnetic resonance imaging in pancreatitis. Top Magn Reson Imaging 2009;20(1):25–30.

28. Hayashi TY, Gonoi W, Yoshikawa T, et al. Ansa pancreatica as a predisposing factor for recurrent acute pancreatitis. World J Gastroenterol 2016;22(40): 8940–8.

29. Hirohashi S, Hirohashi R, Uchida H, et al. Pancreatitis: evaluation with MR cholangiopancreatography in children. Radiology 1997;203(2):411–5.

30. Darge K, Anupindi S. Pancreatitis and the role of US, MRCP and ERCP. Pediatr Radiol 2009;39(Suppl 2): S153–7.

31. Freeman ML. Complications of endoscopic retrograde cholangiopancreatography: avoidance and management. Gastrointest Endosc Clin N Am 2012;22(3):567–86.

32. Morgan DE, Baron TH, Smith JK, et al. Pancreatic fluid collections prior to intervention: evaluation with MR imaging compared with CT and US. Radiology 1997;203(3):773–8.

33. Nadkarni NA, Kotwal V, Sarr MG, et al. Disconnected pancreatic duct syndrome: endoscopic stent or surgeon's knife? Pancreas 2015;44(1):16–22.

34. Tirkes T, Sandrasegaran K, Sanyal R, et al. Secretin-enhanced MR cholangiopancreatography: spectrum of findings. Radiographics 2013;33(7): 1889–906.

35. Hocaoglu E, Aksoy S, Akarsu C, et al. Evaluation of diffusion-weighted MR imaging in the diagnosis of mild acute pancreatitis. Clin Imaging 2015;39(3): 463–7.

36. Iranmahboob AK, Kierans AS, Huang C, et al. Preliminary investigation of whole-pancreas 3D histogram ADC metrics for predicting progression of acute pancreatitis. Clin Imaging 2017; 42:172–7.

37. Barral M, Sebbag-Sfez D, Hoeffel C, et al. Characterization of focal pancreatic lesions using normalized apparent diffusion coefficient at 1.5-Tesla: preliminary experience. Diagn Interv Imaging 2013; 94(6):619–27.

38. Li X, Zhuang L, Zhang X, et al. Preliminary study of MR diffusion tensor imaging of pancreas for the diagnosis of acute pancreatitis. PLoS One 2016; 11(9):e0160115.

39. Shi Y, Liu Y, Liu YQ, et al. Early diagnosis and severity assessment of acute pancreatitis (AP) using MR elastography (MRE) with spin-echo echo-planar imaging. J Magn Reson Imaging 2017;46(5): 1311–9.

40. Pozzessere C, Porter KK, Kamel IR. Surveillance liver MRI for monitoring patients with known or suspected chronic liver disease. Clin Radiol 2017; 72(1):93.e7-13.

Chronic Pancreatitis
What the Clinician Wants to Know from MR Imaging

Temel Tirkes, MD

KEYWORDS

- Pancreas • Chronic pancreatitis • MR imaging • Magnetic resonance cholangiopancreatography
- Computerized tomography

KEY POINTS

- MR imaging, CT, and EUS are the best imaging methods for establishing a diagnosis of CP. ERCP is reserved for therapeutic purposes.
- The diagnosis of chronic pancreatitis remains challenging in early stages of the disease. T1 signal intensity changes of the parenchyma may precede ductal abnormalities and detect early CP.
- The use of secretin increases the diagnostic potential of MRCP in the evaluation of patients with known or suspected CP.
- There is a need for an MR imaging/MRCP-based diagnostic criteria for CP, combining the ductal findings with the parenchymal changes secondary to fibrosis.
- Genetic discoveries are rapidly uncovering new susceptibility factors. Knowledge of gene and gene-environment interactions may translate into new diagnostic and treatment paradigms.

INTRODUCTION

Chronic pancreatitis (CP) is a low prevalence disease.[1–3] In 2006, there were approximately 50 cases of definite CP per 100,000 population in Olmsted County, Minnesota,[3] translating to a total of 150,000 to 200,000 cases in the US population. Clinical features of CP are highly variable and include minimal or no symptoms of debilitating pain, repeated episodes of acute pancreatitis, pancreatic exocrine and endocrine insufficiency, and pancreatic cancer. CP profoundly affects the quality of life, which can be worse than other chronic conditions and cancers.[4]

Natural history studies for CP originated mainly from centers outside the United States[5–11] conducted during the 1960s to 1990s and consisted primarily of men with alcoholic CP. Only one large retrospective longitudinal cohort study has been conducted in the United States for patients seen at the Mayo Clinic from 1976 to 1982.[12] Although these data provide general insights into disease evolution, it is difficult to predict the probability of outcomes or disease progression in individual patients. Few data exist on the risk of progression in patients with recurrent acute pancreatitis, or in the early stage disease when definitive morphologic features of CP are not evident. There are no longitudinal prospective cohort studies of CP in the United States.

In the past two decades, new knowledge has broadened the etiologic profile of CP to highlight

Disclosure: T. Tirkes receives support from National Cancer Institute and National Institute of Diabetes and Digestive and Kidney Diseases of the National Institutes of Health under award number U01DK108323. The content is solely the responsibility of the author and does not necessarily represent the official views of the National Institutes of Health.
Department of Radiology and Imaging Sciences, Indiana University School of Medicine, IU Health University Hospital, 550 North University Boulevard, UH0663, Indianapolis, IN 46202, USA
E-mail address: atirkes@iupui.edu

contributions from genetic,[13] autoimmune,[14] and environmental (smoking)[15] factors. Improvement in imaging techniques has enabled better recognition of morphologic and functional changes in the pancreas.[16] The clinical significance of type 3c diabetes mellitus in patients with diagnosed or undiagnosed pancreatic disease is increasingly recognized.[17,18] The impact of these developments on the natural history of CP is unknown.

The evaluation of chronic abdominal pain costs an estimated $30 billion in health care and lost wages annually.[19] Patients with suspected or definite CP comprise a significant fraction of these patients. Although diagnosing moderate-severe CP is often straightforward, detection of early stage CP remains difficult because of the absence of reliable morphologic and functional diagnostic methods. Biopsy of the pancreas is not usually performed because it may not provide a definite diagnosis and entails a risk of biopsy-related pancreatitis. Patients often undergo an exhaustive array of costly studies (endoscopic, radiologic) with their attendant risks. Pancreatic function testing (PFT) is usually performed as a clinical test in patients with chronic abdominal pain or suspected CP to assess for the presence of early stage disease, but this practice varies between centers,[20–22] and limited data suggest a high negative predictive value of PFT. However, it is cumbersome to perform, has low positive predictive value (~50%),[23] and has not gained widespread use (<20 centers in the United States).

Because treatment options for definite CP are limited, patients with early stage CP or at high-risk of developing CP are ideally suited for interventions (eg, anti-inflammatory or antifibrotic medications) to prevent the development of definite CP and its associated morbidity. It is desirable to have a practical, fast, and cost-efficient test to exclude CP with high certainty, to reliably rule-in early stage CP or help predict disease progression in these patients, to identify patients suitable for intervention (eg, medication, surgery), and to monitor their effects to slow or reverse disease progression.

ETIOLOGY

The cause of CP is determined after a thorough patient investigation considering all known risk factors, including alcohol consumption and smoking, laboratory values (triglyceride levels, Ca^{2+} levels for ruling out elevated primary hyperparathyroidism, carbohydrate-deficient transferrin/phosphatidylethanol levels), and family medical history.

The most common risk factor for CP is alcohol abuse, with a logarithmic risk increase, although the type of alcohol consumed is irrelevant.[24] The amount and duration of alcohol consumption required to develop CP have not been unequivocally defined. Some authors suggest at least 80 g/d for at least 6 years is a threshold for developing CP. Smoking is probably an independent risk factor, and smoking cessation is advisable for patients with CP.[25]

Autoimmune pancreatitis should be ruled out following current consensus guidelines and when no other cause is found in patients (See Nima Hafezi-Nejad and colleagues' article, "Magnetic Resonance Imaging of Autoimmune Pancreatitis," in this issue for information on typical imaging and clinical findings of autoimmune pancreatitis.)

Cholecystolithiasis and choledocholithiasis are not considered independent risk factors for the development of CP. Whether anatomic anomalies, such as pancreas divisum, increase the CP risk is a matter of debate; however, with additional risk factors, pancreas divisum might lead to CP development. If no etiologic factor is identified, genetic screening for predisposing variants is offered.

Genetic factors also contribute to CP development. The most important genetic risk factors are variants in cationic trypsinogen (PRSS1), serine protease inhibitor Kazal-type 1 (SPINK1), and carboxypeptidase A1. Further genetic susceptibility genes are cystic fibrosis transmembrane conductance regulator (CFTR), chymotrypsinogen C, and carboxyesterlipase.[13]

CLINICAL FEATURES

Abdominal pain is a dominant feature of CP. The pain is typically epigastric, often radiates to the back, is occasionally associated with nausea and vomiting, and may be partially relieved by sitting upright or leaning forward. The pain is usually worse 15 to 30 minutes after eating. Early in the course of CP, the pain may occur in discreet attacks; as the condition progresses, the pain tends to become more continuous.

The pain in CP varies among patients. This pattern was illustrated in a prospective cohort of 207 patients with alcoholic CP in which two typical pain patterns were observed.[26] The first was characterized by episodes of pain (usually lasting less than 10 days) with pain-free intervals lasting from months to more than a year. The second pattern was characterized by prolonged periods of daily pain or clusters of severe pain exacerbations often requiring repeated hospitalizations. Also, although abdominal pain is the most consistent finding in patients with CP, it may be absent in some cases.

In one series, for example, 20% of patients with CP presented with evidence of pancreatic exocrine or endocrine dysfunction in the absence of pain.[12]

Patients with severe pancreatic exocrine dysfunction cannot correctly digest complex foods or absorb partially digested breakdown products. Nevertheless, clinically significant protein and fat deficiencies do not occur until more than 90% of pancreatic function is lost.[27]

Steatorrhea usually occurs before protein deficiencies because lipolytic activity decreases faster than proteolysis.[28] The clinical manifestations of fat malabsorption include loose, greasy, foul-smelling stools that are difficult to flush. Malabsorption of the fat-soluble vitamins (A, D, E, and K) and vitamin B_{12} may also occur, although clinically symptomatic vitamin deficiency is rare.[29]

Glucose intolerance occurs with some frequency in CP, but overt diabetes mellitus usually occurs late in the course of the disease. Patients with calcifying CP, particularly those who develop it early, may develop diabetes more frequently than those with noncalcifying CP.[30] Diabetes is also more likely to occur in patients with a family history of type 1 or type 2 diabetes; this observation suggests a role for an underlying decrease in pancreatic reserve or insulin responsiveness. Pancreatic surgery (including drainage or pancreaticoduodenectomy) does not seem to increase the risk of diabetes. Exceptions include distal pancreatectomy and significant pancreatic resection in the setting of extensive pancreatic fibrosis.[30] Diabetes that develops in patients with CP is usually insulin-requiring. However, it is different from typical type 1 diabetes in that the pancreatic alpha cells, which produce glucagon, are also affected; as a result, there is an increased risk of treatment-related and spontaneous hypoglycemia. Diabetic ketoacidosis and nephropathy are rare; neuropathy and retinopathy occur more frequently.[28]

HISTOPATHOLOGY

Histologically, the two most common features of CP are the loss of acinar tissue (atrophy) and fibrosis. The fibrosis may surround the lobules (perilobular or interlobular fibrosis) or extend into the lobules of acinar tissue (intralobular fibrosis).[31] Chronic inflammatory infiltrate may be present, but this feature is highly variable and disappears late in the course of CP. A diagnosis of CP may be made by atrophy and fibrosis in the absence of other changes. CP can be a patchy or localized process with regional involvement. This feature is best understood by considering the mechanisms of pathogenesis, in particular the necrosis-fibrosis hypothesis, which posits that CP develops as a result of multiple episodes of acute pancreatitis with necrosis and scarring. This process may be patchy at first, progressing to a diffuse pattern after multiple episodes. This is commonly considered to be the mechanism in alcoholic CP, paraduodenal CP, and likely hereditary pancreatitis. However, duct obstruction can lead to progressive fibrosis and loss of acinar tissue that may be localized or segmental, as in the presence of an obstructing neoplasm, or may be diffuse as is characteristic of cystic fibrosis.

IMAGING STUDIES

Imaging studies that may be useful in CP include plain abdominal films, transabdominal ultrasound (US), computed tomography (CT) scan, MR imaging combined with magnetic resonance cholangiopancreatography (MRCP), endoscopic retrograde cholangiopancreatography (ERCP), and endoscopic ultrasound (EUS).

Calcifications within the pancreatic duct are present on plain film in approximately 30% of patients with CP. Calcium deposition is most common with alcoholic pancreatitis but can also be seen in the hereditary and tropical forms of the disorder; it is rare in idiopathic pancreatitis.

Transabdominal ultrasonography, CT scan, and MR imaging/MRCP may show ductal dilatation, enlargement of the pancreas, calcifications, and postinflammatory fluid collections adjacent to the gland. The sensitivity and specificity of US for the diagnosis of CP are 60% to 70% and 80% to 90%, respectively.[32] The corresponding values for CT scanning are 75% to 90% and 85%, respectively.[33] Most common CT imaging features of CP are listed in **Table 1**.[33]

MRCP is becoming the diagnostic test of choice because MR imaging/MRCP is a more sensitive imaging tool for the diagnosis of CP by evaluating parenchymal and ductal changes. Most common findings of CP seen by MR imaging and MRCP are listed in **Table 2**. Ductal abnormalities are specific and reliable MR imaging signs of CP; however, signal intensity changes either by T1-weighted gradient echo or T1 mapping may precede ductal abnormalities and detect early CP.[34-38] One study investigated the association between the bicarbonate level of the pancreatic juice and the T1-weighted gradient echo signal and reported a significant direct correlation. The signal intensity ratio of 1.2 yielded sensitivity of 77% and specificity of 83% for detection of pancreatic exocrine dysfunction (area under the curve, 0.89).[34] This imaging finding is helpful information to the clinician who

Table 1
Imaging features of CP observed by CT

CT Features of CP	Incidence
Ectatic pancreatic duct	68%
Atrophy	54%
Calcifications	50%
Fluid collections	30%
Focal pancreatic enlargement	30%
Biliary ductal dilatation	29%
Alterations in peripancreatic fat	16%
Others	Contiguous organ invasion, large cavities, focal acute pancreatitis, intraductal filling defects, disconnected/disrupted pancreatic duct

is evaluating a patient whose symptoms are suspected of CP but has normal ductal findings.

MRCP can also be performed by using the hormone secretin, which stimulates a normal

Table 2
Features of CP seen by MR imaging/MRCP with or without secretin

MR imaging and MRCP Features of CP	
Main pancreatic duct and side branches	Strictures Ductal filling defects Ectatic side branches Ductal contour irregularity Disconnected/disrupted main pancreatic duct Congenital anomalies (eg, pancreas divisum)
Parenchyma	Atrophy Steatosis
Fluid collections	Walled-off necrosis vs pseudocyst
Secretin MRCP specific findings	Increase in diameter of main pancreatic duct Decreased duodenal filling by the pancreatic juice
T1 signal change	Decrease T1 signal in precontrast phase
Biliary system	Dilatation/strictures
Duodenum	Obstruction/stricture

pancreas to secrete a significant amount of fluid while transiently increasing the tone of the sphincter of Oddi. Transient increase in the diameter of the duct improves the depiction of the anatomy, which is useful in cases where detailed evaluation of the pancreatic duct is most desired in patients with the suspected pancreatic disease.[39,40] Improved visualization of the ductal anatomy is important in differentiating side-branch intraductal papillary mucinous neoplasms from other cystic neoplasms; diagnosis and classification of CP; disconnected pancreatic duct syndrome; and ductal anomalies, such as anomalous pancreaticobiliary junction and pancreas divisum. In the postpancreatectomy patients, stimulation by secretin can give information about the patency of the pancreaticoenteric anastomosis. Duodenal filling during the postsecretin phase of the MRCP can estimate the excretory reserve of the pancreas.[41] It is expected that with increasing severity of CP there is a decrease in the number of acinar cells and the fluid output, which is detected with secretin MRCP. Current consensus is that duodenal filling during secretin MRCP does not help to evaluate the grade of severity of CP, because a substantial number of patients with severe CP may still have a normal duodenal filling.

Diffusion-weighted MR imaging measures the restriction of free water molecules in the gland. The more fibrosis there is, the more likely there is less diffusion of water molecules (which is measured as apparent diffusion coefficient). The apparent diffusion coefficient value is expected to be lower in patients with pancreatic fibrosis than in normal patients. Exploiting this idea, one can evaluate the gland using diffusion MR imaging after intravenous secretin stimulation and enhance the sensitivity to depict subtle abnormalities in diffusion restriction and separate normal patients from those with early CP.[42]

Magnetic resonance elastography has been shown to be a reliable marker of hepatic fibrosis in patients with the chronic liver disease. Although there are no controlled data evaluating this technique in patients with CP, there is room for optimism because recent data demonstrated the feasibility of using magnetic resonance elastography to determine pancreatic stiffness in healthy volunteers. Reproducible stiffness measurements were noted throughout the pancreas, with imaging parameters and equipment different than that used for liver imaging. Preliminary data suggest that pancreatic magnetic resonance elastography can provide promising and reproducible stiffness measurements throughout the pancreas, potentially allowing for assessment of pancreatic fibrosis.[43]

ERCP had been used to identify ductal abnormalities or obstructions; to clarify ductal anatomy before surgical intervention; and to confirm the patency of postsurgical anastomoses, including pancreaticojejunostomies.[44] Guidelines published by the American Society for Gastrointestinal Endoscopy in 2006 recommend that ERCP should be reserved for patients in whom the diagnosis remains unclear after PFT or other noninvasive (CT or MR imaging) or less invasive imaging studies (EUS) have been performed.[45] Characteristic beading of the main pancreatic duct and ectatic side branches is diagnostic of CP. The Cambridge classification has divided patients into normal, equivocal, mild, moderate, and severe CP categories based on ductal changes on ERCP.[46,47] Today, ERCP is rarely used for diagnostic purposes.

EUS may be as sensitive as ERCP or PFT, but requires a highly skilled gastroenterologist to perform[48] and multicenter studies showed the interobserver agreement to be less than optimal for the diagnosis of CP.[49] The most predictive endosonographic feature is the presence of stones. Other suggestive features include visible side branches, cysts, lobularity, an irregular main pancreatic duct, hyperechoic foci and strands, dilation of the main pancreatic duct, and hyperechoic margins of the main pancreatic duct. Many endosonographers consider the presence of four or more of these features to be highly suggestive of CP.[48]

Several invasive and noninvasive PFTs are available for the diagnosis of pancreatic insufficiency, which is classified as direct or indirect. Direct tests involve the stimulation of the pancreas through the administration of a meal or hormonal secretagogues, after which duodenal fluid is collected and analyzed to quantify normal pancreatic secretory content (ie, enzymes and bicarbonate). Only a few specialized centers perform these tests. Their main role is in the diagnosis of early CP in patients with compatible clinical features but without characteristic radiographic findings. The estimated sensitivity and specificity of secretin PFT in diagnosing CP are 82% and 86%, respectively.[23] Indirect tests measure the consequences of pancreatic insufficiency and are more widely available. However, they depend on the consequences of pancreatic maldigestion, which are not apparent until normal enzyme secretory output has declined by more than 90%. Thus, they are insensitive to early pancreatic insufficiency.

LABORATORY

Serum concentrations of amylase and lipase may be slightly elevated in patients with CP. However, these enzymes are more commonly normal because CP is a patchy, focal disease, leading to a minimal increase in pancreatic enzymes within the blood and there is frequently significant fibrosis, resulting in a decreased abundance of these enzymes within the pancreas. Thus, serum measurements of amylase or lipase should be reserved only for the diagnosis of acute pancreatitis and not CP where they are neither diagnostic nor prognostic. It is not unusual that a patient with elevated amylase or lipase values less than three times the upper limit of normal is labeled as having CP when, in fact, these are nondiagnostic.

The complete blood count, electrolytes, and liver function tests are typically normal. Elevations of serum bilirubin and alkaline phosphatase suggest compression of the intrapancreatic portion of the bile duct by edema, fibrosis, or pancreatic cancer. Markers of chronic autoimmune pancreatitis include an elevated erythrocyte sedimentation rate, IgG4, rheumatoid factor, antinuclear antibodies, and anti–smooth muscle antibody titer.

Steatorrhea should no longer be diagnosed qualitatively by Sudan staining of feces because it is nonspecific. A 72-hour quantitative fecal fat determination is the gold standard. The quantitative test is usually performed over 72 hours; excretion of more than 7 g of fat per day is diagnostic of malabsorption, although patients with steatorrhea often have values greater than 10 g/d. In the proper clinical setting (eg, in a patient with typical symptoms of abdominal pain), confirmation of increased fecal fat excretion may be sufficient to diagnose CP.

Given the cumbersome nature of the 72-hour fecal fat test, measurement of fecal elastase is helpful for evaluating pancreatic exocrine dysfunction, and it is considered the test of choice. Among PFTs, fecal elastase measurement is the most sensitive and specific, especially in the early phases of pancreatic insufficiency. Also, its values are independent of pancreatic enzyme replacement therapy and require only a single random stool sample. According to unpublished data from the manufacturer, values less than 200 µg/g are suggestive of pancreatic insufficiency (sensitivity and specificity of 93%).[50]

GENETIC TESTING

In the past few years, genetic mutations have been associated with CP. These genes include the CFTR gene responsible for cystic fibrosis; SPINK-1, which encodes for trypsin inhibitor; and the PRSS-1 gene linked to hereditary pancreatitis. In a study where extensive sequencing of the CFTR gene was performed in conjunction with functional analyses, 44% of patients with idiopathic CP were found to have at least one variant in the CFTR gene, which was associated with CFTR dysfunction.[51] That 22% of healthy control subjects had at least one variant in that study combined with the data that more than 2000 variants (ie, not disease-proven mutations and thus of unknown significance) have been detected in the CFTR gene by extensive sequencing, indicates that CF genotyping should not be performed routinely to diagnose a patient with CP. Alternatively, sweat chloride testing may be of benefit because it assesses CFTR function and does not rely on full gene sequencing.[52] Up to 10% of patients have abnormal results, which should prompt further investigation of occult male infertility or lung disease and may warrant professional genetic counseling. SPINK-1 mutations are present in 23% of patients with CP but are seen in 2% of healthy individuals.[53] In conjunction with the finding that homozygous mutations are found in healthy individuals, testing for this gene is presently not of diagnostic or therapeutic benefit and hence not recommended. PRSS-1 mutations are diagnostic of hereditary pancreatitis, which can present with recurrent acute episodes of pancreatitis and progress to the chronic form.

CLASSIFICATION

CP has been classified into different forms (calcifying, obstructive, autoimmune, and groove). These classifications are based on clinical features, morphologic characteristics, and response to treatment. In calcifying CP, for example, perilobular fibrosis and acinar destruction with infiltration of acute and chronic inflammatory cells are present. Obstructive CP develops as a secondary complication caused by an area of obstruction with dilatation of the pancreatic duct proximal to the stenosis, atrophy of acinar cells, and fibrosis. Finally, groove pancreatitis affects the groove between the pancreatic head, duodenum, and the bile duct.

Classification systems are of great importance for guiding management strategies, because treatment strategies cannot rely solely on the type and degree of morphologic changes in the pancreas, but need to include clinical, functional, and imaging findings. So far, no globally accepted classification system has been established. Classification systems for CP are the Cambridge classification, Manchester classification, ABC classification, M-ANNHEIM, TIGAR-O, and Rosemont classification.

There is no MR imaging/MRCP-, CT-, or US-specific classification criteria for CP. Radiologists often interpret MRCP using Cambridge classification, which was designed for ERCP more than three decades ago.[46] There is a need for a new staging system for CP, specifically designed for CT, MR imaging, and MRCP combining the ductal and the parenchymal changes secondary to pancreatic fibrosis. The American Pancreatic Association released a morphology characterization imaging guide for the current imaging modalities (Table 3).[47]

The Manchester classification system uses imaging modalities and clinical signs of CP.[54] The degree of severity is mostly influenced by the presence of exocrine and endocrine insufficiency or the presence of complications, whereas imaging findings are of minor importance. The ABC classification recommends similar findings to the Manchester classification system.[55,56] The Rosemont classification was developed to diagnose CP using EUS.[57]

Two major classification systems have been established to help assess risk factors in the development of CP (TIGAR-O and M-ANNHEIM), and are helpful in guiding providers as to when to initiate testing for CP. Etiologic factors in the M-ANNHEIM system are alcohol consumption, nutrition, hereditary factors, ductal factors, immunology, and miscellaneous and rare metabolic disorders (eg, hypercalcemia, hyperparathyroidism, chronic renal failure, drugs, toxins).[58] The M-ANNHEIM system includes the stage, severity, and clinical findings of CP and offers a severity index. Different guidelines recommend using the TIGAR-O classification. This system comprises six etiologic groups: (1) toxic/metabolic, (2) idiopathic, (3) genetic, (4) autoimmune, (5) recurrent acute pancreatitis, and (6) obstructive.[59]

DIFFERENTIAL DIAGNOSIS

Pancreatic cancer is the primary diagnosis that must be considered in patients suspected of having CP. An endoscopic sampling of the pancreatic juice might be necessary to differentiate CP from the main or mixed-type intraductal papillary mucinous neoplasm. Acute pancreatitis may also be difficult to distinguish from CP in some patients.

There are data to suggest that CP is associated with an increased risk of developing pancreatic carcinoma.[60,61] In a report from the International Pancreatitis Study Group, 2015 patients with CP were followed for a mean of 7.4 years.[60] A total of 56 pancreatic cancers were identified. The expected number of cases of cancer calculated from country-specific incidence data and adjusted for age and sex was 2.13, yielding a standardized

Table 3
Cambridge classification adapted for findings seen on MRCP, CT, and US

Cambridge Classification	MRCP/ERCP Findings	US/CT/MR Findings
0 Normal	No abnormal signs	No abnormal signs
I Equivocal	<3 abnormal branches	One of the following • Dilated main pancreatic duct (2–4 mm) • Slight gland enlargement • Heterogeneous parenchyma • Small cavities (<10 mm) • Irregular ducts • Focal pancreatitis • Increased echogenicity of main duct wall • Irregular head/body contour
II Mild	≥3 abnormal branches	≥2 of the following • Dilated main duct (2–4 mm) • Gland enlargement • Heterogeneous parenchyma • Small cavities (<10 mm) • Irregular ducts • Focal acute pancreatitis • Increased echogenicity of main duct wall • Irregular head/body contour
III Moderate	>3 abnormal side branches and abnormal main duct	Same as above
IV Severe	All above and 1 or more of • Large cavity >10 mm • Intraductal filling defects • Duct obstruction (stricture) • Duct dilatation or irregularity	Above changes and 1 or more of • Large cavity >10 mm • Gland enlargement • Intraductal filling defects/calculi • Duct obstruction/stricture/or gross irregularity

Data from Conwell DL, Lee LS, Yadav D, et al. American Pancreatic Association Practice Guidelines in chronic pancreatitis: evidence-based report on diagnostic guidelines. Pancreas 2014;43(8):1143–62.

incidence ratio (the ratio of observed to expected cases) of 26.3.

Findings suggestive of possible pancreatic cancer in a patient thought or known to have CP include older age, the absence of a history of alcohol use, weight loss, a protracted flare of symptoms, and the onset of significant constitutional symptoms. Supporting data for malignancy include a pancreatic duct stricture greater than 10 mm in length on ERCP.[62] Markers, such as CA 19-9 and carcinoembryonic antigen, are helpful if abnormal, but normal values do not rule out pancreatic cancer.

Radiologists sometimes encounter lesions that show focal enlargement or distortion of the normal contour of the pancreas while still lacking pathognomonic features of pancreatic carcinomas. In such cases, a small percentage of patients with such focal enlargements of the pancreas have a conventional pancreatic carcinoma, whereas a small percentage of the patients may have an inflammatory pancreatic mass. Despite these

histories that suggest the presence of CP, one may not usually be certain whether a mass appearing at the pancreas is related to inflammatory pancreatic mass or cancer. The duct-penetrating sign on MRCP images (a smoothly stenotic or normal main pancreatic duct penetrating a mass) was seen more frequently in inflammatory pancreatic mass than in pancreatic cancer (**Fig. 1**).[63]

Paraduodenal pancreatitis, also known as groove pancreatitis, is a rare form of CP that masquerades as pancreatic adenocarcinoma affecting the pancreaticoduodenal groove, a potential space between the head of the pancreas, duodenum, and common bile duct (**Fig. 2**). Imaging findings of groove pancreatitis often overlap with primary duodenal, ampullary, or pancreatic neoplasms, which often results in a diagnostic challenge.[64] Also, paraduodenal pancreatitis is mistaken for cystic pancreatic lesions, especially when there is involvement of the duodenal wall. Preoperative recognition of this entity is essential

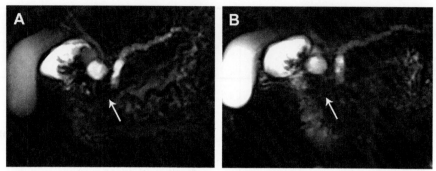

Fig. 1. Penetrating duct sign. (*A*) Coronal MRCP image in a 49-year-old patient with abdominal pain. There is obstruction of the pancreatic duct in the pancreatic head (*arrow*). Differential diagnosis includes CP given the history; however, also concerning for pancreatic cancer. (*B*) Coronal MRCP image obtained after administration of secretin. The pancreatic duct became visible (*arrow*) following stimulation of the pancreas with secretin. There is a smoothly narrowed pancreatic duct from the level of obstruction to the sphincter compatible with penetrating duct sign. This finding favors a benign cause of obstruction rather than malignancy.

to avoid unnecessary procedures, although surgery, such as pancreaticoduodenectomy, may still be required to relieve obstructive symptoms.

COMPLICATIONS

There are several potential complications of CP that require active surveillance by clinicians, including diabetes, exocrine pancreatic

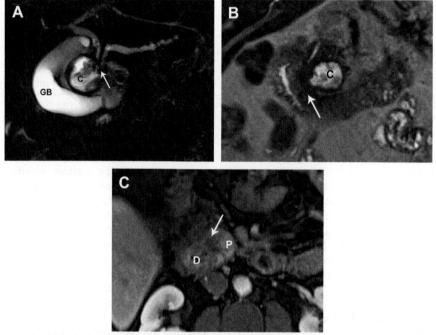

Fig. 2. Paraduodenal/groove pancreatitis. (*A*) Coronal MRCP image in a 36-year-old man with a history of alcohol abuse. There is obstruction of the pancreatic duct and the biliary tree in the region of the pancreaticoduodenal junction (*arrow*). The patient presented with acute pancreatitis and developed a postinflammatory cyst. (*B*) Coronal T2-weighted image shows a T2 hypointense tissue (*arrow*) causing stricture of the pancreatic duct. (*C*) Axial T1-weighted image after contrast administration is shown. There is a hypoenhancing lesion (*arrow*) corresponding to T2 hypointense soft tissue in the pancreaticoduodenal junction concerning for necrotizing pancreatitis and possibly a malignancy. There are acute inflammatory changes in and around the duodenum and pancreatic head in addition to the history of acute CP. Combination of the clinical and imaging findings favors a nonmalignant cause, such as paraduodenal, also called groove, CP. C, postinflammatory cyst; D, duodenum; GB, gallbladder; P, pancreas.

Table 4
Common complications of CP

Endocrine insufficiency (type 3c diabetes mellitus)	Up to 80%
Exocrine insufficiency	30%–80%
Metabolic bone disease	66%
Splenic vein thrombosis	10%–20%
Biliary obstruction	Up to 25%
Pancreatic cancer	4%
Duodenal stricture	1%

insufficiency, metabolic bone disease, and pancreatic cancer (**Table 4**).[65] Most common complications of CP are endocrine/exocrine insufficiencies, and metabolic bone disorders are not diagnosed by imaging studies. Those seen by cross-sectional imaging include but are not limited to postinflammatory cyst formation, bile duct or duodenal obstruction, pancreatic ascites or pleural effusion, splenic vein thrombosis, and pancreatic cancer.[5] Patients may also develop acute attacks of pancreatitis, particularly alcoholics who continue drinking.

SUMMARY

The diagnosis of CP is challenging because biopsy of the pancreas is not performed, and laboratory studies and imaging procedures may be normal during the early stage of the disease. The diagnosis of advanced CP is confirmed if there are calcifications within the pancreas on plain abdominal films or CT scan, an abnormal pancreatogram, or an abnormal secretin PFT in subtle cases of early pancreatitis. Identification of early stage CP and its treatment may delay or prevent morbidity secondary to CP. In settings where MR imaging/MRCP is available and of high quality, it may be the imaging test of choice, allowing for assessment of ductal changes and potentially obviating an invasive procedure. Stimulation of the pancreas using intravenous secretin may improve diagnostic accuracy in the detection of ductal and parenchymal abnormalities seen in CP. T1 signal intensity changes in the pancreatic parenchyma may precede ductal abnormalities and may detect early CP. US and CT are best for the late findings of CP but are limited in the diagnosis of early or mild pancreatitis. Contrast-enhanced CT scan can rule out other causes of pain that mimic CP and is helpful for the diagnosis and complications of CP. There is a need for an EUS-like MR imaging staging system for CP, combining the ductal findings with the parenchymal changes.

REFERENCES

1. Hirota M, Shimosegawa T, Masamune A, et al. The seventh nationwide epidemiological survey for chronic pancreatitis in Japan: clinical significance of smoking habit in Japanese patients. Pancreatology 2014;14(6):490–6.
2. Levy P, Dominguez-Munoz E, Imrie C, et al. Epidemiology of chronic pancreatitis: burden of the disease and consequences. United European Gastroenterol J 2014;2(5):345–54.
3. Yadav D, Timmons L, Benson JT, et al. Incidence, prevalence, and survival of chronic pancreatitis: a population-based study. Am J Gastroenterol 2011; 106(12):2192–9.
4. Amann ST, Yadav D, Barmada MM, et al. Physical and mental quality of life in chronic pancreatitis: a case-control study from the North American Pancreatitis Study 2 cohort. Pancreas 2013;42(2): 293–300.
5. Ammann RW, Akovbiantz A, Largiader F, et al. Course and outcome of chronic pancreatitis. Longitudinal study of a mixed medical-surgical series of 245 patients. Gastroenterology 1984;86(5 Pt 1):820–8.
6. Ammann RW, Buehler H, Muench R, et al. Differences in the natural history of idiopathic (nonalcoholic) and alcoholic chronic pancreatitis. A comparative long-term study of 287 patients. Pancreas 1987;2(4):368–77.
7. Cavallini G, Frulloni L, Pederzoli P, et al. Long-term follow-up of patients with chronic pancreatitis in Italy. Scand J Gastroenterol 1998;33(8):880–9.
8. Lankisch PG, Lohr-Happe A, Otto J, et al. Natural course in chronic pancreatitis. Pain, exocrine and endocrine pancreatic insufficiency and prognosis of the disease. Digestion 1993;54(3):148–55.
9. Maisonneuve P, Lowenfels AB, Mullhaupt B, et al. Cigarette smoking accelerates progression of alcoholic chronic pancreatitis. Gut 2005;54(4): 510–4.
10. Dani R, Mott CB, Guarita DR, et al. Epidemiology and etiology of chronic pancreatitis in Brazil: a tale of two cities. Pancreas 1990;5(4):474–8.
11. Marks IN, Bank S, Louw JH. Chronic pancreatitis in the Western Cape. Digestion 1973;9(5):447–53.
12. Layer P, Yamamoto H, Kalthoff L, et al. The different courses of early- and late-onset idiopathic and alcoholic chronic pancreatitis. Gastroenterology 1994; 107(5):1481–7.
13. Whitcomb DC. Genetic risk factors for pancreatic disorders. Gastroenterology 2013;144(6):1292–302.
14. Hart PA, Zen Y, Chari ST. Recent advances in autoimmune pancreatitis. Gastroenterology 2015;149(1): 39–51.
15. Greer JB, Thrower E, Yadav D. Epidemiologic and mechanistic associations between smoking and pancreatitis. Curr Treat Options Gastroenterol 2015; 13(3):332–46.

16. Akisik MF, Jennings SG, Aisen AM, et al. MRCP in patient care: a prospective survey of gastroenterologists. AJR Am J Roentgenol 2013;201(3):573–7.

17. Andersen DK. The practical importance of recognizing pancreatogenic or type 3c diabetes. Diabetes Metab Res Rev 2012;28(4):326–8.

18. Ewald N, Kaufmann C, Raspe A, et al. Prevalence of diabetes mellitus secondary to pancreatic diseases (type 3c). Diabetes Metab Res Rev 2012;28(4):338–42.

19. Hulisz D. The burden of illness of irritable bowel syndrome: current challenges and hope for the future. J Manag Care Pharm 2004;10(4):299–309.

20. Chowdhury R, Bhutani MS, Mishra G, et al. Comparative analysis of direct pancreatic function testing versus morphological assessment by endoscopic ultrasonography for the evaluation of chronic unexplained abdominal pain of presumed pancreatic origin. Pancreas 2005;31(1):63–8.

21. Conwell DL, Wu BU. Chronic pancreatitis: making the diagnosis. Clin Gastroenterol Hepatol 2012; 10(10):1088–95.

22. Conwell DL, Zuccaro G Jr, Vargo JJ, et al. An endoscopic pancreatic function test with synthetic porcine secretin for the evaluation of chronic abdominal pain and suspected chronic pancreatitis. Gastrointest Endosc 2003;57(1):37–40.

23. Ketwaroo G, Brown A, Young B, et al. Defining the accuracy of secretin pancreatic function testing in patients with suspected early chronic pancreatitis. Am J Gastroenterol 2013;108(8):1360–6.

24. Lin Y, Tamakoshi A, Hayakawa T, et al, Research Committee on Intractable Pancreatic Diseases. Associations of alcohol drinking and nutrient intake with chronic pancreatitis: findings from a case-control study in Japan. Am J Gastroenterol 2001; 96(9):2622–7.

25. Talamini G, Bassi C, Falconi M, et al. Alcohol and smoking as risk factors in chronic pancreatitis and pancreatic cancer. Dig Dis Sci 1999;44(7):1303–11.

26. Ammann RW, Muellhaupt B. The natural history of pain in alcoholic chronic pancreatitis. Gastroenterology 1999;116(5):1132–40.

27. DiMagno EP, Go VL, Summerskill WH. Relations between pancreatic enzyme outputs and malabsorption in severe pancreatic insufficiency. N Engl J Med 1973;288(16):813–5.

28. Mergener K, Baillie J. Chronic pancreatitis. Lancet 1997;350(9088):1379–85.

29. Toskes PP, Hansell J, Cerda J, et al. Vitamin B 12 malabsorption in chronic pancreatic insufficiency. N Engl J Med 1971;284(12):627–32.

30. Malka D, Hammel P, Sauvanet A, et al. Risk factors for diabetes mellitus in chronic pancreatitis. Gastroenterology 2000;119(5):1324–32.

31. Kloppel G. Chronic pancreatitis, pseudotumors and other tumor-like lesions. Mod Pathol 2007;20(Suppl 1):S113–31.

32. Bolondi L, Li Bassi S, Gaiani S, et al. Sonography of chronic pancreatitis. Radiol Clin North Am 1989; 27(4):815–33.

33. Luetmer PH, Stephens DH, Ward EM. Chronic pancreatitis: reassessment with current CT. Radiology 1989;171(2):353–7.

34. Tirkes T, Fogel EL, Sherman S, et al. Detection of exocrine dysfunction by MRI in patients with early chronic pancreatitis. Abdom Radiol (NY) 2017;42(2): 544–51.

35. Tirkes T, Lin C, Fogel EL, et al. T1 mapping for diagnosis of mild chronic pancreatitis. J Magn Reson Imaging 2017;45(4):1171–6.

36. Balci C. MRI assessment of chronic pancreatitis. Diagn Interv Radiol 2011;17(3):249–54.

37. Balci NC, Smith A, Momtahen AJ, et al. MRI and S-MRCP findings in patients with suspected chronic pancreatitis: correlation with endoscopic pancreatic function testing (ePFT). J Magn Reson Imaging 2010;31(3):601–6.

38. Choueiri NE, Balci NC, Alkaade S, et al. Advanced imaging of chronic pancreatitis. Curr Gastroenterol Rep 2010;12(2):114–20.

39. Hellerhoff KJ, Helmberger H 3rd, Rosch T, et al. Dynamic MR pancreatography after secretin administration: image quality and diagnostic accuracy. AJR Am J Roentgenol 2002;179(1):121–9.

40. Sherman S, Freeman ML, Tarnasky PR, et al. Administration of secretin (RG1068) increases the sensitivity of detection of duct abnormalities by magnetic resonance cholangiopancreatography in patients with pancreatitis. Gastroenterology 2014;147(3):646–54.e2.

41. Cappeliez O, Delhaye M, Deviere J, et al. Chronic pancreatitis: evaluation of pancreatic exocrine function with MR pancreatography after secretin stimulation. Radiology 2000;215(2):358–64.

42. Akisik MF, Aisen AM, Sandrasegaran K, et al. Assessment of chronic pancreatitis: utility of diffusion-weighted MR imaging with secretin enhancement. Radiology 2009;250(1):103–9.

43. Shi Y, Glaser KJ, Venkatesh SK, et al. Feasibility of using 3D MR elastography to determine pancreatic stiffness in healthy volunteers. J Magn Reson Imaging 2015;41(2):369–75.

44. NIH state-of-the-science statement on endoscopic retrograde cholangiopancreatography (ERCP) for diagnosis and therapy. NIH Consens State Sci Statements 2002;19(1):1–26.

45. Adler DG, Lichtenstein D, Baron TH, et al. The role of endoscopy in patients with chronic pancreatitis. Gastrointest Endosc 2006;63(7):933–7.

46. Sarner M, Cotton PB. Classification of pancreatitis. Gut 1984;25(7):756–9.

47. Conwell DL, Lee LS, Yadav D, et al. American pancreatic association practice guidelines in chronic pancreatitis: evidence-based report on diagnostic guidelines. Pancreas 2014;43(8):1143–62.

48. Wallace MB, Hawes RH, Durkalski V, et al. The reliability of EUS for the diagnosis of chronic pancreatitis: interobserver agreement among experienced endosonographers. Gastrointest Endosc 2001; 53(3):294–9.

49. Stevens T, Lopez R, Adler DG, et al. Multicenter comparison of the interobserver agreement of standard EUS scoring and Rosemont classification scoring for diagnosis of chronic pancreatitis. Gastrointest Endosc 2010;71(3):519–26.

50. Keim V, Teich N, Moessner J. Clinical value of a new fecal elastase test for detection of chronic pancreatitis. Clin Lab 2003;49(5–6):209–15.

51. Bishop MD, Freedman SD, Zielenski J, et al. The cystic fibrosis transmembrane conductance regulator gene and ion channel function in patients with idiopathic pancreatitis. Hum Genet 2005;118(3–4): 372–81.

52. Ooi CY, Gonska T, Durie PR, et al. Genetic testing in pancreatitis. Gastroenterology 2010;138(7):2202–6, 2206.e1.

53. Witt H, Luck W, Hennies HC, et al. Mutations in the gene encoding the serine protease inhibitor, Kazal type 1 are associated with chronic pancreatitis. Nat Genet 2000;25(2):213–6.

54. Bagul A, Siriwardena AK. Evaluation of the Manchester classification system for chronic pancreatitis. JOP 2006;7(4):390–6.

55. Bank S, Singh P, Pooran N. Proposal for a new grading system for chronic pancreatitis: the ABC system. J Clin Gastroenterol 2002;35(1):3–4.

56. Buchler MW, Martignoni ME, Friess H, et al. A proposal for a new clinical classification of chronic pancreatitis. BMC Gastroenterol 2009;9:93.

57. Catalano MF, Sahai A, Levy M, et al. EUS-based criteria for the diagnosis of chronic pancreatitis: the Rosemont classification. Gastrointest Endosc 2009;69(7):1251–61.

58. Schneider A, Lohr JM, Singer MV. The M-ANNHEIM classification of chronic pancreatitis: introduction of a unifying classification system based on a review of previous classifications of the disease. J Gastroenterol 2007;42(2):101–19.

59. Etemad B, Whitcomb DC. Chronic pancreatitis: diagnosis, classification, and new genetic developments. Gastroenterology 2001;120(3):682–707.

60. Lowenfels AB, Maisonneuve P, DiMagno EP, et al. Hereditary pancreatitis and the risk of pancreatic cancer. International Hereditary Pancreatitis Study Group. J Natl Cancer Inst 1997;89(6):442–6.

61. Bang UC, Benfield T, Hyldstrup L, et al. Mortality, cancer, and comorbidities associated with chronic pancreatitis: a Danish nationwide matched-cohort study. Gastroenterology 2014;146(4):989–94.

62. Shemesh E, Czerniak A, Nass S, et al. Role of endoscopic retrograde cholangiopancreatography in differentiating pancreatic cancer coexisting with chronic pancreatitis. Cancer 1990;65(4):893–6.

63. Ichikawa T, Sou H, Araki T, et al. Duct-penetrating sign at MRCP: usefulness for differentiating inflammatory pancreatic mass from pancreatic carcinomas. Radiology 2001;221(1):107–16.

64. Mittal PK, Harri P, Nandwana S, et al. Paraduodenal pancreatitis: benign and malignant mimics at MRI. Abdom Radiol (NY) 2017;42(11):2652–74.

65. Ramsey ML, Conwell DL, Hart PA. Complications of chronic pancreatitis. Dig Dis Sci 2017;62(7): 1745–50.

MR Imaging of Autoimmune Pancreatitis

Nima Hafezi-Nejad, MD[a], Vikesh K. Singh, MD, MSc[b,c], Christopher Fung, MD[d], Naoki Takahashi, MD[e], Atif Zaheer, MD, FSAR[a,b,*]

KEYWORDS

- Autoimmune • Pancreatitis • IgG4 • MR imaging • Computed tomography

KEY POINTS

- AIP is a fibro-inflammatory disorder with 2 distinct subtypes that may be differentiated based on clinical, histologic, and radiologic features.
- Type 1 is a multi-organ IgG4-related disease with the pancreas being the most commonly involved organ.
- Type 2 AIP typically involves younger patients and possible concomitant inflammatory bowel disease with significant overlap with pancreatic findings of type 1 disease.
- Differentiation between the two entities may be based on clinical grounds, and histology and is important due to different treatment strategies and overall prognostication.

INTRODUCTION

Definition and Epidemiology

Autoimmune pancreatitis (AIP) is characterized by inflammatory destruction of the pancreatic tissue.[1] The autoimmune nature of pancreatic destruction was first proposed by Yoshida and colleagues[2] in 1995, though an association between pancreatitis and increased serum globulin levels was reported in the early 1960s.[3] Investigations by Kamisawa and colleagues[4] highlighted several extrapancreatic manifestations that were associated with AIP and had similar abundant infiltration of immunoglobulin G4 (IgG4)-positive plasma cells on histology. Further studies during the last decade explored and identified the spectrum of IgG4-related disease,[5,6] with the pancreas being the most commonly involved organ in IgG4-

related disease.[7,8] However, not all AIPs fall under the category of IgG4-related disease and not all patients with the IgG4-related disease have pancreatic involvement or AIP.[9–11] The terms *type 1 AIP* and *lymphoplasmacytic sclerosing pancreatitis* (LPSP) are used interchangeably for this disease. Type 2 or idiopathic duct-centric chronic pancreatitis (IDCP) is a related disease that shares some histopathologic and clinical features with the type 1 disease with differences in the diagnostic criteria and treatment approach.

Limited studies have attempted to estimate the annual incidence of AIP in the general population. A landmark 2002 national survey of randomly selected hospitals in Japan revealed a point prevalence of 0.82 per 100,000.[12] The overall prevalence rate in 2007 and 2011 was estimated at 2.2 and 4.6 per 100,000, respectively.[13,14]

Conflict of Interest: The authors have nothing to disclose.
[a] The Russell H. Morgan Department of Radiology and Radiological Science, Johns Hopkins University, 600 North Wolfe Street, Baltimore, MD 21287, USA; [b] Department of Internal Medicine, Pancreatitis Center, Johns Hopkins Medical Institutions, 1800 Orleans Street, Sheikh Zayed Tower, Baltimore, MD 21287, USA; [c] Division of Gastroenterology, Johns Hopkins University, School of Medicine, 1800 Orleans Street, Sheikh Zayed Tower, Baltimore, MD 21287, USA; [d] Department of Radiology and Diagnostic Imaging, University of Alberta, 2J2.00 WC Mackenzie Health Sciences Centre, 8440 112 Street Northwest, Edmonton, Alberta T6G 2R7, Canada; [e] Department of Radiology, Mayo Clinic, 200 First Street Southwest, Rochester, MN 55905, USA
* Corresponding author. The Russell H. Morgan Department of Radiology and Radiological Science, Johns Hopkins University, 600 North Wolfe Street, Hal B164, Baltimore, MD 21287.
E-mail address: azaheer1@jhmi.edu

Magn Reson Imaging Clin N Am 26 (2018) 463–478
https://doi.org/10.1016/j.mric.2018.03.008

Approximately 3% to 4% of cases with suspected chronic pancreatitis may be related to AIP.[15,16] Likewise, 4% of patients undergoing pancreatico-duodenectomy for pancreatic head mass may have AIP on histopathology.[17]

Histologic and Clinical Findings

AIP is subdivided into 2 distinct entities based on clinical manifestations and histology, type 1 and 2.[18,19] Most of the primary studies evaluating and proposing AIP type 1 as a distinct diagnosis were performed in Asian populations.[18] AIP type 1 is now recognized as a systemic disease with IgG4-positive plasma cell infiltration of virtually every organ system that can be associated with fibrosis.[20] Elevated serum IgG4 may be seen in about two-thirds of patients but has a low positive predictive value because of its elevation in patients with pancreatic adenocarcinoma, chol-angiocarcinoma, and primary sclerosing cholangi-tis.[19] Endoscopic-guided or surgical core biopsy helps obtain a histologic diagnosis and is preferred over fine-needle aspiration (FNA), which has a var-iable yield.[21] Type 1 AIP or LPSP demonstrates infiltration of IgG4-positive plasma cells in the peri-ductal and interlobular areas, leading to fibrosis, pancreatic duct narrowing, and acinar atrophy on histology.[22–24] Although nonspecific, the presence of IgG4 as greater than 40% of the total IgG-positive plasma cells and an IgG4/IgG ratio of greater than 0.4 on immunostaining of the pancre-atic tissue favors a diagnosis of type 1 AIP.[25,26] The clinical presentation of AIP is highly variable, pertaining to the inflammation and fibrosis of the pancreas. In a study of 235 patients, the median age was 67 years (range 35–86) and the most common involved organ was the pancreas (60%) followed by the salivary glands (34%), kidneys, lacrimal glands (23%), and the retroperitoneum (20%).[27] In another study of 57 patients with type 1 AIP, epigastric pain or discomfort (58%), jaun-dice (54%), weight loss (51%), and new-onset dia-betes (38%) were the most common disease presentations.[22,27] Other extrapancreatic manifes-tations of IgG4-related disease include but are not limited to thyroiditis, interstitial pneumonia, lymph-adenopathy, cholangitis, and cholecystitis.[20]

In contrast, type 2 AIP or IDCP was introduced in studies on Western populations as chronic pancreatitis histologically recognized by neutrophil infiltration and epithelial destruction (granulocytic epithelial lesions).[28] Unlike type 1, there is no increased incidence of elevated serum IgG4 levels[29] and number of IgG4-positive cells in the pancreatic tissue (<10 per high power field [HPF], <40% of IgG-positive plasma cells[30]). It typically affects younger patients with a median age of 31 years (range 23–49), and the most common clinical presentation is of acute recurrent pancreatitis with concurrent in-flammatory bowel disease seen in up to 44% of pa-tients.[31] Patients may also present with obstructive jaundice secondary to the presence of a focal mass. One important reason for differentiating these two entities is the risk of relapse after induction cortico-steroid therapy, which is 30% to 33% in type 1 and only 9% to 11% in type 2 AIP.[32]

Diagnostic Criteria

Given the diffuse and systemic nature of the IgG4-related disease that includes type 1 AIP and the distinct histopathology of type 2 AIP demonstrating granulocytic epithelial lesions, diagnostic criteria were proposed to facilitate the analysis of AIP. The International Association of Pancreatology pub-lished its consensus diagnostic criteria for AIP diag-nosis in 2011.[33] Five cardinal components were considered: imaging features of the ducts and the pancreatic parenchyma, serology, histology, sys-temic involvement, and significant response to corticosteroid therapy.[33] Additional population-specific studies tried to validate and propose enhanced algorithms for AIP diagnosis.[34,35] Of note, the Unifying-Autoimmune-Pancreatitis-Criteria (U-AIP) was recently introduced to unify the AIP diagnosis, improve the diagnostic accuracy, and embrace the AIP diagnosis within the frame-work of the broader M-ANNHEIM classification scheme for chronic pancreatitis.[36] U-AIP criteria consist of negative pancreatic cancer workup in addition to disease features, including histology (typical histology; either LPSP or IDCP), imaging and serology (computed tomography [CT]/MR im-aging/endoscopic retrograde cholangiopancrea-tography (ERCP) in addition to elevated serum IgG4 or autoimmune antibodies), and response to corticosteroid therapy.[36] U-AIP was developed in an effort to unify different criteria, including the Jap-anese, Korean, Mayo-HISORt (Histology, Imaging features, Serology, Other organ involvement, and Response to steroid treatment), and Italian criteria for the diagnosis of AIP[33,36] (Table 1).

Imaging Modalities

Imaging plays an essential role in the evaluation of AIP by characterizing the pancreatic paren-chyma, main pancreatic duct (MPD), peripancre-atic lymph nodes, and fatty tissue.[37] Imaging modalities, including CT and MR imaging; endo-scopic techniques, including ERCP and endo-scopic ultrasonography (EUS); and functional imaging, including PET, have all been investigated for the evaluation of AIP.[37] CT is often the first, and

Table 1
International Consensus Diagnostic Criteria for autoimmune pancreatitis

AIP Diagnosis	Criteria
Histology	Histologic evaluation from resection or core biopsy demonstrating AIP type I (LPSP): 1. >10 IgG4-positive cells in HPF 2. Periductal lymphoplasmacytic infiltrate and absence of granulocytic infiltration 3. Obliterative phlebitis 4. Storiform fibrosis • Level 1: >2 out of 4 items; level 2: 2 out of 4 items AIP type II (IDCP): • Level 1: granulocytic infiltration of duct wall (+/− acinar inflammation) and 2–10 IgG4-positive cells in HPF • Level 2: granulocytic and lymphoplasmacytic acinar infiltration and 2–10 IgG4-positive cells in HPF
Imaging	Parenchymal evaluation: • Level 1: diffuse enlargement of the pancreas with delayed enhancement with or without rimlike enhancement • Level 2: focal or segmental enlargement of the pancreas with delayed enhancement Ductal evaluation: • Level 1: single, long stricture of the main pancreatic duct without significant upstream dilation • Level 1: multiple strictures of the main pancreatic duct without significant upstream dilation • Level 2: focal or segmental narrowing of small pancreatic ducts without significant upstream dilation
Serology	AIP type I: Serum IgG4 level greater than the upper limit of normal • Level 1 >2×; level 2 >1× and <2×
Other organs	AIP type I: Level 1: histology of an extrapancreatic organ involvement with 3 of the following items 1. >10 IgG4-positive cells in HPF 2. Periductal lymphoplasmacytic infiltrate and absence of granulocytic infiltration 3. Obliterative phlebitis 4. Storiform fibrosis Level 2: histology of an extrapancreatic organ involvement with endoscopic bile duct biopsy showing 2 of the following items 1. >10 IgG4-positive cells in HPF 2. Periductal lymphoplasmacytic infiltrate and absence of granulocytic infiltration Level 1 radiologic evidence: 1. Multiple segmental proximal (including hilar or intrahepatic) or proximal and distal bile duct stricture 2. Retroperitoneal fibrosis Level 2 clinical/radiologic evidence: 1. Symmetrically enlarged salivary/lachrymal glands 2. Renal involvement in association with AIP AIP type II: Level 2 evidence: Clinically diagnosed inflammatory bowel disease
Response to steroids	Diagnostic steroid trial: Radiological resolution or significant clinical improvement in response to steroid therapy in <2 wk

Following the International Consensus Diagnostic Criteria for AIP,[33] each feature was categorized as level 1 or level 2 based on the strength that each specific finding adds to the likelihood of AIP diagnosis. Definitive diagnosis of AIP type I can be established by imaging evidence and histologic confirmation of lymphoplasmacytic sclerosing pancreatitis, or typical imaging evidence and any level 1 or 2 criteria, or indeterminate imaging evidence and at least 2 level 1 criteria or indeterminate imaging evidence and level 1 serology/other organ criteria and steroid response, or indeterminate imaging evidence and level 1 ductal and level 2 serology/other organ/histology criteria and steroid response. Probable diagnosis of AIP type I can be established by indeterminate imaging evidence and level 2 serology/other organ/histology criteria and steroid response. Definitive AIP type II diagnosis can be established by imaging evidence of AIP and histologic confirmation or imaging evidence and clinical inflammatory bowel disease and level 2 histology criteria and response to steroid. Probable AIP type II diagnosis can be established by imaging evidence of AIP and level 2 histology/clinical inflammatory bowel disease criteria and response to steroid.

most commonly used, modality[38] and can be used to categorize changes in pancreatic morphology as diffuse, focal, or multifocal as well as the detection of the extrapancreatic findings seen in the head, neck, and chest. Diffuse enlargement of the pancreas is the most common finding, followed by focal enlargement of the pancreatic head in type 1 AIP.[38,39] Swelling and loss of lobular structures may lead to the characteristic appearance of a sausage-shaped pancreas. Peripancreatic fat stranding and a capsulelike low attenuation rim with delayed postcontrast enhancement may be present in up to 80% of patients with AIP.[40–42] Likewise, pancreatic parenchyma may show arterial and venous phase hypoattenuation[40] that becomes iso-attenuating (or hyperattenuating, due to fibrosis) in the delayed phase.[43,44] Pancreatic ducts are either small and nondilated or diffusely narrowed. Although mild ductal dilation proximal to the area of pancreatic enlargement may be secondary to a focal inflammatory mass, significant dilation of the pancreatic duct with an abrupt cutoff can be a sign of pancreatic ductal adenocarcinoma (PDAC).[45] ERCP may be used to further examine pancreatic duct narrowing and irregularity.[46] When evaluated independently from other modalities, ERCP has limited sensitivity (as low as 44%) and excellent specificity (as high as 92%). Knowledge of specific AIP features like the presence of a long stricture (more than one-third of the pancreatic duct), absence of upstream dilatation, presence of multiple strictures, and presence of strictures that result in side branch ectasia (more commonly observed in type 1 AIP) can improve the diagnostic accuracy of ERCP. ERCP is not usually performed for diagnostic purposes because of its relatively high rate of complications and is substituted with MRCP. EUS may reveal diffuse enlargement of the pancreas or presence of a focal pancreatic mass, especially in the pancreatic head.[47] EUS can also assess the echotexture of the pancreas and presence of surrounding enlarged lymph nodes. However, no reliable feature on EUS is pathognomonic for AIP[40]; it is used primarily to diagnose a focal mass and for tissue sampling.

MR Imaging of Autoimmune Pancreatitis

MR imaging protocol
MR imaging protocols for the assessment of AIP are designed to evaluate the pancreatic parenchyma on T1-weighted, T2-weighted, and diffusion-weighted imaging (DWI); the presence of ductal abnormalities within the pancreatic duct and the biliary tree on MRCP; and hypovascularity and delayed enhancement on postcontrast imaging. Standardized MR imaging protocol for pancreas evaluation can be performed using a phased-array torso coil. Axial T2-weighted fat-saturated images are obtained as well as coronal and transverse T2-weighted images (single-shot fast spin echo imaging repetition time: 4500 milliseconds; echo time 92 milliseconds; field of view: 320 mm; matrix: 256 × 180; section thickness: 6 mm; slice gap: 1.2 mm; receiver bandwidth: 543 Hz per pixel; flip angle: 150°). MRCP images can be constructed by acquiring at least 6 thick slab (40–50 mm; repetition time: 4500 milliseconds; echo time: 500–700 milliseconds) heavily T2-weighted images. Precontrast and postcontrast T1-weighted fat-suppressed spoiled gradient-echo images (field of view: 320–400 mm; matrix: 192 × 160; slice thickness: 2.5 mm; repetition time: 5.77 milliseconds; echo time: 2.77 milliseconds; received bandwidth: 64 kHz; flip angle: 10°) can be obtained in the arterial (20 seconds), portal (70 seconds), and delayed (3 minutes) phases. Gadopentetate (0.1 mmol/kg) can be used for intravenous contrast. DWI is obtained as single-shot echo-planar imaging with respiratory triggering; the b values of 0, 100, and 800 s/mm^2; and the acquisition time of 3 to 4 minutes (according to respiratory rhythm). The apparent diffusion coefficient (ADC) values are calculated with b values of 0 and 800 s/m^2 as follows: $ADC = (1/(b1–b0)) \ln(S0/S1)$. S0 and S1 are the signal intensities obtained from diffusion sensitized T2 images with low (b0) and high (b1) values for the gradient factor b.

Common features of autoimmune pancreatitis
Changes in pancreatic parenchyma Pancreatic parenchymal changes can be appreciated on MR imaging and include enlargement of the entire gland, focal enlargement presenting as a mass, and focal or diffuse signal abnormalities of the pancreas seen on multiple MR imaging sequences. Because of the overlap in imaging findings within the pancreas in patients with type 1 and 2 diseases, differentiation may be difficult based on the pancreatic findings alone; extrapancreatic findings, when present, may help in the differentiation of the two types. Although diffuse pancreatic enlargement and loss of lobular morphology of the gland is the most classic and common appearance of AIP (**Fig. 1**), focal mass-like enlargement and a mixture of focal and diffuse enlargement are also frequently seen and are reported in up to 57% of cases[48,49] (**Fig. 2**). Involved areas usually demonstrate hypointensity on T1-weighted imaging and mild hyperintensity on T2-weighted imaging.[40] Absence of pancreatic enlargement has been reported in up to 14% of

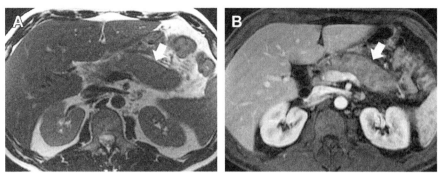

Fig. 1. A 68-year-old man with type 1 autoimmune pancreatitis. Axial T2-weighted image shows an enlarged pancreas with loss of the normal feathery appearance and a sausagelike appearance (*arrow, A*). There is diffuse hypoenhancement seen on the T1-weighted postcontrast image (*arrow, B*).

patients and does not exclude the presence of AIP.[48,50] In such cases, the aforementioned signal abnormalities may be the only parenchymal findings (**Fig. 3**). Pancreatic lymphoma may be considered in the differential diagnosis, presenting as a diffuse or focal lesion with low signal intensity on T1- and low to intermediate signal intensity on T2-weighted imaging.[51]

Recent studies have assessed DWI to study tissue cellularity and to aid the diagnosis of non-neoplastic pancreatic disorders, including AIP.[52] Like neoplastic lesions with high cellularity impeding cellular diffusion, AIP can similarly show restricted diffusion (see **Figs. 2** and **3**; **Fig. 4**). Previous studies have suggested a lower average ADC value in patients with AIP when compared with

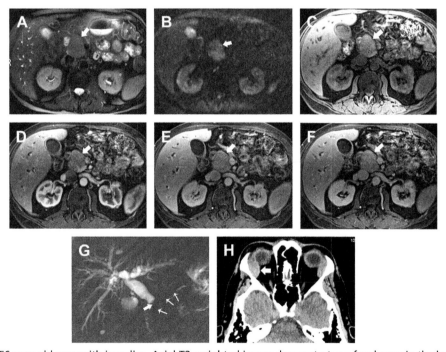

Fig. 2. A 56-year-old man with jaundice. Axial T2-weighted image demonstrates a focal mass in the head of the pancreas (*arrow, A*). The mass demonstrates restricted diffusion on DWI ($b = 800$ s/mm^2) (*arrow, B*). The mass is hypointense compared to the signal intensity of the liver on the precontrast T1-weighted image (*arrow, C*) and demonstrates hypoenhancement on the T1-weighted arterial phase postcontrast image (*arrow, D*). There is progressive enhancement seen on the venous- and delayed-phase images (*arrows, E, F*). Severe diffuse intrahepatic and extrahepatic biliary dilation is present on the MRCP image with a focal stricture of the distal common bile duct (*thick arrow, G*). Skip strictures in the MPD are also present (*thin arrows, G*). A noncontrast head CT demonstrates asymmetric enlargement of the right lacrimal gland (*arrow, H*) consistent with dacryoadenitis, and biopsy showed lymphoplasmacytic infiltrates and greater than 100 IgG4-positive plasma cells per HPF. The constellation of findings is consistent with type 1 AIP, and the patient responded well to corticosteroid therapy.

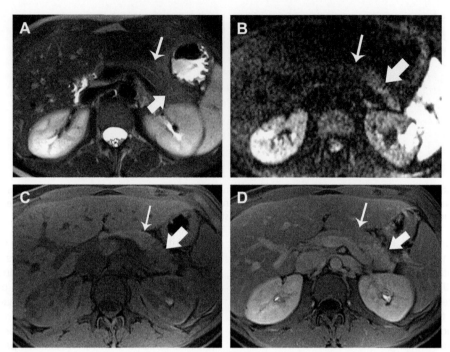

Fig. 3. A 32-year-old woman with acute abdominal pain with elevated lipase (4000 range). Axial T2-weighted image demonstrates slight hyperintensity of the pancreatic tail (*thick arrow, A*) and restricted diffusion (b = 800 s/mm²) (*thick arrow, B*) compared with the normal signal in the pancreatic body (*thin arrow, A*) and absence of diffusion restriction (*thin arrow, B*). There is corresponding decreased signal in the pancreatic tail on the T1-weighted precontrast image (*thick arrow, C*) with delayed enhancement (*thick arrow, D*) compared with the normal parenchyma (*thin arrows, C, D*). Serum IgG4 and cancer antigen 19-9 were not elevated, and EUS with FNA did not reveal malignancy. A diagnosis of type 2 AIP was made, and the patient responded well to corticosteroid treatment with resolution of symptoms and imaging findings.

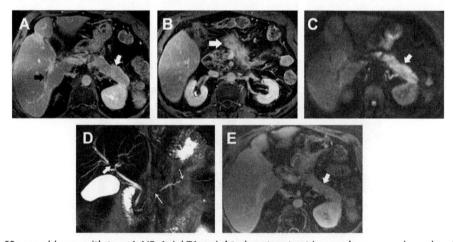

Fig. 4. A 69-year-old man with type 1 AIP. Axial T1-weighted postcontrast image shows an enlarged and feature-less pancreas (*white arrow, A*) and intrahepatic biliary dilation (*black arrow, A*) due to a common bile duct stric-ture. Enhancing soft tissue mass is seen in the mesentery (*arrow, B*) consistent with sclerosing mesenteritis. Note the presence of restricted diffusion (*arrow, C*) on diffusion weighted imaging (b = 800 s/mm²). MRCP image shows the presence of skip strictures in the MPD (*thin arrows, D*) and the presence of a high-grade intrahepatic biliary stricture (*thick arrow, D*) with upstream biliary dilation. Axial postcontrast T1-weighted image obtained 18 months later demonstrates resolution of the pancreatic enlargement (*arrow, E*) after corticosteroid treatment.

PDAC; however, ADC values of these diagnoses may significantly overlap.[53,54] ADC values can be related to patients' symptoms,[54] follow-up status,[55] and corticosteroid treatment[53] and have limited accuracy when used alone.[54,55] For example, asymptomatic patients who receive corticosteroid treatment have higher ADC values, especially in follow-up examinations.[53–55] Thus, it is important to interpret the results of DWI studies along with conventional imaging findings.[52] A specificity of 99% has been shown in differentiating AIP from PDAC when a cutoff of 0.9407×10^{-3} mm^2/s was used in combination with homogeneous enhancement and duct penetrating sign (discussed later).[56]

Changes in pancreatic ducts and biliary structures

Pancreatic parenchymal swelling leads to compression and nonvisualization of the pancreatic duct in many cases[57] (see Fig. 1). MRCP is used to provide an additional assessment of the MPD. In AIP, the MPD is typically irregularly narrowed.[22] The accuracy of MRCP for the evaluation of the pancreatic duct is usually assessed against ERCP.[58,59] Previous studies suggest that MRCP cannot replace ERCP, as it does not accurately visualize and sometimes overestimates the areas of narrowing of the MPD.[58,59] However, MRCP can be useful in the detection of skipped strictures in the MPD as well as the presence of concurrent biliary involvement if present[58] (see Fig. 2). In addition, MRCP imaging plays an important role in the evaluation of the response to therapy for resolution of ductal changes, which may be easier to assess as a marker for response than parenchymal changes. Furthermore, MRCP can help differentiate AIP from PDAC with high specificity (up to 100%) by demonstrating the presence of a duct penetrating sign and icicle sign (smooth, tapered narrowing of the upstream pancreatic duct) within inflammatory masses of the pancreas[50,56,60] (see

Fig. 4) and upstream dilation of the MPD along with an abrupt cutoff in the presence of PDAC.[56,61] In contrast, pancreatic lymphoma may present as bulky lesions without significant MPD dilation. Common bile duct dilation can be more common than MPD dilation in lymphomas.[51,62]

Lesions of the biliary tract are the second most common site of involvement in IgG4-related disease after the pancreas.[20,41,63] Up to 80% of AIP type 1 cases may have hepatobiliary lesions (see Fig. 4; Fig. 5). Although not common, hepatobiliary involvement without type 1 AIP has conversely been reported[41,63] (Fig. 6). The pancreatic portion of the common bile duct is most often involved when associated with AIP due to pancreatic edema, and this is not considered extrapancreatic involvement.[64] Infiltration of the IgG4-positive plasma cells results in ductal thickening resulting in strictures, irregularities, stenosis, and upstream dilation anywhere along the biliary tree (see Figs. 4 and 5). The gallbladder may also be involved, typically showing decreased signal intensity on T2-weighted images and delayed postcontrast enhancement.[22,61]

Changes after contrast administration

The pattern of postcontrast enhancement is a key feature for the diagnosis of AIP. Affected parenchyma remains hypointense in the early arterial phase after contrast administration and shows progressive enhancement on the venous and delayed phase due to the presence of fibrosis[40,49] (see Figs. 2 and 3; Figs. 7 and 8). PDAC can have a similar pattern of delayed enhancement and is always considered in the differential diagnosis of focal AIP.[61] In such cases, recognition of other imaging and clinical findings may be necessary to make a diagnosis. Surgical excision is performed in equivocal cases. On the other hand, pancreatic lymphomas can present with a faint, homogenous contrast enhancement.[51,62]

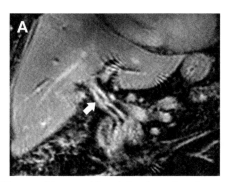 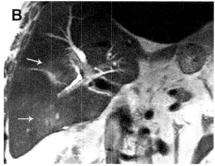

Fig. 5. A 66-year-old man with painless jaundice. Coronal T1-weighted postcontrast image demonstrates diffuse thickening of the common bile duct (*arrow*, A). Patchy areas of increased signal in the peribiliary regions are seen on the coronal T2-weighted image (*arrows*, B) representing edema secondary to inflammation. ERCP with brushings revealed chronic inflammation and 20 IgG4 cells per HPF. A diagnosis of IgG4-related disease was made, and the patient responded well to induction of remission using oral corticosteroids.

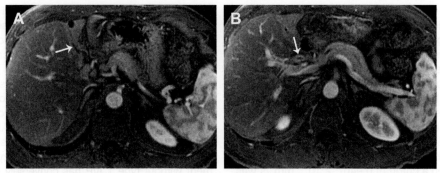

Fig. 6. A 57-year-old man with isolated IgG4 sclerosing cholangitis. On axial T1-weighted postcontrast image there is focal biliary dilation (*arrow, A*) with surrounding enhancement. There is diffuse thickening of common bile duct seen on the axial T1-weighted postcontrast image (*arrow, B*). Patient underwent resection, which confirmed the diagnosis.

Peripancreatic findings Infiltration of the adipose tissue surrounding the pancreas by inflammatory cells may result in the classic halo sign on MR imaging (**Figs. 9** and **10**).[49] However, peripancreatic fat planes are often normal or demonstrate minimal fat stranding.[65] Peripancreatic fluid collections and lymph node enlargement are 2 uncommon findings that suggest superimposed acute pancreatitis.[22,66] Other peripancreatic findings of AIP are relatively uncommon and include large vessel infiltration or pseudocysts, present in 11% and 8% of AIP cases, respectively.[49] The presence of vascular encasement or pancreatic calcification is atypical for AIP and should prompt evaluation for other differential diagnoses, including PDAC.[38,40] Vascular involvement is less common in pancreatic lymphomas. An intact fat plane differentiating the pancreatic tissue may not be present in diffuse

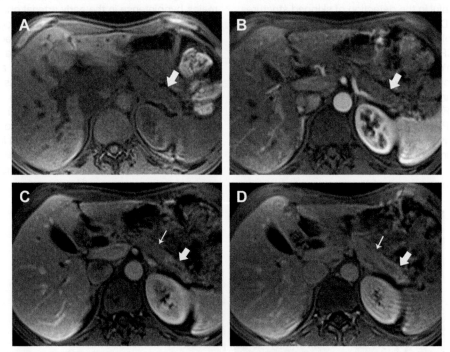

Fig. 7. A 50-year-old man with painless jaundice. Axial T1-weighted precontrast image demonstrates loss of normal hyperintense signal of the pancreas (*arrow, A*). On the arterial-phase postcontrast image there is diffuse low enhancement of the pancreatic tail (*arrow, B*). On the postcontrast venous and delayed phases (*C, D*) there is progressive enhancement of the pancreatic tail (*thick arrows*) compared with the more proximal pancreatic tail (*thin arrows*) indicating fibrosis. Patient had elevated serum IgG4, and a diagnosis of type 1 AIP was made. The patient responded well to oral corticosteroid therapy with resolution of the clinical and imaging findings on subsequent imaging studies.

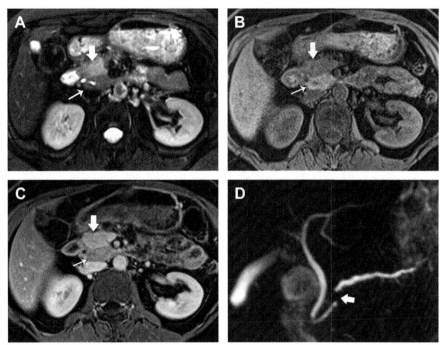

Fig. 8. A 53-year-old woman with epigastric pain. Axial T2-weighted image demonstrates a mass in the head of the pancreas (*thick arrow, A*) and normal signal in the ventral anlage of the pancreas (*thin arrow, A*). There is decreased signal in the mass on the T1-weighted precontrast image (*thick arrow, B*) compared to the normal bright signal in the ventral anlage (*thin arrow, B*). Delayed enhancement is seen in the mass on the delayed post-contrast image (*thick arrow, C*) compared with the normal adjacent pancreas (*thin arrow, C*). Note the presence of a stricture at the site of the mass in the MPD (*arrow, D*) with upstream dilation of the duct. Serum IgG4 and cancer antigen 19-9 were not elevated. A malignancy was excluded on EUS-guided FNA. A diagnosis of type 2 AIP was made, and the patient responded well to corticosteroid treatment.

infiltrative lymphomas, leading to poor definition of the pancreatic tissue and an appearance similar to acute pancreatitis.[51,62] **Table 2** compares common features of AIP, PDAC, and lymphoma.

Extrapancreatic findings: head and neck

Involvement of the head and neck is relatively common in type 1 AIP or IgG4-related disease.[67]

Involvement of the salivary, lacrimal, thyroid, and pituitary glands as well as orbital, sino-nasal, and laryngeal lesions are among the most commonly reported head and neck manifestations.[67] Involvement of the lacrimal and salivary glands may result in Mikulicz disease or Kuttner tumor (chronic sclerosing sialadenitis of the submandibular glands) (see **Fig. 2**). In Mikulicz disease, symmetric

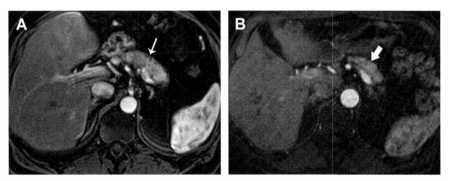

Fig. 9. A 60-year-old man with type 1 AIP presenting with abdominal pain for 3 weeks, mildly elevated lipase, and an elevated IgG4. On the T1-weighted arterial-phase postcontrast image there is enlargement of the pancreatic gland with a peripheral enhancing rim (*arrow, A*). The MPD was not visualized. MR imaging obtained 6 months after treatment with oral corticosteroids shows normalization of the pancreatic parenchyma and resolution of the peripancreatic halo (*arrow, B*).

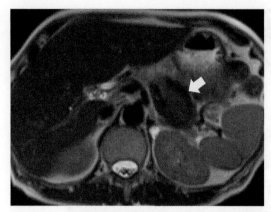

Fig. 10. A 75-year-old man with type 1 AIP. T2-weighted image demonstrates an enlarged pancreas with a surrounding hypointense rim (*arrow*).

bilateral swelling can be visualized on MR imaging.[68,69] Lesions are usually homogenous, have low signal intensity on T1 (similar to muscle) and T2, and show uniform postcontrast enhancement.[48] Similarly, lesions in Kuttner disease have intermediate signal intensity on T1 and low to intermediate signal intensity on T2 and show homogenous postcontrast enhancement.[70] The sino-nasal mucosa may also be affected with lesions that have low T1 and T2 signal intensity and show homogenous postcontrast enhancement.[71] Similar lesions may be seen in the thyroid or pituitary glands, resulting in Riedel thyroiditis (or a subset of Hashimoto thyroiditis) and hypophysitis, respectively.[67,72]

Extrapancreatic findings: chest
Although uncommon, the lungs and their pleural membranes can be involved in the course of IgG4-related disease.[73] Lung involvement can be categorized into 4 groups and may be accompanied by hilar and mediastinal lymphadenopathy. The 4 distinct categories of lung involvement include masslike, ground-glass, alveolar/interstitial, and broncho-vascular opacities.[20,74]

Extrapancreatic findings: abdomen and pelvis
Multiple abdominal and pelvic structures can be involved in patients with type 1 AIP.[20,22] Renal involvement may be seen in 35% of patients, primarily involving the renal cortex.[75] Four common patterns of renal parenchymal involvement included cortical nodules, wedge-shaped, round, or diffuse ill-defined lesions.[75,76] These lesions typically demonstrate low signal intensity on T1- and T2-weighted images, diffusion restriction and show limited postcontrast enhancement (**Fig. 11**). Regression of the signal abnormalities and abnormal

Table 2
Comparing common features of autoimmune pancreatitis, pancreatic ductal adenocarcinoma, and pancreatic lymphoma

	AIP	PDAC	Lymphoma
CT evaluation			
Parenchymal involvement	Diffuse but may be focal	Focal	Diffuse but may be focal
Ductal involvement	Without upstream MPD dilation	Significant dilation of the upstream MPD	Mild dilation of the MPD
Presence of a capsulelike rim or halo of low attenuation	May be present	N/A	N/A
Contrast enhancement	Delayed	Poor enhancement compared with surrounding tissue	Hypoenhancement
Vascular invasion	Uncommon	Common	Uncommon
MR imaging evaluation			
MR imaging signal	Hypointense on T1, minimally increased on T2 with delayed parenchymal enhancement	Hypointense on T1 and variable on T2 with hypoenhancement	Low signal intensity on T1 and T2 with homogenous enhancement
Treatment	Resolution with corticosteroids	Surgery and/or chemotherapy	Chemotherapy

Abbreviation: N/A, not applicable.

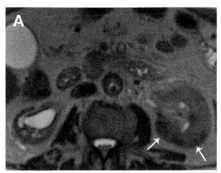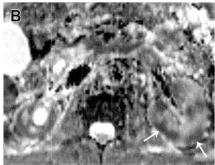

Fig. 11. An 85-year-old man with type 1 AIP. Axial T2-weighted image demonstrates patchy areas of decreased signal intensity in the left kidney (*arrows, A*), which correspond to areas of diffusion restriction on the ADC map ($b = 800$ s/mm^2) (*arrows, B*) representing tubulointerstitial nephritis.

diffusion restriction is common in follow-up studies after treatment with corticosteroids.[77]

Retroperitoneal fibrosis is seen in up to 20% of patients with type 1 AIP presenting as a fibrotic mass that can encase adjacent structures, including the ureters and the aorta (**Fig. 12**).[78,79] IgG4-related periaortic lesions have irregular margins, demonstrate late enhancement on MR imaging, and may be associated with aortic dilation and aneurysms.[80,81]

Although uncommon, inflammatory fibrosis of the bowel mesentery (sclerosing mesenteritis) can also be associated with the IgG4-related disease (see **Fig. 4**). Histopathologic features of IgG4-related disease have been reported in up to 61% of patients with sclerosing mesenteritis.[82] It may be asymptomatic or present with abdominal pain and even an acute abdomen, prompting surgical intervention. MR imaging can aid in differentiating mesenteritis from mass-forming neoplasms and carcinomatosis by documenting preserved fat planes surrounding the mesenteric vessels.

The Role of Imaging in Treatment Response

Corticosteroids serve as the cornerstone for confirmation of diagnosis and treatment of both type 1 and 2 AIP.[43,83] The aim of the treatment is symptom control and to prevent further damage of the pancreatic parenchyma. Treatment is usually initiated with high-dose corticosteroid therapy for 4 weeks followed by gradual taper. Imaging may be performed after this period to assess the treatment response (~2 months). The resolution of diffuse pancreatic swelling, surrounding halo and biliary and pancreatic ductal strictures serve as a radiographic marker for treatment response[84,85] (see **Fig. 4**; **Fig. 13**). However, the atrophy secondary to fibrous changes is typically permanent and may even worsen after treatment (see **Fig. 4**). Conversely, persistent clinical symptoms and imaging findings after high-dose corticosteroid treatment should prompt the search for an alternative

diagnosis, such as chronic pancreatitis or an underlying PDAC. It has been postulated that diffuse swelling and a peripancreatic halo may represent an inflammatory phase of the disease and are more responsive to medical therapy compared with the presence of a focal mass and strictures, which may be secondary to fibrosis and may require surgical intervention for symptom control.[84] Continued maintenance therapy may be effective in preventing disease relapse in patients with type 1 AIP.[86] Relapse may occur in up to 53% patients after steroid withdrawal,[87] and up to 46% of patients may fail to wean off corticosteroids.[88] Maintenance therapy is advocated to prevent relapse, and imaging may help predict high-risk patients. Some of the imaging predictors of relapse include proximal biliary strictures and diffuse pancreatic swelling.[89] Lower-dose corticosteroids and azathioprine are commonly used for maintenance therapy. Methotrexate and mycophenolate mofetil are among common alternative options after relapse or, in rare cases, those who are resistant to corticosteroid therapy.[87] Newer agents, including rituximab, have also been shown to be effective in depleting the B-cell activity, controlling disease progression, and maintaining remission.[90] Disease relapse is uncommon in patients with type 2 AIP, and long term-maintenance therapy is not advocated.

Long-term sequelae of AIP include both endocrine and exocrine insufficiency secondary to glandular atrophy (**Box 1**).[26] Endocrine insufficiency is common and is related to the duration of the disease. Glandular atrophy does not correlate with the presence of exocrine insufficiency, and the diagnosis is made on clinical grounds and by measuring stool fat. Although limited studies have suggested an increased long-term risk of PDAC in patients with AIP,[18,91,92] the two diseases may coexist; PDAC should be suspected in patients unresponsive to corticosteroid therapy (**Box 1**).

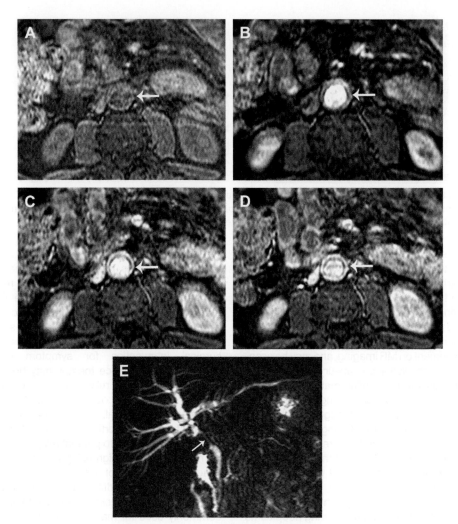

Fig. 12. A 67-year-old man with IgG4-related disease. Axial T1-weighted precontrast (*A*), arterial- (*B*), venous- (*C*), and delayed-phase (*D*) MR imaging demonstrates the presence of a para-aortic ring of tissue, which shows progressive enhancement (*arrows, A–D*) representing IgG4-related retroperitoneal fibrosis. MRCP image shows a long segment, smooth stricture in the proximal common bile duct (*arrow, E*). The pancreas (not shown) was normal on imaging. Patient had elevated serum IgG4 levels and responded well to corticosteroid treatment.

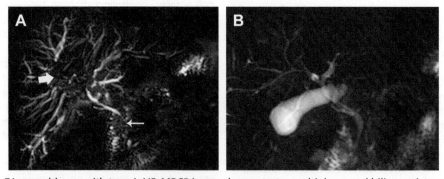

Fig. 13. A 71-year-old man with type 1 AIP. MRCP image demonstrates multiple central biliary strictures (*thick arrow, A*) as well as a distal bile duct stricture (*thin arrow, A*). Patient also had renal cortical lesions and para-aortic soft tissue on imaging and had an elevated serum IgG4. MRCP image obtained after 2 months of oral corticosteroid treatment demonstrates complete resolution of the biliary strictures (*B*). Because proximal biliary strictures are associated with a high risk of relapse, the patient has been continued on azathioprine for maintenance and has not experienced relapse to the present time.

SUMMARY

AIP is a fibro-inflammatory disorder with 2 distinct subtypes that may be differentiated based on clinical, histologic, and radiologic features. Differentiation between the two entities is important because of the difference in treatment strategies and overall prognostication. Imaging plays a vital role in the diagnosis of the disease, differentiation of the two subtypes, and assessment of response to therapy. MR imaging can be used to assess the pancreatic parenchymal changes, whereas MRCP can assess pancreaticobiliary ductal involvement. Type 1 is a multi-organ IgG4-related disease with the pancreas being the most commonly involved organ. Type 2 AIP typically involves younger patients and affects primarily the pancreas with significant overlap in the imaging findings of the pancreas with type 1 disease; differentiation may be based on clinical grounds, concomitant inflammatory bowel disease, and histology. Corticosteroids are the mainstay treatment of both types. However, maintenance therapy may only be needed for type 1 disease because of the lower incidence of relapse in type 2 disease. Endocrine and exocrine insufficiencies may occur as long-term sequelae due to glandular atrophy.

REFERENCES

1. Kawaguchi K, Koike M, Tsuruta K, et al. Lymphoplasmacytic sclerosing pancreatitis with cholangitis: a variant of primary sclerosing cholangitis extensively involving pancreas. Hum Pathol 1991;22(4): 387–95.
2. Yoshida K, Toki F, Takeuchi T, et al. Chronic pancreatitis caused by an autoimmune abnormality. Proposal of the concept of autoimmune pancreatitis. Dig Dis Sci 1995;40(7):1561–8.
3. Sarles H, Sarles JC, Muratore R, et al. Chronic inflammatory sclerosis of the pancreas–an autonomous pancreatic disease? Am J Dig Dis 1961;6: 688–98.
4. Kamisawa T, Funata N, Hayashi Y, et al. A new clinicopathological entity of IgG4-related autoimmune disease. J Gastroenterol 2003;38(10):982–4.
5. Zen Y, Harada K, Sasaki M, et al. IgG4-related sclerosing cholangitis with and without hepatic inflammatory pseudotumor, and sclerosing pancreatitis-associated sclerosing cholangitis: do they belong to a spectrum of sclerosing pancreatitis? Am J Surg Pathol 2004;28(9):1193–203.
6. Hamano H, Kawa S, Uehara T, et al. Immunoglobulin G4-related lymphoplasmacytic sclerosing cholangitis that mimics infiltrating hilar cholangiocarcinoma: part of a spectrum of autoimmune pancreatitis? Gastrointest Endosc 2005;62(1):152–7.
7. Stone JH, Zen Y, Deshpande V. IgG4-related disease. N Engl J Med 2012;366(6):539–51.
8. Finkelberg DL, Sahani D, Deshpande V, et al. Autoimmune pancreatitis. N Engl J Med 2006;355(25): 2670–6.
9. Deshpande V, Gupta R, Sainani N, et al. Subclassification of autoimmune pancreatitis: a histologic classification with clinical significance. Am J Surg Pathol 2011;35(1):26–35.
10. Kamisawa T, Okamoto A. IgG4-related sclerosing disease. World J Gastroenterol 2008;14(25): 3948–55.
11. Tanabe T, Tsushima K, Yasuo M, et al. IgG4-associated multifocal systemic fibrosis complicating sclerosing sialadenitis, hypophysitis, and retroperitoneal fibrosis, but lacking pancreatic involvement. Intern Med 2006;45(21):1243–7.
12. Nishimori I, Tamakoshi A, Otsuki M, et al. Prevalence of autoimmune pancreatitis in Japan from a nationwide survey in 2002. J Gastroenterol 2007; 42(Suppl 18):6–8.
13. Kanno A, Nishimori I, Masamune A, et al. Nationwide epidemiological survey of autoimmune pancreatitis in Japan. Pancreas 2012;41(6):835–9.
14. Kanno A, Masamune A, Okazaki K, et al. Nationwide epidemiological survey of autoimmune pancreatitis in Japan in 2011. Pancreas 2015;44(4):535–9.
15. Sah RP, Pannala R, Chari ST, et al. Prevalence, diagnosis, and profile of autoimmune pancreatitis presenting with features of acute or chronic pancreatitis. Clin Gastroenterol Hepatol 2010;8(1):91–6.
16. van Heerde MJ, Biermann K, Zondervan PE, et al. Prevalence of autoimmune pancreatitis and other benign disorders in pancreatoduodenectomy for presumed malignancy of the pancreatic head. Dig Dis Sci 2012;57(9):2458–65.
17. de Castro SM, de Nes LC, Nio CY, et al. Incidence and characteristics of chronic and lymphoplasmacytic sclerosing pancreatitis in patients scheduled

to undergo a pancreatoduodenectomy. HPB (Oxford) 2010;12(1):15–21.

18. Hart PA, Kamisawa T, Brugge WR, et al. Long-term outcomes of autoimmune pancreatitis: a multicentre, international analysis. Gut 2013;62(12):1771–6.

19. Hart PA, Zen Y, Chari ST. Recent advances in autoimmune pancreatitis. Gastroenterology 2015;149(1): 39–51.

20. Martinez-de-Alegria A, Baleato-Gonzalez S, Garcia-Figueiras R, et al. IgG4-related disease from head to toe. Radiographics 2015;35(7):2007–25.

21. Majumder S, Chari ST. EUS-guided FNA for diagnosing autoimmune pancreatitis: does it enhance existing consensus criteria? Gastrointest Endosc 2016;84(5):805–7.

22. Vlachou PA, Khalili K, Jang HJ, et al. IgG4-related sclerosing disease: autoimmune pancreatitis and extrapancreatic manifestations. Radiographics 2011;31(5):1379–402.

23. Ectors N, Maillet B, Aerts R, et al. Non-alcoholic duct destructive chronic pancreatitis. Gut 1997;41(2): 263–8.

24. Van Moerkercke W, Verhamme M, Doubel P, et al. Autoimmune pancreatitis and extrapancreatic manifestations of IgG4-related sclerosing disease. Acta Gastroenterol Belg 2010;73(2):239–46.

25. Deshpande V, Zen Y, Chan JK, et al. Consensus statement on the pathology of IgG4-related disease. Mod Pathol 2012;25(9):1181–92.

26. Majumder S, Takahashi N, Chari ST. Autoimmune pancreatitis. Dig Dis Sci 2017;62(7):1762–9.

27. Inoue D, Yoshida K, Yoneda N, et al. IgG4-related disease: dataset of 235 consecutive patients. Medicine (Baltimore) 2015;94(15):e680.

28. Zamboni G, Luttges J, Capelli P, et al. Histopathological features of diagnostic and clinical relevance in autoimmune pancreatitis: a study on 53 resection specimens and 9 biopsy specimens. Virchows Arch 2004;445(6):552–63.

29. Kamisawa T, Chari ST, Giday SA, et al. Clinical profile of autoimmune pancreatitis and its histological subtypes: an international multicenter survey. Pancreas 2011;40(6):809–14.

30. Kloppel G, Detlefsen S, Chari ST, et al. Autoimmune pancreatitis: the clinicopathological characteristics of the subtype with granulocytic epithelial lesions. J Gastroenterol 2010;45(8):787–93.

31. Hart PA, Levy MJ, Smyrk TC, et al. Clinical profiles and outcomes in idiopathic duct-centric chronic pancreatitis (type 2 autoimmune pancreatitis): the Mayo Clinic experience. Gut 2016;65(10):1702–9.

32. Sah RP, Chari ST, Pannala R, et al. Differences in clinical profile and relapse rate of type 1 versus type 2 autoimmune pancreatitis. Gastroenterology 2010;139(1):140–8 [quiz: e112–43].

33. Shimosegawa T, Chari ST, Frulloni L, et al. International consensus diagnostic criteria for autoimmune pancreatitis: guidelines of the International Association of Pancreatology. Pancreas 2011;40(3):352–8.

34. Chang MC, Liang PC, Jan IS, et al. Comparison and validation of International Consensus Diagnostic Criteria for diagnosis of autoimmune pancreatitis from pancreatic cancer in a Taiwanese cohort. BMJ Open 2014;4(8):e005900.

35. Sumimoto K, Uchida K, Mitsuyama T, et al. A proposal of a diagnostic algorithm with validation of International Consensus Diagnostic Criteria for autoimmune pancreatitis in a Japanese cohort. Pancreatology 2013;13(3):230–7.

36. Schneider A, Michaely H, Ruckert F, et al. Diagnosing autoimmune pancreatitis with the unifying-autoimmune-pancreatitis-criteria. Pancreatology 2017;17(3):381–94.

37. Lee LK, Sahani DV. Autoimmune pancreatitis in the context of IgG4-related disease: review of imaging findings. World J Gastroenterol 2014;20(41): 15177–89.

38. Kawamoto S, Siegelman SS, Hruban RH, et al. Lymphoplasmacytic sclerosing pancreatitis (autoimmune pancreatitis): evaluation with multidetector CT. Radiographics 2008;28(1):157–70.

39. Van Hoe L, Gryspeerdt S, Ectors N, et al. Nonalcoholic duct-destructive chronic pancreatitis: imaging findings. AJR Am J Roentgenol 1998;170(3):643–7.

40. Sahani DV, Kalva SP, Farrell J, et al. Autoimmune pancreatitis: imaging features. Radiology 2004; 233(2):345–52.

41. Kamisawa T, Egawa N, Nakajima H, et al. Clinical difficulties in the differentiation of autoimmune pancreatitis and pancreatic carcinoma. Am J Gastroenterol 2003;98(12):2694–9.

42. Zaheer A, Singh VK, Akshintala VS, et al. Differentiating autoimmune pancreatitis from pancreatic adenocarcinoma using dual-phase computed tomography. J Comput Assist Tomogr 2014;38(1):146–52.

43. Wakabayashi T, Kawaura Y, Satomura Y, et al. Clinical study of chronic pancreatitis with focal irregular narrowing of the main pancreatic duct and mass formation: comparison with chronic pancreatitis showing diffuse irregular narrowing of the main pancreatic duct. Pancreas 2002;25(3):283–9.

44. Wakabayashi T, Kawaura Y, Satomura Y, et al. Clinical and imaging features of autoimmune pancreatitis with focal pancreatic swelling or mass formation: comparison with so-called tumor-forming pancreatitis and pancreatic carcinoma. Am J Gastroenterol 2003;98(12):2679–87.

45. Kawamoto S, Siegelman SS, Hruban RH, et al. Lymphoplasmacytic sclerosing pancreatitis with obstructive jaundice: CT and pathology features. AJR Am J Roentgenol 2004;183(4):915–21.

46. Takuma K, Kamisawa T, Tabata T, et al. Utility of pancreatography for diagnosing autoimmune pancreatitis. World J Gastroenterol 2011;17(18):2332–7.

47. Farrell JJ, Garber J, Sahani D, et al. EUS findings in patients with autoimmune pancreatitis. Gastrointest Endosc 2004;60(6):927–36.

48. Carbognin G, Girardi V, Biasiutti C, et al. Autoimmune pancreatitis: imaging findings on contrast-enhanced MR, MRCP and dynamic secretin-enhanced MRCP. Radiol Med 2009;114(8):1214–31.

49. Rehnitz C, Klauss M, Singer R, et al. Morphologic patterns of autoimmune pancreatitis in CT and MRI. Pancreatology 2011;11(2):240–51.

50. Kim HJ, Kim YK, Jeong WK, et al. Pancreatic duct "icicle sign" on MRI for distinguishing autoimmune pancreatitis from pancreatic ductal adenocarcinoma in the proximal pancreas. Eur Radiol 2015;25(6): 1551–60.

51. Low G, Panu A, Millo N, et al. Multimodality imaging of neoplastic and nonneoplastic solid lesions of the pancreas. Radiographics 2011;31(4):993–1015.

52. Lee NK, Kim S, Kim DU, et al. Diffusion-weighted magnetic resonance imaging for non-neoplastic conditions in the hepatobiliary and pancreatic regions: pearls and potential pitfalls in imaging interpretation. Abdom Imaging 2015;40(3): 643–62.

53. Kamisawa T, Takuma K, Anjiki H, et al. Differentiation of autoimmune pancreatitis from pancreatic cancer by diffusion-weighted MRI. Am J Gastroenterol 2010;105(8):1870–5.

54. Oki H, Hayashida Y, Oki H, et al. DWI findings of autoimmune pancreatitis: comparison between symptomatic and asymptomatic patients. J Magn Reson Imaging 2015;41(1):125–31.

55. Klauss M, Maier-Hein K, Tjaden C, et al. IVIM DW-MRI of autoimmune pancreatitis: therapy monitoring and differentiation from pancreatic cancer. Eur Radiol 2016;26(7):2099–106.

56. Choi SY, Kim SH, Kang TW, et al. Differentiating mass-forming autoimmune pancreatitis from pancreatic ductal adenocarcinoma on the basis of contrast-enhanced MRI and DWI findings. AJR Am J Roentgenol 2016;206(2):291–300.

57. Manfredi R, Frulloni L, Mantovani W, et al. Autoimmune pancreatitis: pancreatic and extrapancreatic MR imaging-MR cholangiopancreatography findings at diagnosis, after steroid therapy, and at recurrence. Radiology 2011;260(2):428–36.

58. Kamisawa T, Tu Y, Egawa N, et al. Can MRCP replace ERCP for the diagnosis of autoimmune pancreatitis? Abdom Imaging 2009;34(3):381–4.

59. Park SH, Kim MH, Kim SY, et al. Magnetic resonance cholangiopancreatography for the diagnostic evaluation of autoimmune pancreatitis. Pancreas 2010; 39(8):1191–8.

60. Ichikawa T, Sou H, Araki T, et al. Duct-penetrating sign at MRCP: usefulness for differentiating inflammatory pancreatic mass from pancreatic carcinomas. Radiology 2001;221(1):107–16.

61. Zaheer A, Fishman EK, Pittman ME, et al. Pancreatic imaging: a pattern-based approach to radiologic diagnosis with pathologic correlation. Switzerland: Springer International Publishing; 2017.

62. Merkle EM, Bender GN, Brambs HJ. Imaging findings in pancreatic lymphoma: differential aspects. AJR Am J Roentgenol 2000;174(3):671–5.

63. Shanbhogue AK, Fasih N, Surabhi VR, et al. A clinical and radiologic review of uncommon types and causes of pancreatitis. Radiographics 2009; 29(4):1003–26.

64. Hirano K, Tada M, Isayama H, et al. Endoscopic evaluation of factors contributing to intrapancreatic biliary stricture in autoimmune pancreatitis. Gastrointest Endosc 2010;71(1):85–90.

65. Furukawa N, Muranaka T, Yasumori K, et al. Autoimmune pancreatitis: radiologic findings in three histologically proven cases. J Comput Assist Tomogr 1998;22(6):880–3.

66. Chari ST, Smyrk TC, Levy MJ, et al. Diagnosis of autoimmune pancreatitis: the Mayo Clinic experience. Clin Gastroenterol Hepatol 2006;4(8):1010–6 [quiz: 1934].

67. Fujita A, Sakai O, Chapman MN, et al. IgG4-related disease of the head and neck: CT and MR imaging manifestations. Radiographics 2012;32(7):1945–58.

68. Takahira M, Kawano M, Zen Y, et al. IgG4-related chronic sclerosing dacryoadenitis. Arch Ophthalmol 2007;125(11):1575–8.

69. Takano K, Yamamoto M, Takahashi H, et al. Clinicopathologic similarities between Mikulicz disease and Kuttner tumor. Am J Otolaryngol 2010;31(6):429–34.

70. Abu A, Motoori K, Yamamoto S, et al. MRI of chronic sclerosing sialoadenitis. Br J Radiol 2008;81(967): 531–6.

71. Ishida M, Hotta M, Kushima R, et al. Multiple IgG4-related sclerosing lesions in the maxillary sinus, parotid gland and nasal septum. Pathol Int 2009;59(9): 670–5.

72. Leporati P, Landek-Salgado MA, Lupi I, et al. IgG4-related hypophysitis: a new addition to the hypophysitis spectrum. J Clin Endocrinol Metab 2011;96(7): 1971–80.

73. Hirano K, Kawabe T, Komatsu Y, et al. High-rate pulmonary involvement in autoimmune pancreatitis. Intern Med J 2006;36(1):58–61.

74. Inoue D, Zen Y, Abo H, et al. Immunoglobulin G4-related lung disease: CT findings with pathologic correlations. Radiology 2009;251(1):260–70.

75. Takahashi N, Kawashima A, Fletcher JG, et al. Renal involvement in patients with autoimmune pancreatitis: CT and MR imaging findings. Radiology 2007; 242(3):791–801.

76. Triantopoulou C, Malachias G, Maniatis P, et al. Renal lesions associated with autoimmune pancreatitis: CT findings. Acta Radiol 2010; 51(6):702–7.

77. Zaheer A, Halappa VG, Akshintala VS, et al. Renal lesions in autoimmune pancreatitis: diffusion weighted magnetic resonance imaging for assessing response to corticosteroid therapy. JOP 2013; 14(5):506–9.

78. Fujinaga Y, Kadoya M, Kawa S, et al. Characteristic findings in images of extra-pancreatic lesions associated with autoimmune pancreatitis. Eur J Radiol 2010;76(2):228–38.

79. Sohn JH, Byun JH, Yoon SE, et al. Abdominal extrapancreatic lesions associated with autoimmune pancreatitis: radiological findings and changes after therapy. Eur J Radiol 2008;67(3):497–507.

80. Inoue D, Zen Y, Abo H, et al. Immunoglobulin G4-related periaortitis and periarteritis: CT findings in 17 patients. Radiology 2011;261(2):625–33.

81. Kasashima S, Zen Y, Kawashima A, et al. A new clinicopathological entity of IgG4-related inflammatory abdominal aortic aneurysm. J Vasc Surg 2009; 49(5):1264–71 [discussion: 1271].

82. Kerdsirichairat T, Mesa H, Abraham J, et al. Sclerosing mesenteritis and IgG4-related mesenteritis: case series and a systematic review of natural history and response to treatments. Immunogastroenterology 2013;2(2):119–28.

83. Uchida K, Miyoshi H, Ikeura T, et al. Clinical and pathophysiological issues associated with type 1 autoimmune pancreatitis. Clin J Gastroenterol 2016;9(1):7–12.

84. Sahani DV, Sainani NI, Deshpande V, et al. Autoimmune pancreatitis: disease evolution, staging, response assessment, and CT features that predict response to corticosteroid therapy. Radiology 2009;250(1):118–29.

85. Manfredi R, Graziani R, Cicero C, et al. Autoimmune pancreatitis: CT patterns and their changes after steroid treatment. Radiology 2008;247(2):435–43.

86. Kamisawa T, Okazaki K, Kawa S, et al. Amendment of the Japanese Consensus Guidelines for Autoimmune Pancreatitis, 2013 III. Treatment and prognosis of autoimmune pancreatitis. J Gastroenterol 2014;49(6):961–70.

87. Ghazale A, Chari ST, Zhang L, et al. Immunoglobulin G4-associated cholangitis: clinical profile and response to therapy. Gastroenterology 2008; 134(3):706–15.

88. Sandanayake NS, Church NI, Chapman MH, et al. Presentation and management of post-treatment relapse in autoimmune pancreatitis/immunoglobulin G4-associated cholangitis. Clin Gastroenterol Hepatol 2009;7(10):1089–96.

89. Wallace ZS, Mattoo H, Mahajan VS, et al. Predictors of disease relapse in IgG4-related disease following rituximab. Rheumatology (Oxford) 2016;55(6):1000–8.

90. Hart PA, Topazian MD, Witzig TE, et al. Treatment of relapsing autoimmune pancreatitis with immunomodulators and rituximab: the Mayo Clinic experience. Gut 2013;62(11):1607–15.

91. Uchida K, Yazumi S, Nishio A, et al. Long-term outcome of autoimmune pancreatitis. J Gastroenterol 2009;44(7):726–32.

92. Ikeura T, Miyoshi H, Uchida K, et al. Relationship between autoimmune pancreatitis and pancreatic cancer: a single-center experience. Pancreatology 2014;14(5):373–9.

Moving?

Make sure your subscription moves with you!

To notify us of your new address, find your **Clinics Account Number** (located on your mailing label above your name), and contact customer service at:

Email: journalscustomerservice-usa@elsevier.com

800-654-2452 (subscribers in the U.S. & Canada)
314-447-8871 (subscribers outside of the U.S. & Canada)

Fax number: 314-447-8029

Elsevier Health Sciences Division
Subscription Customer Service
3251 Riverport Lane
Maryland Heights, MO 63043

Moving?

Make sure your subscription
moves with you!

To notify us of your new address, find your Clinics Account Number (located on your mailing label above your name), and contact customer service at:

Email: JournalsCustomerService-usa@elsevier.com

800-654-2452 (subscribers in the U.S. & Canada)
314-447-8871 (subscribers outside of the U.S. & Canada)

Fax number: 314-447-8029

Elsevier Health Sciences Division
Subscription Customer Service
3251 Riverport Lane
Maryland Heights, MO 63043

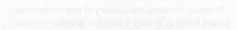

To ensure uninterrupted delivery of your subscription, please notify us at least 4 weeks in advance of move.

Printed and bound by CPI Group (UK) Ltd, Croydon, CR0 4YY

08/05/2025

01864727-0005